Mometrix
TEST PREPARATION

AF901584

Neonatal CCRN® Exam Secrets Study Guide Part 2 of 2

DEAR FUTURE EXAM SUCCESS STORY

First of all, **THANK YOU** for purchasing Mometrix study materials!

Second, congratulations! You are one of the few determined test-takers who are committed to doing whatever it takes to excel on your exam. **You have come to the right place.** We developed these study materials with one goal in mind: to deliver you the information you need in a format that's concise and easy to use.

In addition to optimizing your guide for the content of the test, we've outlined our recommended steps for breaking down the preparation process into small, attainable goals so you can make sure you stay on track.

We've also analyzed the entire test-taking process, identifying the most common pitfalls and showing how you can overcome them and be ready for any curveball the test throws you.

Standardized testing is one of the biggest obstacles on your road to success, which only increases the importance of doing well in the high-pressure, high-stakes environment of test day. Your results on this test could have a significant impact on your future, and this guide provides the information and practical advice to help you achieve your full potential on test day.

Your success is our success

We would love to hear from you! If you would like to share the story of your exam success or if you have any questions or comments in regard to our products, please contact us at **800-673-8175** or **support@mometrix.com**.

Thanks again for your business and we wish you continued success!

Sincerely,
The Mometrix Test Preparation Team

Need more help? Check out our flashcards at:
http://MometrixFlashcards.com/CCRN

Written and edited by the Mometrix Exam Secrets Test Prep Team
Printed in the United States of America

TABLE OF CONTENTS

Clinical Judgment: Multisystem

Life-Threatening Maternal/Fetal Complications

Preeclampsia and Eclampsia

Preeclampsia is a disorder that develops in approximately 5% of all pregnancies. It is defined as a new onset of elevated blood pressure of at least 140/90 on two occasions at least 4 hours apart. In addition to elevated BP, diagnosis requires one or more of the following complications after the 20th week of pregnancy: proteinuria, new-onset headaches or visual disturbances, thrombocytopenia, impaired liver or kidney function, or pulmonary edema. Proteinuria is a common feature of preeclampsia, but diagnostically, it is possible to have preeclampsia without proteinuria when there is evidence of significant end-organ dysfunction. Preeclampsia is more commonly seen after 34 weeks gestation. Delivery is the only cure for preeclampsia. If it is not severe, patients are often induced after 37 weeks gestation. In patients with severe features, induction should be considered after 34 weeks gestation. Antihypertensive treatment, such as thiazide, hydralazine, propranolol, labetalol, nifedipine, and methyldopa, is recommended for severe hypertension, as well as anticonvulsants if seizures occur. Magnesium sulfate is given prophylactically for severe preeclampsia and for treatment of seizures. **Eclampsia** is a complication of severe preeclampsia in which seizures occur. The main detrimental effect on the fetus occurs when longstanding hypertension leads to uteroplacental vascular insufficiency, which impairs the transfer of nutrients and oxygen to the fetus, resulting in intrauterine growth restriction (IUGR). Placental abruption also occurs more frequently. The IUGR is usually asymmetric (fetal head size is normal for gestational age). Infants who are born with IUGR and/or prematurity have increased morbidity and mortality.

Superimposed Preeclampsia

Superimposed preeclampsia is a condition in which preeclampsia is concurrent with already existing chronic hypertension or a condition that predisposes the pregnant woman to hypertension, such as kidney disease and autoimmune disorders (e.g., diabetes, lupus erythematous), or in which preeclampsia develops prior to 20 weeks of gestation. Superimposed preeclampsia occurs in approximately 20% of pregnant women and tends to be more severe than *de novo* preeclampsia, carrying a greater risk of complications. Symptoms of superimposed preeclampsia usually occur after 20 weeks of gestation and include:

- Proteinuria (new onset): ≥300 mg in 24-hour urine, protein/creatinine ratio ≥0.3, urine dipstick reading of ≥1+
- Sudden increase in previously stable blood pressure: ≥160/110 mmHg
- Indications of end-organ damage: Thrombocytopenia <100,000/μL, liver enzymes of twice the normal level, serum creatinine >1.1 mg/dL, pulmonary edema, neurological impairments (e.g., headache, scotoma, blurred vision)
- Eclampsia: Seizures

Maternal complications can also include HELLP syndrome (i.e., **h**emolysis, **e**levated **l**iver enzymes, and **l**ow **p**latelets), stroke, intracranial hemorrhage, liver rupture, disseminated intravascular coagulation (DIC), acute kidney injury, and placental abruption. Treatment includes antihypertensive medications (e.g., labetalol, nifedipine), magnesium sulfate to prevent seizures, fetal monitoring with serial ultrasounds, Doppler studies (umbilical artery flow), and planned delivery at 37 weeks or ≤34 weeks if the maternal or fetal status deteriorates. Fetal complications can include intrauterine growth restriction (IUGR), preterm birth, stillbirth, low birth weight, and respiratory distress syndrome.

HELLP SYNDROME

HELLP syndrome occurs in 4-12% of those with preeclampsia, most often during weeks 27-37, but it may develop within 24 hours postpartum. It is characterized by the following:

- **H**—hemolysis
- **EL**—elevated liver enzymes
- **LP**—low platelet count

HELLP syndrome is most common in older multiparous mothers. Hypertension may be less pronounced than in others with preeclampsia. Pain in the right upper quadrant related to liver dysfunction may be misdiagnosed as gastrointestinal upset or gall bladder disease. Mothers often present with flu-like nonspecific symptoms, including headache, nausea and vomiting, and visual disturbances. Prompt diagnosis and treatment are necessary because of high mortality. Platelet transfusions are given if platelet counts are <20,000/mm³ before vaginal delivery or <50,000/mm³ before Cesarean section. The primary treatment is immediate delivery of the fetus as the mother may develop hepatic hemorrhage or permanent liver damage. Both the mother and the fetus are at risk. Neonates are at increased risk and may require mechanical ventilation. Complications include abruptio placentae, DIC, and postpartum hemorrhage.

CLASSES I TO IV CARDIAC DISEASE IN PREGNANCY

Maternal heart disease complicates approximately one percent of all pregnancies, with congenital heart disease accounting for more than half of the cases. Pre-pregnancy cardiac function is an excellent predictor of cardiac complications in pregnancy and is based on the New York Heart Association classification:

I. No cardiac insufficiency or activity limitations
II. Slight activity limitations: symptoms present with ordinary physical activity
III. Marked activity limitations: mild activity causes symptoms
IV. Inability to carry out physical activities without severe symptoms

The **maternal classification** affects the fetus. There is minimal danger to the fetus for mothers in Class I or Class II, but increased risk to both the mother and the fetus for Classes III and IV. Most medications cross the placenta, and the degree of safety during pregnancy has not been established for all of these. The most common drugs—heparin, digitalis glycosides, antiarrhythmics, thiazide, and loop diuretics—are not **teratogenic**. For Classes III and IV, delivery may be facilitated by low forceps or vacuum assistance, and Cesarean may be done if the mother or the fetus is in danger. Labor and delivery are particularly dangerous to the fetus because of inadequate oxygen and blood supply, so continuous fetal monitoring is essential.

PREGNANCY WITH CONGENITAL HEART DEFECTS

With improved surgical repair techniques for **congenital heart defects,** many women survive to childbearing age. These are common **maternal defects**:

- Tetralogy of Fallot
- Ventricular and atrial septal defects
- Patent ductus arteriosus
- Coarctation of the aorta

If surgical correction was successful, there is no added **fetal risk**, but if the condition has not been completely repaired or involves cyanosis, pregnancy can put the fetus at risk because of inadequate oxygen supply. Mothers with cardiac disease have a 5-10% increased risk of having a baby with cardiac anomalies. Fetal echocardiography is recommended in pregnancy to evaluate the structure and function of the fetus' heart.

Marfan syndrome poses severe risks to the mother, with mortality rates of 25-50% because of possible rupture of the aorta, which also puts the fetus at risk. Additionally, because this is an autosomal dominant disorder, there is a 50% chance that an infant will inherit the syndrome.

Mitral valve prolapse usually does not pose a risk to the fetus.

Severe maternal cardiopulmonary disorders can result in death of the mother and/or fetus. However, the most common fetal complications are premature labor/birth and a fetus that is small for gestational age.

Maternal Respiratory Disorders

Asthma

Maternal asthma, which complicates 4–8% of pregnancies, can negatively affect the development of the fetus; therefore, controlling asthma during pregnancy is essential. Asthma management is the same for pregnant women as for nonpregnant women. Typically, approximately one-third of those with asthma experience worsening of symptoms during pregnancy, one-third are stable, and one-third improve. Maternal asthma can result in fetal hypoxia if the maternal oxygen saturation drops too low. Additionally, asthma may impair glucocorticoid signaling, which is critical for the maturation of fetal lungs and the production of surfactant, which is necessary for alveolar expansion and gas exchange. The pregnant woman with asthma is at an increased risk of preeclampsia, Cesarean section birth, pregnancy-induced hypertension, preterm labor, and respiratory compromise. Fetal risks include IUGR, preterm birth, low birth weight, congenital anomalies, seizures, neonatal hypoglycemia, asphyxia, being small for gestational age, and stillbirth. The neonate is at risk for transient tachypnea of the newborn, respiratory distress syndrome (RDS), and impaired lung function and has an increased risk of developing asthma and wheezing as the child ages.

Pulmonary Edema

Pulmonary edema, (i.e., retention of fluid in the interstitial spaces and alveoli of the lungs) during pregnancy most often occurs in the first 24 hours after delivery, although it can occur during pregnancy as well. The most common cause is preeclampsia, but pulmonary edema can also result from the use of beta-agonists (such as terbutaline) for tocolysis and from fluid overload (especially during labor and delivery), peripartum cardiomyopathy, PE, sepsis, and acute respiratory distress syndrome (ARDS). Because of hemodynamic changes during pregnancy, the pregnant woman is at an increased risk of fluid overload from even minor procedures. Symptoms include dyspnea, weight gain, rapid irregular heart rate, cough, and frothy sputum or hemoptysis. Pulmonary edema results in an increased maternal risk of respiratory failure, need for mechanical ventilation, exacerbation of hypertensive disorders, and death. Because pulmonary edema negatively affects maternal oxygenation, the fetus is at risk for hypoxia, acidosis, fetal distress, preterm birth, low Apgar score (used to measure the infant's condition), and stillbirth. Treatment for the woman with pulmonary edema includes supplemental oxygen, diuretics (furosemide), head elevation, fluid restriction, and treatment of the underlying cause.

Pulmonary Embolism (PE)

Pregnant women are at risk for pulmonary embolism (PE) because of the increased clotting factors, reduced fibrinolysis, and impaired circulation associated with venous stasis, resulting in clots dislodging and traveling to the lungs. PE is responsible for 11% of maternal deaths. PE most often occurs after labor and delivery because of endothelial injury, but it can also occur during pregnancy. Symptoms of PE may include sudden dyspnea, tachycardia, tachypnea, cough, hemoptysis or frothy sputum, syncope, hypotension, and indications of DVT. Maternal complications include hypoxemia, cardiovascular collapse, cardiac arrythmias, cardiac arrest, and death. If PE occurs during pregnancy, the fetus is particularly vulnerable to maternal hypoxia and unstable hemodynamics. Risks to the fetus may include acute fetal hypoxia, nonreassuring fetal heart rate, preterm birth, IUGR (if PE is recurrent or subclinical), and stillbirth. Maternal treatment includes supplemental oxygen, anticoagulation (low-molecular-weight heparin during pregnancy and unfractionated heparin near delivery), and thrombolysis or embolectomy. The fetus must be monitored carefully, and delivery may be expedited for fetal or maternal compromise.

Infants of a Diabetic Mother (IDM)

Infants of a diabetic mother (IDM) suffer from increased morbidity and mortality. Glucose crosses the placenta, so when the mother has elevated blood glucose, the infant also has elevated blood glucose. Insulin does not cross the placenta. The pancreas of the fetus begins to produce insulin at about 20 weeks of gestation. Prior to the fetus producing insulin, the infant is exposed to elevated levels of glucose that restrict fetal growth. After week 20, the fetus responds to hyperglycemia with elevated production of insulin. The combination of elevated blood glucose and elevated insulin triggers rapid fetal growth, with increased fat and glycogen stores, hepatosplenomegaly, cardiomegaly, and increased head size. Sudden withdrawal from the consistent maternal source of glucose after birth, combined with the continued production of insulin by the newborn, result in hypoglycemia shortly after birth.

Maternal Hematologic Disorders

Sickle Cell Anemia

Sickle cell disease is a recessive genetic disorder of chromosome 11, causing hemoglobin to be defective so that red blood cells (RBCs) are sickle-shaped and inflexible, resulting in their accumulating in small vessels and causing painful blockage. There are 5 variations of sickle cell disease, with **sickle cell anemia** the most severe. Pregnant women with sickle cell anemia are at risk for urinary and pulmonary infections, congestive heart failure, and acute renal failure, all of which can trigger a vaso-occlusive crises that puts the fetus at risk. Perinatal mortality rates are about 18%, caused by sickling in the placenta. Neonates are at increased risk for prematurity and intrauterine growth restriction. Maternal infections must be treated promptly to avoid dehydration and/or fever that can trigger sickling. Steps to shorten the second stage of labor (oxytocin, forceps, episiotomy) may be necessary to protect the fetus if sickling occurs during labor.

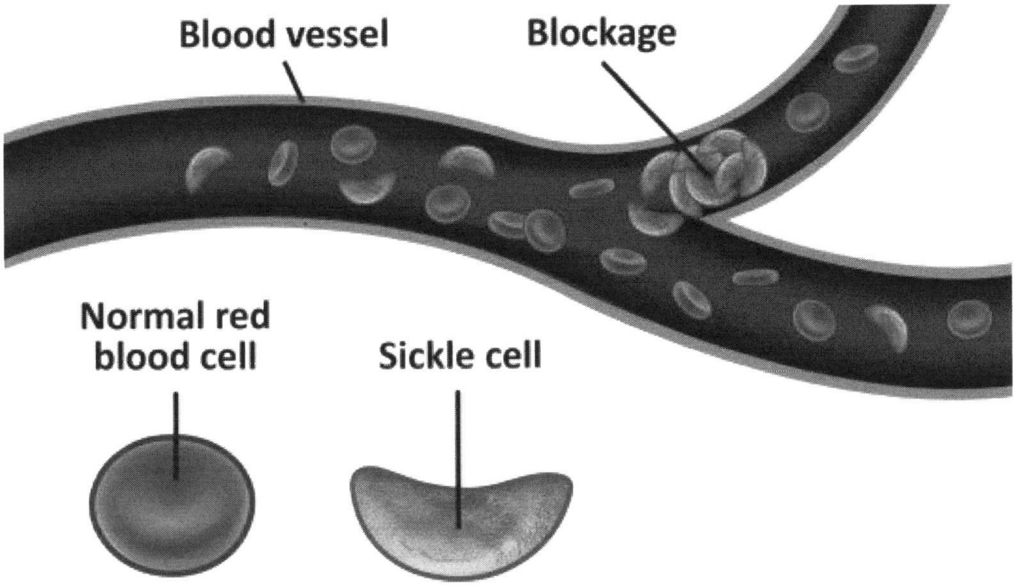

Review Video: Sickle Cell Disease
Visit mometrix.com/academy and enter code: 603869

IRON-DEFICIENCY ANEMIA

Iron is necessary for the development of red blood cells. During pregnancy, the mother's plasma volume increases by about 50% but red cell mass increases less, so the **hematocrit** drops from a normal of 38-47% to as low as 30% (physiologic/iron deficiency anemia of pregnancy). Because the fetus takes iron from the mother, the mother's iron intake must compensate for this loss. When **hemoglobin** falls <10 g/dL, the mother is at increased risk of infection, preeclampsia, and postpartal hemorrhage, with associated dangers to the fetus. If hemoglobin falls <6 g/dL, the mother may suffer cardiac failure, and the fetus is at high risk, with increased rates of miscarriage, stillbirth, low birth weight, and neonatal death. Initial symptoms of iron deficiency include pallor, glossitis, headache, and pica, progressing to weakness, lethargy, confusion, ataxia, and cardiovascular abnormalities. Recommended treatment for iron-deficiency anemia is 60-120 mg daily of elemental iron. To promote absorption, it is best to avoid caffeine and dairy products within an hour of taking the iron supplement and to take some source of vitamin C with the iron.

FOLATE/FOLIC ACID DEFICIENCY ANEMIA

Folate/folic acid deficiency can result in **megaloblastic anemia**. Folate is the naturally occurring form of vitamin B9 and is necessary for DNA synthesis and the formation and maturation of red blood cells. Folic acid is the synthetic form of vitamin B9, used in supplements and added to processed foods. Causes of folate deficiency include inadequate diet, malabsorption syndromes (especially of the small intestine), medications that interfere with absorption (oral contraceptives, methotrexate, phenobarbital, and diphenylhydantoin), anorexia, alcoholism, and dialysis. Diagnostic findings include decreased hemoglobin, hematocrit, and folate (normal value is 3-25 mg/mL), as well as increased MCV and MCHV. Cobalamin level is normal and gastric analysis is positive for hydrochloric acid. Other blood studies are usually within normal range. RBCs are macrocytic and normochromic. Folate deficiency is associated with **neural tube defects**, such as myelomeningocele, spina bifida, and anencephaly in the fetus.

Signs and symptoms include:

- Asymptomatic (initially)
- GI disturbances, such as indigestion, anorexia, and weight loss
- Red, beefy-appearing tongue
- Pallor
- Weakness, fatigue
- Forgetfulness, impaired concentration

Treatment:

- Diet high in folate: green leafy vegetables, liver, citrus fruits, legumes, nuts, and grains
- Oral supplementation: L-Methylfolate 600-1000 mcg daily or folic acid 1-5 mg per day

THROMBOCYTOPENIA

Thrombocytopenia is a platelet count <150,000/µL. Thrombocytopenia occurs in up to 11% of pregnant women. Although there are many causes for thrombocytopenia in pregnancy, the most common include:

- **Gestational thrombocytopenia (75%):** Most often occurs in the third trimester and is generally asymptomatic and poses little threat to the parent or fetus.
- **Preeclampsia thrombocytopenia (20%):** Most often occurs in the second and third trimesters and in approximately half of preeclamptic mothers. Increases the maternal risk of hypertension, HELLP syndrome, liver failure, kidney failure, cerebral hemorrhage, and stroke. Fetal risks include IUGR, preterm birth, stillbirth, and neonatal death.
- **Immune thrombocytopenia (4%):** Most often present before pregnancy or during the first trimester. Increases the risk of maternal hemorrhage, especially during delivery. Fetal risks include neonatal alloimmune thrombocytopenia, intracranial hemorrhage, and visceral hemorrhage. With neonatal alloimmune thrombocytopenia, the neonate may need corticosteroids to increase the platelet count or transfusions if the platelet count is <25,000/µL (in a stable infant) or <50,000/µL (in an unstable infant).
- **Disseminated intravascular coagulation (DIC)/thrombocytopenia (0.3–0.35%):** Increases the maternal risks of hemorrhage, organ dysfunction, placental abruption, and death. Fetal risks include preterm birth and fetal demise.

THROMBOPHILIA

Pregnancy produces a hypercoagulable state with increased clotting factors, and this can be exacerbated by **thrombophilia**, which is a predisposition to develop blood clots (such as deep vein thrombosis [DVT]). Changes in hemodynamics and hormones during pregnancy can result in hemostasis with a reduced velocity of the venous blood flow, which is more pronounced on the left side, the reason that most DVTs occur in the left leg in pregnant women. Types of thrombophilia include:

- **Inherited**: Factor V Leiden mutation (DVT), prothrombin G20-210A mutation (which increases clot formation), protein C deficiency (brings the risk of uncontrolled clotting), protein S deficiency (which increases the risk of clotting), and antithrombin III deficiency (has a high risk of clotting).
- **Acquired**: Antiphospholipid syndrome (highest risk for clotting), prolonged immobilization (has a risk of DVT), and hormone therapy (has an increased risk of DVT).

Regardless of the underlying cause, thrombophilia in the pregnant woman increases the risk of thromboembolism, including DVT and pulmonary embolism (PE) and it increases the risk of preeclampsia and recurrent miscarriage (especially in the first trimester). Risks to the fetus include IUGR, acute fetal distress, and stillbirth.

Hemolytic Disease

In addition to common cause of **hemolytic disease**, such as sickle cell disease and Rh incompatibility, a number of different hemolytic diseases may affect the pregnant woman and the developing fetus:

Disorder	Maternal Effects	Management	Fetal Effects
Hereditary spherocytosis	RBCs become spherical, increased destruction in the spleen	Folic acid, transfusions, splenectomy (rare)	Asymptomatic (common), fetal anemia, neonatal jaundice
Autoimmune hemolytic anemia	Body produces antibodies against RBCs	Corticosteroids, intravenous immunoglobulin, immunosuppressants, rituximab (rare)	Hemolytic anemia, hyperbilirubinemia, hydrops fetalis (rare)
Alpha and beta thalassemia	Causes microcytic anemia and hemolysis	Folic acid, transfusions, chelation therapy (rare)	Severe anemia, hydrops fetalis, hydrops fetalis, stillbirth
G6PD deficiency	Causes episodic hemolysis	Hydration, oxygen, folic acid, transfusions	Asymptomatic (common), neonatal jaundice, hemolysis
Paroxysmal nocturnal hemoglobinuria	Increases the risk of thrombosis and hemolysis	Eculizumab, prophylactic heparin, transfusions	IUGR, miscarriage, stillbirth, fetal anemia

Maternal effects of hemolytic disease can include anemia, jaundice, HELLP syndrome, infections, and thromboembolism. Because hemolytic disease may impair oxygenation and nutrient transfer to the placenta, the fetus is generally at risk for fetal anemia, hydrops fetalis, IUGR, and hyperbilirubinemia, regardless of the type of maternal hemolytic disease.

Disseminated Intravascular Coagulation (DIC)

Disseminated intravascular coagulation (DIC) is a secondary disorder triggered by another disorder such as postpartum hemorrhage (especially massive rapid loss of blood), placental abruption, preeclampsia, HELLP syndrome, amniotic fluid embolism (a major cause of DIC), sepsis, and acute fatty liver of pregnancy. DIC causes widespread activation of the coagulation system with release of procoagulant substances (the placenta being a primary source) into the blood, resulting in the formation of blood clots in small vessels, but DIC also consumes both clotting factors and platelets, resulting in an increased risk of bleeding. As platelets adhere to the clots, they block the microvascular system and can lead to ischemia and tissue necrosis. Maternal complications associated with DIC include hemorrhage (most common), organ dysfunction (e.g., liver, kidneys, lungs) from microvascular thrombosis, retained stillbirth, sepsis (e.g., systemic inflammatory response syndrome), placental abruption, and death. Fetal risks associated with DIC include preterm birth, intrauterine fetal death (resulting from disrupted blood supply), fetal acidosis, and IUGR. Neonates that survive maternal DIC may have respiratory distress syndrome and neurological impairment (e.g., cerebral palsy).

Rh Incompatibility

If the pregnant woman is Rh– and the father is Rh+ (**Rh incompatibility**), then their infant is at risk for hemolytic disease of the newborn. The baby can develop erythroblastosis fetalis, characterized by jaundice, fever, generalized edema, cyanosis, and hepatosplenomegaly. Hyperbilirubinemia and jaundice occur from red blood cell (RBC) destruction, leading to neurological impairment (i.e., kernicterus). Erythroblastosis fetalis can lead to hydrops fetalis, in which the production of interstitial fluid and lymphatic return are not balanced, so fluid accumulates. Treatment includes an exchange transfusion in utero or after birth. Pregnant women who are Rh– with an Rh+ mate should receive the serum RhoGAM, containing anti-Rh+ antibodies, which agglutinate any fetal RBCs that pass over into the pregnant woman's circulatory system. This prevents the mother from forming antibodies against them that will attack the fetus and will also sensitize the pregnant woman for future pregnancies:

- Pregnancy: 300 μg RhoGAM (Rho[D] immune globulin [RhIg]) intramuscularly at 26–28 weeks of pregnancy and again within 72 hours after the delivery.
- Miscarriage, ectopic, abortion: At ≤12 weeks, 50 μg of MICRhoGAM. At ≥13 weeks, RhoGAM as for pregnancy.

Maternal Acidosis

Maternal pH directly impacts the pH of the fetus, particularly in the case of **metabolic acidosis**. Because the fetus is extremely vulnerable to even minor changes in pH, this can be a very threatening condition. Maternal acidosis is linked with decreased fetal pH (fetal acidosis), resulting in lower Apgar scores for these neonates. Maternal causes of acidosis include uncontrolled diabetes (leading to diabetic ketoacidosis), renal dysfunction, and severe diarrhea. Fetal acid-base balance should be closely monitored in mothers with these conditions. Should the fetus show signs of distress (FHR abnormalities, decreased fetal movement, etc.) and acidosis in the fetus be suspected, the mother should immediately be tested in the case that fetal acidosis is secondary to maternal acidosis.

Acute Fatty Liver of Pregnancy (AFLP)

Acute fatty liver of pregnancy (AFLP) (the most common cause of liver failure during pregnancy) is characterized by micro-vesicular fat deposits throughout the liver that crowd out hepatocytes and interfere with liver function. AFLP, which is associated with genetic mutations, occurs in the third trimester or postpartal period. Women may exhibit nausea and vomiting, upper GI hemorrhage, coagulopathy, pancreatitis, hypoglycemia, hepatic encephalopathy (with confusion and altered mental status), hypertension, jaundice, general malaise, and renal and hepatic failure. Neonates may exhibit fatty acid oxidation defects that affect multiple body systems: cardiomyopathy, liver failure, myopathy, neuropathy, and hypoglycemia (nonketotic). Some may die *in utero* and 15% die after birth. The key to treatment of AFLP is immediate delivery of the fetus through labor induction or Cesarean (although coagulopathy may pose risks). Supportive care may include IV fluids, blood products, coagulation factors, and/or plasma exchange or plasmapheresis with continuous renal replacement therapy. Some women may require liver transplantation.

Maternal Systemic Lupus Erythematosus (SLE)

Systemic lupus erythematosus (SLE), a systemic reaction to collagen or connective tissue in the body, is believed to be triggered by an antibody-antigen immune response to an environmental agent, resulting in widespread damage of vessels and organs, primarily in females. Symptoms may include: malar and discoid rash; photosensitivity; oral ulcers; arthritis; serositis; and renal (proteinuria/nephritis), neurological (seizures, psychosis), and immunological disorders. Pregnant women with SLE have high rates of hypertension (up to 30%) and preeclampsia, especially with lupus nephritis, so they may need to continue immunosuppressive drugs during pregnancy. Women must be monitored carefully during pregnancy for flare-ups of SLE. Impaired circulation to the fetus may result from maternal decidual vasculopathy with placental infarction. Fetal risks include preterm delivery, fetal growth restriction, spontaneous abortion, and stillbirths. The newborn may inherit neonatal lupus, with symptoms appearing up to 4 weeks after birth. Indications include congenital heart block, autoimmune hemolysis, thrombocytopenia, and lupus dermatitis.

Review Video: Systemic Lupus Erythematosus
Visit mometrix.com/academy and enter code: 657082

Cholelithiasis and Cholecystitis

Pregnancy increases the risk of a woman developing **cholelithiasis** and **cholecystitis** because of increased levels of estrogen and increased biliary sludge (forerunner to gallstones). Symptoms occur when stones block the bile duct and may include RUQ pain, nausea, vomiting, low-grade fever, and mildly elevated white blood cell count. Some may have clay-colored stools and jaundice. Medical management has been most common in the first and third trimesters and surgical repair in the second trimester (when it is safest). However, early cholecystitis often recurs later in the pregnancy, increasing the risk of pre-term delivery and making surgery more difficult because of the size of the uterus, so some authorities advise against conservative treatment. Surgical procedures include laparoscopic cholecystectomy and endoscopic retrograde cholangiopancreatography for stones in the common bile duct. The fetus is usually unimpaired if the blockage is resolved.

Maternal Hypothyroidism and Hyperthyroidism

Maternal hypothyroidism threatens the development of the fetal brain and spinal cord. T4 is needed for proper development, and the fetus is not capable of T4 production during the critical period of growth. Decreased mental capacity or fetal death can occur.

Hyperthyroidism is difficult to detect since symptoms mimic normal pregnancy problems. The pregnant woman may have temporary hyperthyroidism in early pregnancy but levels should return to normal by the beginning of the second trimester. Continued high levels can cause thyroid crisis and result in fetal death or premature birth.

Review Video: What is Hyperthyroidism?
Visit mometrix.com/academy and enter code: 923159

Maternal Hyperemesis Gravidarum (HG)

Approximately 60–80% of pregnant women suffer from nausea and vomiting (NV), especially during the first trimester, but only approximately 2% suffer severe (sometimes intractable) NV, known as **hyperemesis gravidarum** (HG). NV may be associated with numerous disorders including cholelithiasis, pancreatitis, hepatitis, and ectopic pregnancy, especially if accompanied by abdominal pain. Diagnosis includes physical examination to rule out other disorders, a complete blood count with serum electrolytes, blood urea nitrogen, creatinine, and urinalysis.

Symptoms: Severe (sometimes intractable) NV, weight loss, malnutrition, dehydration, hypokalemia, ketonemia, ketonuria (from inadequate nutrition). Treatment includes:

- Intravenous fluids with 5% glucose in normal saline or Ringer's lactate
- Oral fluids after NV is controlled
- Antiemetic drugs
    - Acute treatment for NV and HG: promethazine (Phenergan), prochlorperazine (Compazine), or chlorpromazine (Thorazine)
    - Maintenance for NV: Doxylamine with pyridoxine (Unisom), diphenhydramine (Benadryl), or cisapride (Propulsid)
    - Maintenance for HG: Metoclopramide (Reglan), trimethobenzamide (Tigan), or ondansetron (Zofran)

Fetal effects can include IUGR, preterm birth, low birth weight, small head circumference (because of maternal malnutrition), and an increased risk for neurodevelopmental impairment and fetal hypoglycemia at birth (resulting from prolonged maternal ketosis).

Maternal Trauma

Maternal trauma can occur at any time during the pregnancy. Motor vehicle accidents are the leading cause of trauma to the pregnant woman. Maternal falls and trauma to the abdomen from domestic abuse are other common causes. Trauma to the abdomen by blunt force can result in abruptio placentae, placental injury, injury to the fetus, or uterine rupture causing fetal death by hemorrhage and hypoxia. Maternal hemorrhage and shock from traumatic injuries can result in both fetal and maternal death from hypoxia. Any trauma that compromises respiration will also cause hypoxia to the mother-fetal unit. Neurological trauma that results in shock, hemorrhage, or damage to the brain will also compromise the fetus when maternal vital functions deteriorate.

Placenta Previa and Abruptio Placentae

Placenta previa: Implantation of the placenta is over or near the internal cervical os. Women with placenta previa have increased incidences of hemorrhage in the third trimester. In infants, placenta previa is associated with poor growth, anemia, and increased risk of congenital anomalies in their central nervous systems, heart, respiratory and gastrointestinal tracts. Placenta previa may also cause premature birth with associated neonatal complications of prematurity.

Abruptio placentae: The placenta prematurely detaches, partially or completely, from the uterus. Abruptio placentae is related to maternal hypertension, and incidence increases with cocaine abuse. Partial detachment interferes with the functioning of the placenta, causing intrauterine growth restriction. Severe bleeding occurs with total detachment. Common fetal complications are preterm labor, hypoxia, and anemia. Fetal mortality is about 25% with partial detachment and 100% with complete. Irreversible brain damage may occur with fetal hypoxia, and neurological deficits occur in about 14% of survivors.

Vasa Previa

Vasa previa is an abnormality where at least one of the fetal blood vessels lies across the internal cervical os. The fetal umbilical vein and arteries lie unprotected on the membrane wall on their way to the placenta. This predisposes the fetus to hemorrhage if one of the vessels is injured during membrane rupture that occurs spontaneously or artificially. The FHR reacts immediately to the vessel damage and death occurs in 56% of all cases. An immediate cesarean section is indicated. Diagnosis may be made prenatally by transvaginal Doppler ultrasound or routine ultrasound that examines placental cord insertion. A planned cesarean increases the fetal survival rate to 97%.

Birth Injuries

Congenital Muscular Torticollis

Congenital muscular torticollis occurs when the infant's sternocleidomastoid muscle is shortened or excessively contracted secondary to trauma. The sternocleidomastoid muscle has its origin on the sternum and the clavicle and inserts at the mastoid process of the temporal bone. It flexes the neck and rotates the head. Torticollis occurs in 0.5-2.0% of live births. Damage to the muscle may occur *in utero* or if the birth process was difficult or traumatic. The muscle may tear, causing fibrosis or scarring. Symptoms of torticollis may not present for several weeks, especially if the trauma occurred during birth. Physical exam shows a head tilt away from the affected side, with limited range of motion. Face and skull asymmetry may be present from lack of position changes. A palpable mass may be felt within the sternocleidomastoid muscle. Treatment involves physical therapy to stretch the tight muscle and strengthening exercises to stimulate symmetry. Torticollis is rarely associated with malformations of the cervical vertebrae.

Fractures

Clavicular fracture is the most common injury during a vaginal birth. They are most commonly seen with high birth weight babies, shoulder dystocia, and forceps delivery. Newborns with a fractured clavicle often exhibit fussiness or crying with movement of the affected arm due to pain in the clavicle. The infant may not be able to move the arm at all if nerve injury occurred. An x-ray or ultrasound image of the clavicle is needed to confirm the fracture. In most cases, birth fractures of the clavicle usually heal in 7-10 days without any problems. Usually no treatment is required, but the parent may need to pin the infant's sleeve of the affected arm to the front of their clothing to immobilize the arm while it heals.

Rib fractures from birth trauma are rare, but may have the same origin as clavicle fractures, caused by the shoulder compression forces to the chest from a high birth weight infant or shoulder dystocia. These fractures may not cause any noticeable symptoms. If there are multiple rib fractures, the infant will show signs of pain when moved or picked up and may develop difficulty breathing that could indicate atelectasis from the fracture. Premature infants can also develop rib fractures after birth from simple handling and chest physiotherapy due to the extremely fragile nature of these bones. A chest x-ray is needed to diagnose a rib fracture.

Birth-Related Nerve Trauma

Cranial Nerve Trauma

Injury to cranial nerves can occur during birth (most commonly the recurrent laryngeal nerve) and is caused by compression of the head against the sacrum during birth or from the use of forceps. Symptoms relate to the specific type of nerve injury but may present as temporary or permanent paralysis. Often asymmetry, drooping of the eye or mouth, or failure of the eyelid to close is noted, especially when the infant cries. Traumatic injury to nerves usually resolves over time, beginning by the end of the first week but symptoms may persist to some degree for months.

An open eye must be protected by the use of synthetic tears and patching to prevent damage. Those with injury to the laryngeal nerve may have dyspnea and dysphagia and may require small frequent feedings or enteral feedings until the condition resolves. In most cases, treatment is symptomatic with careful observation so that complications can be treated promptly.

Brachial Plexus Trauma

Trauma to the brachial plexus may cause a full-term infant to hold his or her arm adducted and internally rotated after a delivery complicated by shoulder dystocia. There is movement in the hands. About 1-3 infants per 1,000 live births suffer **trauma to the brachial plexus**. The brachial plexus is a collection of nerve tissue located in the shoulder area that is the pathway for nerves traveling from the spine to the arm and shoulder. These nerves control the movement of the shoulder and arm. Most commonly, the upper portion of this plexus is damaged, leading to weak arm muscles (Erb's palsy). When examined, the infant holds the arm adducted and internally rotated. The startle reflex is abnormal on the affected side, but the grasp reflex is normal. If the lower portion of the plexus is damaged, the hand is paralyzed also, and the grasp reflex is absent (Klumpke's paralysis). Most infants recover fully, but recovery depends on the degree of damage to the brachial plexus (complete tear vs. stretching).

Infectious Diseases

Immunity

Infants (especially preterm) have **increased susceptibility to infection** when compared to older children and adults because of immaturity or deficiencies in their immune systems:

- **Cellular immunity**: Neutrophils and macrophages in the neonate are deficient in chemotaxis and not as effective in killing invading bacteria. Reserves of neutrophils are easily depleted in neonates.
- **Humoral immunity**: Some passage of immunoglobulin G (IgG) occurs from the mother to the fetus, but mostly during the third trimester. In general, immunoglobulin levels are low. The neonate does not produce IgA until 2-5 weeks after birth. Complement activity is also immature in newborns, leaving them especially susceptible to Gram-negative organisms.
- **Barrier function**: The skin and mucous membranes, which normally act as barriers, are less effective in newborns. Prolonged invasive instrumentation (central lines or endotracheal tubes) associated with infants who are premature or those with complex congenital deformities are other routes for infection.

Humoral Immunity

Humoral immunity in neonates is mainly mediated by maternal transfer of **Immunoglobulin G (IgG)** that greatly increases after 32 weeks of gestation. Infants born prior to 32 weeks have a significantly lower immunoglobulin level than term infants. Endogenous production of immunoglobulins does not begin until 24 weeks after birth, allowing serum immunoglobulin levels to trough until production begins. This trough further lowers the premature infant's ability to fight infections. The lower the infant's gestational age, the higher the incidence of neonatal sepsis. The risk of neonatal sepsis is 10 times higher in infants who weigh less than 2,500 grams, when compared to full term infants. Boost the premature infant's immunoglobulin level with intravenous IgG (IVIG) to prevent the acquisition of nosocomial infections or as adjunctive therapy in neonates with early onset sepsis. (Studies have shown mixed results with only minimal benefits.)

Sources of Neonatal Infection

For the neonate there are three main categories of sources of infection:

- **Transplacental (Intrauterine)** infection is a direct infection from the mother to the fetus prior to birth. Infections such as AIDS, Cytomegalovirus, Rubella, Syphilis and Toxoplasmosis are the most common types in this category.
- **Perinatal acquisition** during labor and delivery occurs at the time of birth rather than *in utero* and is a direct result of contact with a pathogen present on the mother at birth. Infections in this category include Chlamydia, Enterovirus, Group B *Streptococcus,* Hepatitis B and Herpes.
- **Hospital acquisition** in the neonatal period is the third category. This is an infection that the infant did not have at birth but acquired from hospital personnel, equipment, the mother, or visitors.

Nosocomial Infections in Neonatal Unit

A nosocomial infection is acquired while in the hospital and is often responsible for late onset sepsis in neonates. The immature or compromised immune systems of premature neonates, combined with the frequent use of invasive ventilators, catheters, ventricular shunts, chest tubes, and IVs make neonates susceptible to nosocomial infections:

- **Peripheral IVs** are very common in neonates and often require restarting because of their small and fragile veins. Appropriate aseptic technique is essential to lessen infections associated with peripheral IVs.
- **Percutaneously inserted central catheters**, most commonly used in the NICU as they are more permanent than peripheral IVs, are also associated with nosocomial infections and should not be left in place longer than 21 days.

Pathogens commonly involved in nosocomial infections include coagulase-negative staphylococci (CoNS), *Klebsiella*, *Serratia*, *Enterobacter*, *Pseudomonas*, and *Candida*. Viral infections, such as respiratory syncytial virus (RSV), are usually introduced by parents and visitors. Frequent use of antibiotics contributes to the development of opportunistic bacteria and drug-resistant infections, such as Vancomycin-resistant *Enterococci* and methicillin-resistant *Staphylococcus aureus*.

Gram-Positive and Gram-Negative Pathogens in the Nursery

The Gram stain is a rapid lab test that divides bacteria into two classes (gram-positive or gram-negative) depending on their staining characteristics. Gram staining narrows the range of likely pathogens so the doctor can choose an antibiotic, pending a culture and sensitivity, which requires several days.

- **Gram-positive**
  - Group B *Streptococcus* (most common)
  - *Staphylococcus aureus* and *S. epidermidis*
  - *Listeria monocytogenes*
- **Gram-negative**
  - *Escherichia coli* (most common)
  - *Klebsiella pneumoniae*
  - *Pseudomonas aeruginosa*
  - *Haemophilus influenzae*
  - *Enterobacter aerogenes*

Antibiotic resistance is increasing among gram-negative bacilli such as *Klebsiella pneumoniae, P. aeruginosa*, and *Enterobacter* spp. Organisms that are deemed significant may vary from one department to another, so that organisms that might prove fatal in the neonatal unit may pose less of a threat to adults.

CANDIDIASIS

Candida albicans is a fungus that can cause late onset sepsis and oral thrush in the neonate. Invasive **candidiasis** is a serious infection and has a mortality rate of 25-30%. The source of infection may be from the mother or from colonized health care workers. It is estimated that up to 30% of health care workers are colonized with *candida*. Immunocompromised patients, such as mothers with AIDS, are especially vulnerable to thrush. **Risk factors for the development** of candidiasis include:

- Birth weight less than 1,500 grams
- Prolonged use of broad-spectrum antibiotics
- TPN with infusion of lipids
- Prolonged urinary catheterization
- History of cutaneous or mucous membrane colonization or infection (thrush or candidal diaper rash)

Amphotericin B is the drug of choice for the treatment of candidiasis. Central lines and catheters may have to be removed.

ENTEROVIRUS

Enteroviruses include coxsackievirus, echovirus, and poliovirus (essentially eradicated in the United States). Most **enterovirus infections** (90%) in adults are asymptomatic or non-specific febrile illness with flu-like symptoms. There is no consensus regarding neonatal infections, but most researchers believe they are not acquired transplacentally but that infection occurs perineally (during delivery) or after birth (≥ 2 weeks) from exposure to a mother with the virus or another infected infant. Neonates are at increased risk of developing sepsis-like conditions, such as aseptic meningitis, myocarditis, and hepatitis. It may be difficult to differentiate enterovirus infection from bacterial sepsis. Because of lack of immune response, neonates <10 days are at increased risk from non-polio enteroviruses. Neonates may be lethargic, feverish, and exhibit signs of hypoperfusion (mottled skin, delay in capillary refill time, and cyanosis) and jaundice. They often feed poorly and cry inconsolably.

BACTERIAL INFECTIONS AFFECTING NEWBORNS

ESCHERICHIA COLI

Newborns who are preterm or low birth weight or whose mothers experienced prolonged labor or fever are at increased risk of ***Escherichia coli (E. coli)* infection**. Early recognition of **symptoms** and alerting the physician is critical. Contact precautions must be utilized.

- **GI infection:** Symptoms include green, watery, and bloody diarrhea, fever, and dehydration.
- **UTI:** Symptoms, such as fever pyuria, poor feeding, and irritability, usually occur in the 2nd to 3rd week but may be earlier in preterm neonates or secondary to bacteremia, so urine and blood cultures are usually done and antibiotics administered.
- **Neonatal sepsis:** Infection usually obtained intrapartum with symptoms within 6 hours of delivery. Symptoms include Low APGAR score, poor sucking, apnea, bradycardia, unstable temperature, vomiting, diarrhea, and dyspnea. Mortality rates are higher in low-birth weight and preterm neonates. Treatment is with antibiotics and supportive therapy.
- **Neonatal meningitis:** May progress from diarrhea or UTI. Onset after 48 hours usually includes neurological impairment, stupor, irritability, seizures, posturing, anterior fontanel bulging, and nuchal rigidity. Treatment is with antibiotics and supportive therapy.

Staphylococcus

Neonates may be exposed to *Staphylococcus* through contact with medical personnel or from contaminated equipment, such as ventilators. Risk factors include preterm birth, VLBW (<1500 g), prolonged hospitalization, and invasive procedures such as insertion of venous catheters. Indications of infection may include fever or hypothermia, cardiac changes (tachycardia, bradycardia), vomiting, lethargy, and skin rash or lesions. If the infection enters the bloodstream, the neonate may develop sepsis, which can progress to meningitis and to neurological compromise or death. *Staphylococcus aureus* is one of the most common infective agents and may be either methicillin-susceptible or methicillin resistant (MRSA), which is much more difficult to treat. *Staphylococcus epidermidis*, which is found on skin and mucosa, and coagulase-negative staphylococci both tend to colonize invasive devices, such as catheters, forming biofilms that lead to sepsis and are naturally resistant to antibiotics. Coagulase-negative staphylococci infections may also occur in preterm neonates receiving TPN.

Bacterial Meningitis

Bacterial meningitis is caused by a wide range of pathogenic organisms, varying with the infant's age:

- ≤1 month: *E.coli,* Group B *Streptococci*, *Listeria monocytogenes*, and *Neisseria meningitidis*
- 1-2 months: Group B *Streptococci*

Bacterial infections usually arise from the spread of distant infections but can enter the CNS from surgical wounds, invasive devices, or nasal colonization. The infective process includes inflammation, exudates, white blood cell accumulation, and tissue damage with the brain showing evidence of hyperemia and edema. Purulent exudate covers the brain and invades and blocks the ventricles, obstructing CSF and leading to increased intracranial pressure. Since antibodies specific to bacteria don't cross the blood-brain barrier, the body's ability to fight the infection is very poor.

Diagnosis

Diagnosis of bacterial meningitis is based on examination of cerebrospinal fluid and symptoms. **Symptoms** may be very non-specific, such as hypo- or hyperthermia, jaundice, irritability, lethargy, irregular respirations with periods of apnea, difficulty feeding with loss of suck reflex, hypotonia, weak cry, seizures, and bulging fontanels (late sign). Nuchal rigidity does not usually occur with neonates. Meningitis is often difficult to diagnose in the neonate because it has early nonspecific clinical findings of irritability, lethargy, poor feeding, temperature instability, and hypotension. The more specific neurological symptoms of seizures or bulging fontanels are seen in late onset infection. Antibiotics given to the mother prior to delivery or to the neonate prior to performing a lumbar puncture inhibit bacterial growth in cerebrospinal fluid (CSF), making the diagnosis dependent on other CSF parameters. **CSF findings** suggestive of bacterial meningitis include:

- Decreased glucose
- Elevated protein
- White blood cells values in CSR greater than 100 WBC/dL

A polymerase chain reaction assay test for Group B strep antigen in CSF is available. Values may be more difficult to interpret in the premature neonate, as their blood brain barrier is more permeable.

Neonatal Cytomegalovirus Infections

Cytomegalovirus is the leading infectious cause of birth defects and neurodevelopmental disabilities. Pregnant women infected with cytomegalovirus are usually asymptomatic. Transmission may be intrauterine, perinatal (contact with infected secretions or through breast milk), or postnatal (less severe unless the infant is preterm or immunocompromised). Ninety percent of infected infants are asymptomatic, but those born at <32 weeks are most at risk for symptomatic disease. Symptoms can be severe and can include IUGR, neonatal jaundice, microcephaly, hepatosplenomegaly, purpura, seizures, sensorineural hearing loss (which is progressive, and 10–15% of those who are asymptomatic develop it over time), intracranial calcifications, thrombocytopenia, seizures, chorioretinitis, hypotonia, neurodevelopmental delays (which develop over time), elevated liver enzymes, and hyperbilirubinemia. Diagnosis is per polymerase chain reaction testing or culture from saliva, urine, or blood (within the first 3 weeks), cytomegalovirus DNA in blood or cerebrospinal fluid, and brain imaging. Treatment with antivirals is generally reserved for symptomatic infants because of significant adverse effects and should begin within the first 4 weeks, but it is not recommended for infants younger than 32 weeks of gestation. Antivirals include ganciclovir and valganciclovir, but valganciclovir poses less risk of adverse effects. A common protocol is valganciclovir 16 mg twice a day for 1 year to reduce hearing loss and improve neurodevelopment outcomes.

Hospital-Acquired Pneumonia

Klebsiella Pneumoniae

Klebsiella pneumoniae is a common cause of hospital-acquired infections of the urinary tract, surgical sites, and lower respiratory tract. *K. pneumoniae* is a gram-negative member of the Enterobacteriaceae family and is part of the normal body flora. It can infect children of all ages but is most common in infants who are premature and/or in neonatal intensive care. Infants with invasive devices, such as those with mechanical ventilation, are at increased risk. There have been a number of outbreaks in neonatal units, especially with multi-drugs resistant forms, with the hands of health staff and the gastrointestinal tract of the infants providing reservoirs of bacteria.

When the infection attacks the lungs, the **symptoms** include inflammatory changes that result in necrosis and hemorrhage, clogging the lungs with thick puro-sanguineous exudate. The disease spreads rapidly, with high fever and dyspnea. Mortality rates are high.

Treatment includes antibiotic therapy (such as 3rd generation cephalosporins or quinolones) based on cultures and sensitivities.

Pseudomonas Aeruginosa

Hospital-acquired pneumonias (HAP) are far more lethal than community-acquired pneumonias (CAP), with HAP death rates of 20-40% and up to 90% if the infant is on mechanical ventilation, with ***Pseudomonas aeruginosa*** one of the most lethal (40-60% mortality) because it can invade blood vessels, resulting in hemorrhage. Most infections are spread by contact with contaminated hands of healthcare staff or from invasive devices, such as endotracheal tubes and mechanical ventilators.

Symptoms include fever, cough, bradycardia, and elevated WBC counts.

Treatment includes:

- Antibiotic therapy: Usually combinations of 2 antibiotics are given, such as piperacillin or ceftazidime and gentamicin or ciprofloxacin (based on cultures). Vancomycin is generally avoided because of the rise of vancomycin-resistant organisms.
- Preventive measures include maintaining ventilated patients in 30° upright positions, universal precautions, and changing ventilator circuits as per protocol.

Sepsis

Early-Onset Sepsis

Early-onset bacterial sepsis usually occurs in the first 24 hours after birth, but may occur any time up to day 6 of life. Infants born prematurely have an increased rate of early-onset sepsis and more rapid onset of symptoms. In early onset sepsis, the source of infection is from the mother, either transplacentally, or a microorganism that colonized the mother's birth canal. Pathogens that most commonly cause early-onset sepsis are Group B *Streptococcus, E. coli, Haemophilus influenzae,* coagulase-negative staphylococci, and *Listeria monocytogenes.* **Risk factors** for the development of early onset sepsis include:

- Premature, preterm, or prolonged rupture of membranes
- Maternal colonization with Group B *Streptococcus*
- Fever in the mother greater than 38 °C during delivery
- Premature birth or low birth weight (<2500 g)
- Maternal urinary tract infection
- Chorioamnionitis
- APGAR score less than 6 at 1 minute or 5 minutes
- Delivery with birth asphyxia or meconium staining

Clinical Manifestations and Diagnosis

The clinical manifestations for **early-onset sepsis** are often vague and nonspecific making it a particular challenge to diagnose early. Sometimes the only noticeable sign is that the mother or nurse will note that the infant just doesn't seem well—nothing that can be specified but general symptoms perhaps starting with a poor feeding or other seemingly minor event. Infection may localize or cause bacteremia and sometimes meningitis. Some **manifestations** that should be noted include:

- The inability of the infant to maintain a normal body temperature
- Apnea, tachypnea
- Vomiting
- Cyanosis
- Lethargy
- Jaundice
- Seizures
- Purpura

If sepsis is suspected, CSF examination is done to evaluate for possible meningitis, a frequent complication of sepsis, especially if the infant is exhibiting symptoms of sepsis, GBS sepsis, or late onset of infection.

LATE-ONSET SEPSIS

Late-onset sepsis occurs after day 6 of life and is more common in preterm infants and those with medical or surgical conditions. The infection is acquired from the environment after birth, rather than from the mother. Infants with indwelling catheters, nasal cannulas, continuous positive airway pressure (CPAP), intubation, ventricular taps, and any other type of prolonged instrumentation are at increased risk. Late onset sepsis generally has a more gradual onset than early onset sepsis, and the site of primary infection relates to the cause. For example, ventilation-associated infection results in pneumonia. **Likely organisms involved in late onset sepsis** include:

- Gram-positive organisms like *Staphylococcus aureus* and Group B *Streptococcus* in 2/3 of cases
- Gram-negative organisms such as *E coli*, *Klebsiella pneumoniae*, *Pseudomonas aeruginosa*, *Serratia*, *Enterobacter*, and *Acinetobacter*
- *Candida*

TREATMENT OF SEPSIS/MENINGITIS

Neonatal sepsis and meningitis are treated with **intravenous antibiotics**. Usually if sepsis is suspected, treatment with broad-spectrum antibiotics (IV aminoglycoside and penicillin) will be started while awaiting the culture results. Once culture results are obtained any adjustment to a more effective medication to treat the now identified organism may be made. Using antibiotics too liberally when not indicated by a confirmed bacterial infection can have serious consequences for the neonate, such as the development of antibiotic resistant strains of bacteria and the killing of the normal flora of organisms that inhabit the intestinal tract leading to digestive problems. These problems must be weighed with the need to quickly treat a suspected sepsis when cultures have not been completed as many of these take days to finish growing. If hydrocephalus occurs with meningitis, then a ventroperitoneal shunt may be inserted surgically. Enteral or parenteral feedings may be necessary to provide adequate nutrition during treatment. Radiant warmers or incubators may be needed for thermoregulation.

RANGE OF SEVERE INFECTIONS

There are a number of terms used to refer to the range of severe infections and often used interchangeably, but they are part of a continuum:

- **Bacteremia** is the presence of bacteria in the blood but without systemic infection.
- **Septicemia** is a systemic infection caused by pathogens (usually bacteria or fungi) present in the blood.
- **Systemic inflammatory response syndrome (SIRS)**, a generalized inflammatory response affecting many organ systems, may be caused by infectious or non-infectious agents, such as trauma, adrenal insufficiency, pulmonary embolism, and drug overdose. If an infectious agent is identified or suspected, SIRS is an aspect of sepsis. Infective agents for infants include a wide range of bacteria and fungi, including *Streptococcus pneumoniae* and *Staphylococcus aureus.* SIRS includes 2 of the following:
    - Elevated (>38 °C) or subnormal rectal temperature (<36 °C)
    - Tachypnea >60 for infants or $PaCO_2$ <32 mmHg
    - Tachycardia >160 for infants
    - Leukocytosis (>12,000) or leukopenia (<4000)

- **Sepsis** is the presence of infection either locally or systemically in which there is a generalized life-threatening inflammatory response (SIRS). It includes all the indications for SIRS as well as one of the following:
    - Hypoxemia (<72 mmHg) without pulmonary disease
    - Elevation in plasma lactate
    - Decreased urinary output <5 mL/kg/hr for ≥1 hour
- **Severe sepsis** includes both indications of SIRS and sepsis as well as indications of increasing organ dysfunction with inadequate perfusion and/or hypotension.
- **Septic shock** is a progression from severe sepsis in which refractory hypotension occurs despite treatment. There may be indications of lactic acidosis.
- **Multi-organ dysfunction syndrome** (MODS) is the most common cause of sepsis-related death. Cardiac function becomes depressed, acute respiratory distress syndrome (ARDS) may develop, and renal failure may follow acute tubular necrosis or cortical necrosis. Thrombocytopenia appears in about 30% of those affected and may result in disseminated intravascular coagulation (DIC). Liver damage and bowel necrosis may occur.

Thermoregulation

Neutral Thermal Environment

A neutral thermal environment (NTE) is a place in which the infant's body temperature is maintained within a normal range without alterations in metabolic rate or increased oxygen consumption (i.e., environmental temperature in which oxygen consumption and glucose consumption are lowest). Infants who are in an NTE are not utilizing energy to maintain their body temperature in the normal range. Just because an infant has a normal body temperature does not mean he/she is in an NTE. The infant may still be utilizing mechanisms, such as non-shivering thermogenesis, to maintain body temperatures, as evidenced by increased oxygen consumption and poor weight gain over time. Charts are commercially available that outline the appropriate NTE for infants based on current weight and birth weight.

Heat Transfer Mechanisms

There are four heat transfer mechanisms to consider when caring for a neonate, especially a premature one:

- **Conduction**: The transfer of heat between solid objects of different temperatures in contact with each other. Heat is transferred from the body of the infant to a cold surface it may come into contact with, such as a scale. Care should be taken to make sure the scales are warmed before use. Conduction can also be used to warm the infant by placing a warmed blanket next to the skin.
- **Convection**: The transfer of heat through air currents moving around and across an infant's body. Incubators use convection of warm air being pumped into the incubator to keep an infant warm. Heat can be lost this way if a cool draft is allowed near the infant.
- **Radiation**: Heat transferred between two objects not in contact with each other. This is the transfer of heat through emission of infrared rays. Radiant warming beds use this mechanism to warm the infant. Heat loss occurs when an infant is in an incubator and the walls of the incubator are cooler than body temperature. The neonate in an incubator with this situation will lose body heat through radiation from its body to the cooler walls despite the warm air being pumped in.

- **Evaporation**: Loss of heat occurs when moisture evaporates from the surface of the skin. Evaporation is the result of the conversion of liquid into a vapor and is a major concern at birth, as a wet infant can experience a 3-degree drop in body temperature in only about 10 minutes. Thus, it is critical to dry the neonate at birth and to replace wet linens with warm, dry ones.

Evaporative Heat Loss and Humidity Related to Preterm Infants

Evaporative heat loss occurs when moisture vaporizes from the skin of an infant. In infants born younger than 31 weeks gestation, **evaporative heat loss** is greatly enhanced by the poor keratinization of the infant's skin. Poor keratinization makes skin highly permeable, which promotes both fluid and heat loss. This permeability decreases 7-10 days after birth. The amount of evaporation is dependent on the relative humidity of the environment. The more **humid the environment**, the more that evaporation and its associated heat loss are suppressed. A dry environment promotes evaporative heat and fluid loss through the skin. An incubator with humidity controls should be used for infants who are vulnerable to evaporative heat loss. Infants prone to temperature instability should be kept in a highly humid environment.

Cold Stress/Hypothermia

Signs of Cold Stress

Cold stress/hypothermia in the neonate is a body temperature measurement of less than 36.5 °C rectally with associated symptoms. Preterm neonates are especially vulnerable to cold stress, as they have limited ability to intrinsically create or conserve body heat. They do not shiver, have limited ability to constrict superficial blood vessels and have limited amounts of both subcutaneous and brown fat. **Signs of cold stress** include:

- Body is cool to touch
- Central cyanosis and acrocyanosis
- Mottling of skin
- Poor feeding, weak suck, increased gastric residuals, and abdominal distension
- Bradycardia
- Shallow respirations with tachypnea
- Restlessness and irritability
- Apnea
- Lethargy and decreased activity
- Weak cry
- Hypoglycemia
- Central nervous system depression with hypotonia
- Edema

Risk Factors in Preterm Infants

Preterm infants have not yet developed many of the features that full term infants use to help protect them from heat loss. The characteristics that make premature infants especially **vulnerable to cold stress** include:

- Larger surface area to body mass ratio that allows for quicker transfer of body heat to the environment
- Decreased amounts of subcutaneous fat that provides insulation from heat loss
- Decreased amounts of brown fat used for non-shivering thermogenesis

- Immature skin that is not completely keratinized is more permeable to evaporative water and heat loss
- Inability to flex the body to conserve heat
- Limited control of skin blood flow mechanisms that conserve heat

Non-Shivering Thermogenesis

Non-shivering thermogenesis (NST) is the major route of rapid increase of body temperature in response to cold stress in the term neonate. NST is the oxidation of brown fat to create heat. Brown adipose tissue contains a high concentration of stored triglycerides, a rich capillary network, and is controlled by the sympathetic nervous system. Brown fat cells have a rich supply of mitochondria that are unique, in that when fat is metabolized ATP is not produced, but instead heat is created. Temperature regulation is controlled by the posterior hypothalamus. When a cold body temperature is detected, the posterior hypothalamus responds by triggering the adrenal glands to release norepinephrine and the pituitary gland to release thyroxine. Both norepinephrine and thyroxine stimulate NST. Brown adipose production begins around 26-28 weeks of gestation and continues until 3-5 weeks after delivery. Premature infants have limited amounts of brown fat and limited ability to create heat via NST.

Thermoregulation to Treat Hypothermia

There are a number of steps in the treatment of hypothermia:

1. Determine if the cause of hypothermia is from an abnormal physiological process in the infant or from environmental conditions.
2. Rewarm the infant slowly, as rewarming too rapidly may result in apnea or hypotension.
3. Maintain the ambient temperature at 1.0-1.5 °C higher than the infant's temperature. Oxygen consumption is not elevated when the difference between the skin temperature and the environmental air temperature is less than 1.5 °C.
4. Increase the air temperature by approximately 1 °C every hour until the infant's temperature is in the normal range and stable.
5. Warm IV fluids with a blood-warming device prior to infusion, to enhance warming of the child.
6. Closely monitor the infant's blood glucose levels, vital signs, and urinary output during rewarming.

Hyperthermia

Hyperthermia (rectal temperature greater than 37.0 °C) can be caused by excessive heat from an external source (such as a radiant warmer set too high) or internally from a hypermetabolic state (such as a fever):

External heat source	Hypermetabolic
Core temperature < skin temperature	Core temperature > skin temperature
Skin warm and flushed	Skin cool to touch

Infants who are physiologically competent attempt to cool themselves when hyperthermia is caused by an external heat source by an extended posture, diaphoresis, and flushed, warm skin. Hyperthermia in the neonate can cause increased metabolic demands, vasodilatation, and increased fluid loss. An increased metabolic demand leads to an increased oxygen requirement, hypoxia, cyanosis, and breathing irregularities, such as tachypnea. Increased glucose consumption leads to hypoglycemia and its associated signs (jitteriness, lethargy, vomiting, or seizures). Peripheral vasodilatation helps cool the infant but may cause tachycardia and hypotension. Increased fluid losses contribute to tachycardia and hypotension. Signs of shock may develop with lethargy and decreased urine output. Dehydration may also cause electrolyte abnormalities.

Minimizing Heat Loss

At delivery, minimize heat loss while evaluating the newborn by following these steps:

- Dry the infant thoroughly (including hair) to minimize evaporative heat loss and remove wet towels.
- Place a cap on the infant's head, as the head is the most significant area of heat loss.
- When the infant is to be weighed, cover the scales with a warm cloth to minimize conductive heat loss.
- Place the infant in a warm environment such as:
    - Skin-to-skin contact with the mother and covered with a warm blanket.
    - Bundled in warm blankets and given to the mother to hold.
    - Underneath a preheated warmer for further evaluation or resuscitation.

Minimizing heat loss is especially important if the newborn is premature or has intrauterine growth restriction, but full-term newborns also suffer if they become chilled.

Kangaroo Care

Dr. Edgar Ray invented kangaroo care in the late 1970's in Bogotá, Colombia, when morbidity and mortality rates rose in his NICU, but he had limited technological resources. **Kangaroo care** consists of placing the infant, after drying and warming, in minimal clothing in an upright position on the mother's bare chest between her breasts. This allows for skin-to-skin contact with the infant's head next to the mother's heart. A precipitous drop was noted in premature infant mortality after this method of care was instigated. The concept is to provide the neonate with closeness similar to that experienced with the mother while in the womb. Kangaroo care is maintained for as long as the neonate allows. Preterm infants attached to ventilators and IV infusions also benefit from kangaroo care. There are physiological and psychological benefits for both the neonate and the mother. Enhanced bonding between the neonate and the mother, shorter hospital stays, low cost, and decreased morbidity and mortality are all documented benefits.

The following are specific **benefits** of kangaroo care for the mother, the neonate, and the institution:

- **Mother's benefits**:
  - Enhanced bonding with the infant
  - Increased production of milk with higher rates of successful breastfeeding
  - Increased confidence in caring for the infant
  - Increased opportunity for teaching and assessing maternal care by nursing staff
- **Neonate's benefits:**
  - Regulation of temperature, heart and respiratory rates
  - Calming effect with decreased stress
  - Decreased episodes of apnea
  - Increased weight gain
  - Enhanced bonding with the mother
  - Fewer nosocomial infections

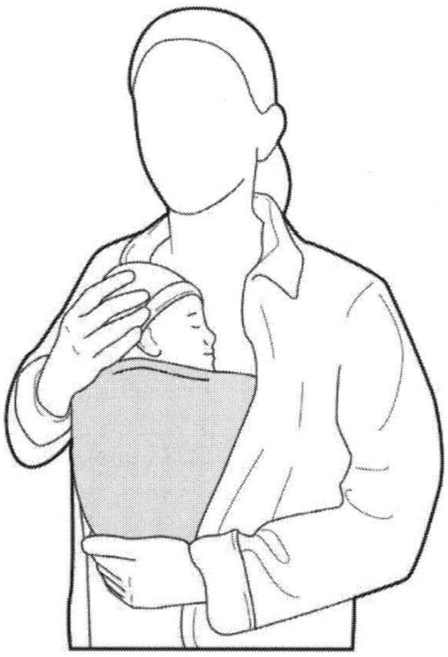

- **Institutional benefits**:
  - Earlier discharge from hospital
  - Decreased morbidity and mortality (especially in developing countries)
  - Decreased use of financial resources

Incubators

The goal of placing an infant in an incubator is to provide a neutral thermal environment (NTE) that places minimal stress on the infant. Most incubators are rigid, box-like structures like an isolette, in which an infant is kept in a controlled environment to receive medical care. The infant is allowed to grow and mature here before being transitioned to the more "uncontrolled" environment of an open crib. Features that incubators possess that enhance the production of an NTE include a heater, a fan to circulate warmed air, and a humidity control system. They also usually have a way to increase the oxygen content of the environment and ports to allow for nursing care without removing the infant. A servo-control is used in conjunction with a temperature-sensing thermistor that is attached to the infant to help regulate the infant's temperature within a set range. Some incubators may have double walls that lessen radiant heat loss. Infants who are in need of close monitoring are not placed in an incubator but instead are placed under a radiant warmer with minimal covering. This allows the nurse to monitor the infant's skin color and breathing patterns more closely.

Radiant Warmers

Radiant warmers are devices that provide overhead heat directly to the infant. Radiant heaters provide an area for direct observation and free access to the infant, which is very useful in the initial evaluation and resuscitation (if necessary) of the newborn or for procedures such as intubation or line placement. Radiant heat devices work best if the room temperature is kept above 25 °C. Two **problems related to radiant warmers** include:

- Promote dehydration if an infant is placed under them for a prolonged amount of time, especially if the infant is premature
- Risk overheating the infant or cause first-degree burns

Temperature sensors must be appropriately placed and the infant's temperature monitored frequently to ensure the infant is not being over or under heated.

SKIN TEMPERATURE PROBES

Skin temperature probes are often used to monitor the temperature of the infant in an isolette or radiant warmer. Incorrect placement of the probe can alter the reading, causing the warming device to deliver too much or too little heat. The temperature probe should not be placed over a bony area of the body or over an area where brown adipose tissue is abundant. Brown adipose tissue is abundant around the neck, the midscapular region of the back, and the mediastinum and organs in the thoracic cavity, kidneys, and adrenal glands. A common probe placement area for an infant who is supine is over the liver. If the probe is not making good skin contact, it will indicate that the infant is cold, and the warmer will deliver increased amounts of heat, possibly causing hyperthermia. If the probe is underneath the infant, it may indicate an artificially warm temperature and decrease heat to the infant, causing hypothermia.

SERVOCONTROL

The servocontrol is a **thermistor probe** used to monitor the temperature of the infant in an incubator or radiant warmer. The servocontrol is essentially the automatic thermostat that adjusts the environmental temperature in response to the infant's body temperature. Typically, the infant's temperature should be maintained at 36.5-37.5°C. Incorrect placement of the probe can alter the reading, causing the warming device to deliver too much or too little heat. The servocontrol should avoid a bony area of the body or an area where brown adipose tissue is abundant (neck, midscapular region, mediastinum, and organs in the thoracic cavity, kidneys, and adrenal glands). If the infant is supine, the probe is placed on the abdomen at the midpoint between the xiphoid process and the umbilicus. If prone, the probe is placed over either flank. If in a radiant warmer, a special foil shield should protect the probe. As mentioned above, the probe must make proper skin contact, and the nurse should be sure that is not reading artificially warm or artificially cool. An incorrect reading can put the infant at risk for hyperthermia or hypothermia.

Toxin/Drug Exposure

FETAL ALCOHOL SYNDROME

Fetal alcohol syndrome (FAS) is a syndrome of birth defects that develop as the result of maternal ingestion of alcohol. Fetal alcohol spectrum disorders (FASD) is an umbrella diagnosis that includes FAS along with infants impacted by alcohol in utero that do not meet the full FAS criteria. Despite campaigns to inform the public, women continue to drink during pregnancy, but no safe amount of alcohol ingestion has been determined. FAS includes:

- **Facial abnormalities**: Hypoplastic (underdeveloped) maxilla, micrognathia (undersized jaw), hypoplastic philtrum (groove beneath the nose), short palpebral fissures (eye slits between upper and lower lids).
- **Neurological deficits**: May include microcephaly, intellectual disability, motor delay, and hearing deficits. Learning disorders may include problems with visual-spatial and verbal learning, attention disorders, delayed reaction times.
- **Growth restriction**: Prenatal growth deficit persists with slow growth after birth.
- **Behavioral problems**: Irritability and hyperactivity. Poor judgment in behavior may relate to deficit in executive functions.

Indication of brain damage without the associated physical abnormalities is referred to as alcohol-related neurodevelopmental disorder (ARND).

Fetal Exposure to Tobacco/Nicotine

Tobacco smoke contains many substances known to be detrimental to a person's health. When a pregnant woman smokes, her fetus is exposed to carbon monoxide, nicotine, and hydrogen cyanide that all cross the placenta. Carbon monoxide displaces oxygen from hemoglobin, resulting in decreased oxygen delivery to the fetus. Exposure increases risk of miscarriage and perinatal death. Infants exposed *in utero* to tobacco may have the following problems:

- Decreased length, weight, and head circumference
- Increased rates of congenital birth defects, such as cleft palate or lip, limb reduction defects, and urinary tract anomalies
- Increased incidence of placenta previa, placental abruption, and preterm birth

If smoking continues after delivery, these further detrimental effects may occur:

- Sudden infant death syndrome
- Increased infant respiratory tract infections and childhood asthma
- Behavioral problems in later childhood

Fetal Exposure to Marijuana, PCP, and MDMA

Marijuana, phencyclidine (PCP), and methylenedioxymethamphetamine (MDMA or ecstasy) are popular club drugs that may be used by some women during pregnancy:

- **Marijuana**: This is often used along with alcohol and tobacco, so effects are difficult to assess, but there do not appear to be teratogenic effects; however, some studies report exposure can result in fine tremors, irritability, and prolonged startle response for the first 12 months after birth.
- **PCP**: One of the biggest problems with PCP is that mothers may have an overdose or psychotic response that can result in hypertension, hyperthermia, and coma, compromising the fetus.
- **MDMA**: Ecstasy is frequently used by teenagers and young adults. There is no clear evidence regarding effects on the fetus although some research suggests it may cause long-term impairments in learning.

Fetal Exposure to Amphetamines

Amphetamines are a class of drugs that cause CNS stimulation. The most commonly abused amphetamine is methamphetamine. Maternal use of these substances causes hypertension and tachycardia, which can cause miscarriage, abruptio placentae, and premature delivery. Vasoconstriction affects placental vessels, decreasing circulation, nutrition, and oxygen to the fetus. Methamphetamines can cross the placental barrier and cause fetal hypertension and prenatal strokes and damage to the heart and other organs. The neonate is commonly small for gestational age, often ≤5 pounds, full term but ≤10 percentile for weight, with shortened length and smaller head circumference. The neonate in withdrawal from maternal amphetamine use will suffer abnormal sleep patterns, often characterized by lethargy and excessive sleeping during the first few weeks, poor feeding, tremors, diaphoresis, miosis, frantic fist sucking, high-pitched crying, fever, excessive yawning, and hyperreflexia.

Fetal Exposure to Heroin

Heroin is a highly addictive, opioid narcotic that is a common drug of abuse. Heroin users are at increased risk of poor nutrition, iron deficiency anemia, and preeclampsia-eclampsia, all negatively affecting the fetus. Infants with prenatal heroin exposure display symmetric intrauterine growth restriction (IUGR) and are often born prematurely. About 60–80% of these infants will undergo neonatal abstinence syndrome (NAS). Heroin has a relatively short half-life and symptoms of NAS typically begin 48–72 hours after delivery. Several different body systems are affected by NAS and include:

- **CNS Dysfunction**
  - High-pitched cry
  - Hyperactive reflexes
  - Irritability
  - Tremors
- **GI Dysfunction**
  - Poor feeding
  - Periods of frantic sucking or rooting
  - Vomiting
  - Loose or watery stools
- **Miscellaneous Signs**
  - Frequent yawning
  - Sneezing multiple times
  - Sweating
  - Fever
  - Tachypnea

Fetal Exposure to Methadone

Methadone is commonly used to treat women who are addicted to opioids, such as heroin or prescriptive narcotics, as it blocks withdrawal symptoms and drug craving. An associated risk is that methadone crosses the placental barrier and exposes the fetus to the drug. Many female heroin users are of reproductive age, and methadone is often administered to pregnant women to decrease dangers associated with heroin, such as fluctuating levels of drug and exposure to hepatitis and HIV from sharing of needles. Exposure to methadone may result in miscarriage, stillbirth, intrauterine growth restriction, fetal distress, and low birth weight, although symptoms are usually less severe than with heroin. However, if the mother takes methadone and other drugs, this can compound the adverse effects. Additionally, sudden withdrawal from methadone may cause preterm labor or death of the fetus, so methadone should be monitored carefully.

Fetal Exposure to Cocaine

Cocaine/crack (freebase cocaine) is a nonopioid substance that readily crosses the placenta through simple diffusion. One of the most potent properties of cocaine is its ability to act as a vasoconstrictor. When a mother uses cocaine, the blood supply to the placenta is severely compromised when the vessels constrict, compromising blood flow and resulting in growth restriction and hypoxia. Cocaine also causes a programmed cell death (known as apoptosis) in the heart muscle cells of the fetus, resulting in cardiac dysfunction for the fetus. Maternal cocaine use increases the risk of premature birth and causes serious consequences for the neonate after birth. Maternal cocaine use can cause cerebral infarctions, non-duodenal intestinal atresia, anal atresia, NEC, defects of the limbs, and genitourinary defects. Cocaine stimulates the central nervous system by limiting the uptake of certain neurotransmitters, such as norepinephrine, serotonin, and dopamine. Cocaine has a direct toxic effect on the nervous system, so the infant will exhibit extreme irritability and tremors followed by sluggish, lethargic behavior.

Neonatal Abstinence Syndrome and Management

Neonatal abstinence syndrome may occur as the result of in utero exposure to legal or illegal drugs, or as a result of fetal or neonatal exposure to opioids for analgesia or sedation. Symptoms are dependent on the drug of exposure. Non-pharmacologic interventions in mild cases may include comfort measures such as contact (e.g., swaddling, skin-to-skin, holding), feeding/non-nutritive sucking, and a quiet environment. Pharmacological management may be required in more severe cases. Scores such as the modified Finnegan NAS score are often used to determine symptom severity and required interventions.

If pharmacologic measures are needed, drug dosages are typically tapered as withdrawal symptoms fade, and treatment is tailored to the individual needs of the neonate. Medications used in the treatment of neonatal abstinence syndrome include the following:

- **Morphine sulfate (oral)**: First-line therapy. Initial dose of 0.04 mg/kg every 3–4 hours. This is the most commonly used drug to reduce withdrawal symptoms (irritability, poor feeding, tremors).
- **Methadone (oral)**: First-line therapy. Initial dose of 0.05–0.01 mg/kg every 6 hours. There are fewer adverse effects than with morphine. It has a longer half-life than morphine.
- **Clonidine (oral)**: Second-line therapy. Initial dose of 0.5–1.0 mcg/kg every 6 hours. This is an adjunctive therapy, usually used with morphine to help relieve irritability, sleep disturbance, and tremors.
- **Phenobarbital (IV or IM)**: Second-line therapy. Initial dose of 20 mg/kg given IV/orally, then maintenance dose of 5 mg/kg per day (orally or IV). It is used for the withdrawal symptoms associated with polydrug use. There is good control of insomnia and irritability.

Fetal Exposure to Prescription/OTC Drugs

Many OTC and prescription drugs have teratogenic effects on the developing fetus and can result in congenital abnormalities, growth restriction, intellectual disability, carcinogenesis, mutagenesis, and miscarriage. The degree of damage relates to multiple factors, such as the amount of drug reaching the fetus, the developmental period during which the drug is taken, and the duration for which the drug was taken. There are some recognizable syndromes:

- **Fetal warfarin (Coumadin) syndrome** (exposure 7–12 weeks): Nasal hypoplasia, laryngomalacia, atrial septal defects, patent ductus arteriosis, eye, ear, and skull abnormalities, intellectual disabilities and growth restriction, brachydactyly, and scoliosis. Exposure during 2nd and 3rd trimester may result in eye abnormalities (cataracts, optic atrophy), microphthalmia (eyes stop developing resulting in abnormally small eyes), fetal/maternal hemorrhage, and microcephaly.
- **Fetal hydantoin (Dilantin) syndrome** (exposure 1st trimester): Facial dysmorphism, microcephaly, underdeveloped nails (hands and feet), cleft left/palate, and developmental delays ranging from mild to severe.
- **Fetal valproate (Depakote) syndrome** (exposure 1st trimester): Facial dysmorphism, spina bifida, CNS and cardiac abnormalities, and delay in development.

Some drugs are classified as high risk (FDA classification D), but use is acceptable if the mother has a life-threatening illness or other drugs are not available, so neonates may exhibit adverse effects.

Drugs with high risk include and their adverse effects on the fetus/infant include:

- **ACE inhibitors** (2nd and 3rd trimesters): skull and pulmonary hypoplasia, renal tubular dysplasia, and oligohydramnios
- **Carbamazepine** (1st trimester): craniofacial defects, neural tube defects, restriction of growth, and hypoplasia of fingernails
- **Antineoplastic alkylating drugs** (1st to 3rd trimesters): eye disorders, including microphthalmia and cataracts, cardiac defects, renal agenesis, and cardiac abnormalities
- **Iodides** (3rd trimester): thyroid disorders, including goiter, and fetal hypothyroidism
- **Methimazole** (1st trimester): aplasia cutis
- **Lithium** (1st trimester): Ebstein anomaly, various cardiac abnormalities
- **Tetracycline** (2nd and 3rd trimesters): yellow discoloration of teeth, weakening of fetal bones, and dysplasia of tooth enamel

Some drugs are classified as extremely high risk (FDA classification X), and these drugs should not be used with women who are pregnant or might become pregnant because fetal risk outweighs benefits to mother:

- **Androgens** (1st trimester): Female fetus will become masculinized.
- **Retinoids**, such as isotretinoin, acitretin, tretinoin, and etretinate (1st trimester): Multiple deformities of heart, ears, face, limbs, & liver, cognitive impairment, thymic hypoplasia, microcephalus, hydrocephalus, microtia, and miscarriage.
- **Thalidomide** (days 34–60): Multiple facial, intestinal, cardiac, limb abnormalities, including lack of limbs and limb reductions, and deafness.
- **Vitamin A** (>18,000 IU/day): Multiple craniofacial deformities, microtia, cardiac abnormalities, atresia of bowel, limb reductions, and defects of urinary tract.

Neonatal Resuscitation and Stabilization

AHA/AAP's Neonatal Resucitation Program

AHA and AAP jointly offer the Neonatal Resuscitation Program to provide a systematic, evidence-based approach to neonatal resuscitation. Key principles include early recognition, a stepwise approach, and team-based care. The steps include:

1. **Initial assessment**: Resuscitation may be needed if the infant's Apgar score is <7.
2. **Resuscitation steps**: Clear airway, position airway (neutral position), dry/warm infant, supplemental O_2.
3. **Assess breathing and heart rate**: If the heart rate is <100, provide positive pressure ventilation (PPV) and possibly chest compressions. If the heart rate remains <60 with PPV, initiate chest compressions.
4. **Ventilation**: No or inadequate respirations, initiate PPV for 30 seconds. Ensure a good bag-valve-mask seal.
5. **Chest compressions**: If the heart rate is <60, initiate compressions in addition to PPV at a rate of 120 compressions per minute at one-third of the chest depth (i.e., the two-thumb or two-finger method).
6. **Medications**: Epinephrine 0.01–0.03 mg/kg IV/intraosseously or via an endotracheal tube.
7. **Additional interventions**: If there is evidence of shock, hypoglycemia, or other complications, provide the necessary support (i.e., IV fluids, thermoregulation).
8. **Ongoing** monitoring: Apgar score at 10 minutes if the 5-minute Apgar score is low, pulse oximetry, blood gases, temperature, heart rate, respiratory status.

Advanced neonatal resuscitation with neonatal endotracheal intubation may be necessary if the infant is not responding to bag-valve-mask ventilation or if a secure airway is needed. Postresuscitation care includes supportive care, monitoring for complications, and transfer to the neonatal intensive care unit.

Minimum Neonatal Resuscitation Equipment

The minimal equipment that should be present for neonatal resuscitation includes the following:

- **Temperature**: Thermometer, warmed drying towels, warmed swaddling blankets, radiant warmer, phototherapy equipment.
- **Respiration**: Oxygen tank and hood, flow meter, humidifier, heater, tubing, nasal prongs. Bag and mask set-up (assorted sizes). Laryngoscope with size 0 and 1 blades. Endotracheal tubes, sizes 2.5 to 4. Bulb syringe, suction catheters (sizes 6, 8, and 10 Fr.), suction canister. Cardiorespiratory monitor, oxygen analyzer.
- **Fluids**: IV needles and tubing, infusion pump, umbilical catheters (sizes 2.5 and 5 Fr.). Blood pressure monitor, pulse oximeter. Isotonic saline, D10W, sodium bicarbonate. If transfusions are done here, blood drainage system, volume expander, and blood warmer.
- **Drugs**: Epinephrine, Naloxone.
- **Procedures**: Various sterile surgical packs, dressings, chest tubes, scalpels, hemostat. Arterial blood gas equipment and portable x-ray machine.

ABCs of Neonatal Resuscitation

The ABCs of resuscitation are a device to help remember in what order to do the steps of the resuscitation process. In this device, the letters stand for the following:

- **Airway**: An airway should be established as the very first thing to tend to. If there is no airway, air cannot be moved during resuscitation attempts. This step includes clearing the mouth and nose of secretions and properly positioning the infant in the "sniff" position.
- **Breathing**: This step involves initiating breathing after the airway has been established. This can be done with stimulation, supplemental oxygen, or through artificial ventilation. Oxygen should be initiated at 21% (up to 30% in preterm neonates) and titrated as needed.
- **Circulation**: Once an airway is open and breathing has been established, then circulation is considered. Chest compressions or the administration of volume expanders may be indicated. Epinephrine is only indicated if the heart rate remains <60 despite warming, ventilation, and chest compressions.

Establishing Airway and Stimulating Respirations

To **establish an airway**, the infant is placed supine with the head slightly extended in the "sniffing" position. A small neck roll may be placed under the shoulders to maintain this position in a very small premature infant. Once the proper position is established, the mouth and nose are suctioned (mouth first, to prevent reflex aspiration of secretions when the nose is suctioned) with a bulb syringe or catheter if necessary. The infant's head can be turned momentarily to the side to allow secretions to pool in the cheek where they can be more easily suctioned and removed to establish the airway. **Stimulating** the newborn is often all that is needed to initiate spontaneous respirations. This tactile stimulation can be accomplished by gently rubbing the infant's back or trunk. Another technique used to provide stimulation is flicking or rubbing the soles of the feet. Slapping neonates as stimulation is no longer practiced and should NOT be used.

ADMINISTRATION OF FREE-FLOW OXYGEN

If an infant remains cyanotic in the chest area (central cyanosis) after the initial steps of resuscitation have taken place, administering **free-flow oxygen** is the next step to take. Free-flow oxygen is administered to the neonate by the use of either a mask hooked up to an oxygen source or by the use of the oxygen tubing itself. If the tubing alone is used, the nurse can hold the tube with a cupped hand to help direct and concentrate the oxygen at the infant's airway. Free flow oxygen should be administered at a rate of 5 L/minute, initiated at 21% (up to 30% in preterm neonates). If the infant starts to turn pink, the oxygen can be carefully and slowly removed while continuing to closely monitor the infant for returning cyanosis. If the infant remains centrally cyanotic after the administration of free-flow oxygen, bag and mask ventilation must be considered as the next step.

BAG AND MASK VENTILATION

Ventilation using a bag and mask is indicated when one or more of the following occurs and has not responded to other resuscitation attempts:

- Apnea that does not respond to tactile stimulation such as rubbing the chest or back or flicking the soles of the feet
- Gasping respirations
- Heart rate of <100 bpm, determined by auscultation at the apex of the heart or palpation of the base of the umbilical cord
- Central cyanosis that persists after administering free-flow oxygen (Acrocyanosis alone is NOT an indication for the need for further oxygenation or ventilation.)

The flowmeter is set at 5–10 L/min, and opening breath pressures of 30–40 cmH_2O are used for full term infants and 20–25 cmH_2O for preterm. Ventilation is done at 40–60 breaths/min with pressure of 15–20 cmH_2O for normal lungs and 20–50 cmH_2O for immature or compromised lungs.

FLOW-INFLATING BAG AND MASK VENTILATION

Bag and mask ventilation is indicated for persistent apnea or gasping respirations, bradycardia (<100 bpm), and persistent cyanosis unrelieved by free-flowing oxygen.

Flow-inflating bag and mask (connected to oxygen flow, which inflates bag) equipment includes:

- Oxygen inlet
- Flow control valve
- Pressure manometer attachment
- Patient outlet for mask attachment

Advantages: Flow-inflating bag and mask ventilation has the ability to deliver anywhere from 21% (room air) to 100% oxygen; any pressure desired can be set. This type of bag and mask also has the ability to maintain positive end-expiratory pressure (PEEP) and CPAP.

Disadvantages: Because this bag must be connected to a gas (oxygen) source to inflate, it can only be used where a gas supply exists. It requires some experience to deliver the desired quantity of air with each breath. The high pressures possible with this type of equipment make overinflation of the lungs possible, resulting in pneumothorax. A complete seal is necessary to deliver a tidal volume.

Self-Inflating Bag and Mask Ventilation

Self-inflating bag and mask (does not require gas source) equipment includes:

- Air inlet
- Oxygen inlet
- Patient outlet for mask attachment
- Valve assembly
- Oxygen reservoir
- Pop-off valve
- Pressure manometer attachment

Advantages: Self-inflating bag and mask ventilation is simple to use and does not require much practice or experience to operate. It can be operated anywhere, even if no oxygen source is near, and can easily deliver a tidal volume.

Disadvantages: These bags usually have a pop-off valve that will open at a pressure set by the manufacturer to prevent over inflation of the lungs. This valve popping off can prevent the ability to deliver enough pressure to ventilate very noncompliant lungs. Another disadvantage is that if 90% or higher oxygen delivery is desired, this equipment must have a reservoir attached to deliver this concentration. The inability to deliver PEEP is also a disadvantage to the self-inflating bag and mask.

Chest Compressions

If **chest compressions** are indicated for resuscitation (for heart rates of less than 60 bpm after ventilating for 30 seconds), these steps should be followed.

1. Position the neonate in the "sniffing" position with the neck slightly extended.
2. Make sure there is firm support for the infant's back.
3. Using a two-finger technique, proceed with the compressions on the lower third of the sternum with a depth of one third of the anterior-posterior diameter of the chest. The compression rate is 90 compressions per minute and 30 breaths per minute, equaling 120 "events" per minute. Essentially, one cycle is 3 compressions and 1 breath every 2 seconds.
4. When performing the compressions, the hands should be placed in a circle around the chest to provide support to the infant's back. The ratio of compressions to breaths should be 3:1.
5. Check the heart rate again after 30 seconds of compressions—about 45 compressions total.
6. If the heart rate is less than 60 beats per minute, continue with another round of compressions, but if the rate is 60 beats per minute or higher, stop compressions.

During chest compressions, oxygen should be delivered at a concentration of 100%.

Sudden Unexpected Postnatal Collapse

Sudden unexpected postnatal collapse **(SUPC)** is the unexpected and sudden deterioration or death of a previously well neonate within the first week after birth. SUPC most often affects neonates of ≥35 weeks. SUPC is associated with skin-to-skin contact while face down, surface sharing (sleeping in an adult's bed), unattended breastfeeding, using supine position for sleeping, swaddling, and when the mother falls asleep while nursing. Risk factors for the neonate include preterm birth at 35–36 weeks, abnormal transition to extrauterine life, hypoglycemia, sepsis, CHD, obstructive apnea, respiratory compromise, and neurological impairment. Indications of SUPC include sudden pallor or cyanosis, apnea, bradycardia, hypotonia, weak or absent, cry, loss of consciousness, and seizures. Treatment includes immediate resuscitation:

- Recognition of early signs
- Clear airway, positive pressure ventilation or intubate if necessary
- Continuous cardiopulmonary monitoring
- Correction of any electrolyte imbalances, acidosis, or hypoglycemia
- Neurological monitoring

Neonates with mild cases of SUPC usually recover well, but prolonged hypoxia may cause hypoxic-ischemic encephalopathy, cerebral palsy, seizure disorder, neurodevelopmental delay, or death. Prevention strategies include avoiding prone position during skin-to-skin contact, ensuring that the neonate's airway is open and the head is positioned properly for breastfeeding, educating parents about the importance of being awake and alert during breastfeeding and skin-to-skin contact, and teaching them the signs of distress (apnea, poor skin tone, cyanosis).

Indications for Stopping or Not Providing Resuscitation to Newborn

The decision to **discontinue or not perform resuscitative efforts** in the newborn (DNR) is very difficult to make. Whenever possible, the decision to withhold or stop resuscitative efforts in the newborn should be made by the attending physician with parental input, especially in situations with variable degrees of morbidity and mortality. Generally, considering the cessation of resusciation efforts should occur if high-quality resuscitation efforts have been ongoing for more than 20 minutes and the infant remains unresponsive despite intubation and the administration of epinephrine. Infants born under these conditions associated with certain death should not be resuscitated:

- Extreme prematurity (less than 23 weeks gestation)
- Extremely low birth weight (less than 400 grams)
- Congenital anomalies that are incompatible with life (anencephaly, trisomy 13 or 18)

Resuscitation Medications

Epinephrine

Epinephrine is a naturally-occurring hormone produced by the adrenal glands. Epinephrine is used to resuscitate both adults and children. It is a sympathomimetic that supports the circulatory system by:

- Increasing heart rate
- Increasing contraction strength
- Vasoconstricting vessels in the skin, mucosa, and circulation of the gastrointestinal tract, causing a rise in blood pressure

If positive pressure ventilation and chest compressions have not caused the neonate's heart rate to rise above 60 beats per minute during resuscitation, then epinephrine is indicated. The recommended IV dose is 0.01–0.03 mg/kg. The usual concentration of epinephrine is 1:10,000 or 0.1 mg/mL. Endotracheal administration is not widely recommended, but may be used if no IV access is available. Higher doses are required for endotracheal administration (0.05–0.1 mg/kg).

Volume Expanders

Volume expanders used in neonatal resuscitation include:

- Normal saline
- Ringer's Lactate
- O- blood, or blood that has been crossmatched with the mother

Prepare 40 mL in a syringe or IV. Give 10 mL/kg over 5–10 minutes. Repeat if necessary. Rapid infusion of a large volume causes intraventricular hemorrhage. (5% albumin in saline is no longer the solution of choice.) Consider volume expanders in instances where neonatal blood loss is suspected and/or the neonate is showing signs of shock that is not responding to other resuscitative efforts. Blood loss occurs due to trauma of the placenta or umbilical cord, or with neonatal hemolysis. Shock is inadequate perfusion in tissues and organs. Signs and symptoms of shock are pallor, cold extremities, neurological depression, and weak pulse.

Naloxone Hydrochloride

Naloxone hydrochloride, an opiate antagonist, is not used in the routine resuscitation of an infant but is used in one very specific situation following birth. Naloxone is considered the antidote for narcotics administered to the mother of the infant within 4 hours of birth if the infant shows signs of serious respiratory depression from secondary absorption. If the mother of the infant has narcotics in her system as a result of an addiction to narcotics rather than as treatment for labor pain, however, naloxone cannot be given to this infant. If naloxone is given to an infant born to a narcotic-addicted mother, the drug will cause a severe abstinence reaction in the newborn that can result in seizure.

Neonatal Transport

An infant that is severely compromised at birth or <32 weeks gestation often requires **transport** to specialized neonatal care units, usually because of respiratory distress, preterm birth, congenital anomalies, and suspected cardiac abnormalities. The infant should be resuscitated and stabilized prior to transport. Communication with the regional center should be immediate and detailed. The **STABLE program** (**s**ugar, **t**emperature, **a**rtificial breathing, **b**lood pressure, **l**ab work, and **e**motional support) can guide efforts to stabilize the infant. The transport team must take copies of all records and lab reports. Transport teams may include NICU nurses, NNPs, physicians, and respiratory therapists. Adequate supplies (similar to those needed for resuscitation) must be available as well as oxygen, air-blended mixtures, monitors, and transport incubators. The incubator must control temperature while allowing access. Insulating material may be needed for very cold environments.

Fluid and Electrolyte Balance

Renal System and Fluid Maintenance

Maintenance of adequate fluid volume can be difficult in neonates. The pediatric renal system matures over the first 3 years of life. The nephrons in the young infant's kidneys are immature and the glomerular filtration rate is low because of impaired ability to filter urine until about 6-12 months of age. Also, the ability to concentrate or dilute urine may not reach adult levels until ages 2-3 years. Premature infants may have additional renal abnormalities, such as decreased creatinine clearance or impaired sodium retention. Infants are less tolerant of both dehydration and fluid overload. The 4-2-1 rule is used to determine maintenance fluid requirements. Sum the following:

- 4 mL/kg/hr for the first 10 kg weight
- 2 mL/kg/hr for the next 10 kg weight
- 1 mL/kg/hr for any remaining weight

Often a programmable infusion pump or buret with microdrip is used to manage fluids because the balance must be maintained within a narrow range.

Body Fluid/Fluid Balance

Body fluid is primarily **intracellular fluid (ICF)** or **extracellular fluid (ECF)**. Infants and children have proportionately more extracellular fluid (ECF) than adults. At birth, more than half of the child's weight is ECF, but by 3 years of age, the balance is more like adults:

- ECF: 20-30% (interstitial fluid, plasma, transcellular fluid)
- ICF: 40-50% (fluid within the cells)

The fluid compartments are separated by semipermeable membranes that allow fluid and solutes (electrolytes and other substances) to move by osmosis. Fluid also moves through diffusion, filtration, and active transport. In fluid volume deficit, fluid is out of balance and ECF is depleted; an overload occurs with increased concentration of sodium and retention of fluid. Signs of **fluid deficit** include:

- Thirsty, restless to lethargic
- Increasing pulse rate, tachycardia
- Fontanels depressed (infants)
- Decreased urinary output
- Normal BP progressing to hypotension
- Dry mucous membranes
- 3-10% decrease in body weight

Total Body Water

Total body water (TBW) content is the percentage of the body composed of water. An extremely premature infant (24-26 weeks of gestation) has a TBW content of 90%. The TBW content drops to 75-80% at full term (40 weeks), compared to 60-65% in adults. Because preterm infants have such a high percentage of TBW, any fluid loss can cause severe problems. Physiological diuresis is fluid loss from the extracellular space, and this is the initial type of fluid loss in neonates. Because intracellular space is relatively small in neonates, there is less fluid available to shift into the extracellular space, so the effects of extracellular fluid loss are much more pronounced on infants than adults. Diuresis continues during the first week after birth, so full term infants lose 5-10% of their weight, and premature infants lose 10-15% of their weight. Diuresis diminishes but slowly continues over the first 1-2 years of life. The typical toddler has a TBW content of 60%.

Sensible and Insensible Water Loss

Sensible water losses occur via urination, stool, and gastric drainage, and can be accurately measured. **Insensible water losses** (IWL) occur as water evaporates from the skin (2/3) or the respiratory tract (1/3). IWL cannot be directly measured. Premature neonates have thin skin that allows for increased amounts of evaporative water loss. As the skin matures and the stratum corneum develops (around 31 weeks of gestation) less water is lost through the skin. A full-term neonate will have an IWL of 12 mL/kg/day at 50% humidity. Factors that increase IWL include prematurity, radiant warmers, phototherapy, fever, low humidity, and tachypnea. Infants who are mechanically ventilated should receive humidified oxygen to negate the IWL through their lungs. The nurse must take into account IWL when providing fluids to neonates.

Fluid Deficit

Fluid deficit must also be carefully estimated and managed. For the neonate, **fluid deficit** should be replaced over 3 hours, with half the first hour and a quarter in each of the remaining 2 hours. Fluid deficit is calculated by first finding the **maintenance fluid requirement** using the 4-2-1 rule (4 mL/kg/hr for the first 10 kg of weight of the neonate, then 2 mL/kg/hr for the next 10 kg, and 1 mL/kg/hr for any remaining kg). Preoperative deficits usually are treated with lactated Ringer's or normal saline (which may cause hyperchloremic acidosis). Glucose-containing fluids may contribute to hyperglycemia.

Fluid replacement must account for both blood loss and third-space loss. Blood loss may be replaced with lactated Ringer's (3 mL for each mL of blood loss) or 5% albumin colloid (1 mL for each mL of blood loss) to maintain hematocrit at a predetermined adequate minimal level:

- Infants and neonates: >30% (may be as high as 40-50%)
- Older children: 20-26%

Blood is replaced with packed red blood cells when the allowable blood loss threshold is exceeded. **Allowable blood loss** is calculated by the following formula based on the infant's average hematocrit:

$$\text{Average hematocrit} = \frac{\text{Initial hematocrit} + \text{Final hematocrit}}{2}$$

$$\text{Allowable blood loss} = \frac{\text{Est. blood volume} \times (\text{Initial hematocric} - \text{Final hematocrit})}{\text{Average hematocrit}}$$

Blood loss should be monitored carefully to determine when it exceeds the allowable blood loss. **Volume of packed red blood cell replacement (PRBC)** is based on the weight, current hematocrit, and desired hematocrit of the patient. If a massive transfusion is required (blood loss exceeds 50% of total blood volume in 3 hours), then the transfusion of platelets and FFP is also indicated.

Third space loss after surgery can only be estimated based on the degree of trauma:

- Minor: 3-4 mL/kg/hr
- Moderate: 5-6 mL/kg/hr
- Severe: 7-10 mL/kg/hr

Lactated Ringer's is most commonly used to replace third space loss.

Preterm Neonatal Fluid Balance

Preterm Neonatal Urinary Output

The pre-term neonate has 3 **phases of urine output**:

1. **Oliguric phase:** Output is lower than intake during the first 12-24 hours after birth. The premature infant's urine output may be less than 1 mL/kg/hr in the oliguric phase.
2. **Diuretic phase:** Output is greater than intake 24-72 hours after birth. The premature infant's urine output may be greater than 5 mL/kg/hr in the diuretic phase, so the infant's weight decreases.
3. **Adaptive phase:** Output is appropriate after 72 hours, as the kidneys adjust to the rate of input. The urine output more closely reflects the real fluid status of the infant.

The appropriate response to decreased fluid intake is to decrease urine output and produce concentrated urine (elevate the specific gravity). The appropriate response to excessive fluids is to increase urine output and produce dilute urine (lower the specific gravity).

Fluid Requirements of Premature Newborns

The nurse must correctly manage fluid for the premature infant, because the infant's immature kidneys have a very limited ability to concentrate or dilute urine. Premature infants are less able to compensate for dehydration or fluid overload than infants who are several months old. **Total fluid requirements** for a newborn are equal to maintenance requirements (sensible plus insensible fluid losses), in addition to the amount required for growth. Typically, the total requirement ranges from 100-150 mL/kg/day of fluid, but many conditions exist that either increase or decrease fluid requirements. Closely monitor these indicators of hydration status: daily weight change, urine output, and urine osmolality. Conditions that increase fluid requirements include:

- Prematurity
- Elevated body and environmental temperatures
- Phototherapy
- Decreased environmental humidity
- Gastroschisis or omphalocele secondary to increased evaporation from exposed tissue

Neonatal Electrolyte Balance

Sodium, Hyponatremia, and Hypernatremia

Sodium (Na) regulates fluid volume, osmolality, acid-base balance, and activity in the muscles, nerves and myocardium. It is the primary cation (positive ion) in ECF, necessary to maintain ECF levels needed for tissue perfusion:

- Normal neonatal value: 133-146 mEq/L
- Hyponatremia: <133 mEq/L (critical value <120)
- Hypernatremia: >146 mEq/L (critical value >160)

Hyponatremia develops with excessive water gain or excessive sodium loss. Late symptoms include apnea, irritability, twitching, and seizures when serum sodium drops below 120 mEq/L, but infants are often asymptomatic. In the first days after birth, hyponatremia is usually secondary to excessive water gain (dilutional hyponatremia), reflected in a weight gain or absence of expected weight loss. Conditions causing dilutional hyponatremia include syndrome of inappropriate antidiuretic hormone (SIADH), renal dysfunction with decreased urine output, and overhydration. **Treatment** involves identifying and treating underlying cause, restricting fluid, and replacing sodium if necessary.

Hypernatremia is caused by dehydration, excess use of sodium-containing solutions, and diabetes insipidus. Late symptoms include seizures. The **underlying cause** must be identified and treated.

Hypocalcemia

The ionized form of **serum calcium** is the only biologically available form in the body.

- Cord: 8.2-11.2 mg/dL
- 0-10 days: 7.6-10.4 mg/dL
- 11 days to 1 yr: 9.0-11.0 mg/dL
- Critical value for hypocalcemia: <7 mg/dL

Signs of **hypocalcemia** include jitteriness, irritability, stridor, tetany, high-pitched cry, seizures, and decreased myocardial contractility, with decreased cardiac output. An electrocardiogram may show a prolonged QT interval and a flattened T-wave. Early-onset hypocalcemia usually presents in the first 3 days of life and is associated with prematurity, birth asphyxia, and infants of diabetic mothers. Late-onset hypocalcemia presents after the first week of life and is associated with DiGeorge syndrome, hyperphosphatemia, vitamin D deficiency, magnesium deficiency, diuretic therapy, and hypoparathyroidism. Hypocalcemia is treated with a slow infusion of calcium gluconate. Rapid infusion may cause bradycardia. Tissue infiltration with calcium causes necrosis, so the administration site must be monitored.

Hypercalcemia

Hypercalcemia (>12 mg/dL) is rare, occurring less often than hypocalcemia. Signs of hypercalcemia include vomiting, constipation, hypertension, hypotonia, lethargy, and seizures. Possible causes of hypercalcemia include congenital hyperparathyroidism, maternal hypoparathyroidism, hypervitaminosis D, hyperthyroidism, hypophosphatasia, subcutaneous fat necrosis, Williams syndrome, and adrenal insufficiency. Idiopathic hypercalcemia is diagnosed when no other cause can be found. Iatrogenic hypercalcemia occurs because of excess administration of calcium or vitamin D or phosphate deprivation. Treatment depends on the exact cause but may include:

- Correction of the underlying cause
- Furosemide (Lasix) after adequate hydration to increase calcium excretion
- Glucocorticoids to inhibit intestinal absorption of calcium
- Use of low calcium and low vitamin D formulas

Magnesium, Hypermagnesemia, and Hypomagnesemia

Magnesium is the second most abundant intercellular cation:

- Normal neonatal value: 1.5-2.2 mg/dL
- Critical values for neonates: <1.2 mg/dL and >3 mg/dL

Hypermagnesemia most commonly results from maternal administration of magnesium prior to delivery. Maternal serum chemistries are reflected in newborn blood values. Magnesium is used in the pregnant woman as a tocolytic agent to stop pre-term labor and also for treatment of pre-eclampsia. Signs of hypermagnesemia in an infant include hypotonia, hyporeflexia, constipation, low blood pressure, apnea, and marked flushing secondary to vasodilatation. Elevated magnesium blocks neurosynaptic transmission by interfering with the release of acetylcholine. Treatment is usually supportive, as the elevated serum magnesium will be cleared by the infant's kidneys. In severe cases, the infant may require respiratory and/or blood pressure support.

Hypomagnesemia in neonates occurs with preterm birth, respiratory distress syndrome, and neonatal hepatitis. **Symptoms** include:

- Neuromuscular excitability/tetany
- Seizure and coma
- Tachycardia with ventricular arrhythmias
- Respiratory depression

Treatment includes diagnosing the underlying cause and administering magnesium replacement.

Serum Potassium Changes After Birth

Electrolyte levels in the newborn reflect those of the mother at birth. Shortly after birth, within the first 24-72 hours, **serum potassium** concentrations are expected to rise without exogenous potassium delivery and with normal renal function, resulting from a shift of potassium from the intracellular space to the extracellular space. **Potassium shift** is more extreme in premature infants and can result in life-threatening hyperkalemia. Over the next several days, the potassium level will fall to normal in an infant with normally functioning kidneys. Preterm infants' serum electrolytes, including potassium, should be carefully monitored in the first 48 hours of life and until values have stabilized.

- Normal neonatal values: 3.7-5.9 mEq/L
- Hyperkalemia: >6 mEq/L (critical value: >6.5 mEq/L)
- Hypokalemia: <3.5 mEq/L (critical value: <2.5 mEq/L)

Hyperkalemia

Hyperkalemia is a serum potassium level greater than 6 mEq/L in a non-hemolyzed blood sample. Squeezing the infant's heel too hard during blood collection can cause the sample to hemolyze and give an artificially elevated laboratory value. Causes of hyperkalemia in the newborn fall into 3 categories:

- Excessive potassium supplementation
- Transcellular shift, where potassium concentrated inside cells moves outside cells, due to low pH, cellular damage, intraventricular hemorrhage, or trauma
- Decreased potassium secretion by the kidneys, due to congenital adrenal hyperplasia with elevated secretion of aldosterone or renal failure

Cardiac manifestations of hyperkalemia include potentially fatal arrhythmias like bradycardia, tachycardia, supraventricular fibrillation, and ventricular fibrillation. EKG shows peaked T waves (earliest sign), and a widened QRS complex.

Hyperkalemia must be treated promptly because it may develop into a lethal cardiac arrhythmia, especially if the blood potassium value is >7 mEq/L and the infant's electrocardiogram shows abnormalities. Follow these steps to lower potassium levels:

- Discontinue all potassium administration.
- Elevate the blood pH by inducing hyperventilation.
- Give sodium bicarbonate to shift extracellular potassium back inside cells.
- Administer insulin and/or inhaled albuterol to enhance the shift of extracellular potassium back inside cells. *Monitor glucose levels closely.*
- Increase excretion of potassium by giving furosemide (Lasix) or sodium polystyrene sulfonate (Kayexalate).

- Give calcium gluconate concurrently to help stabilize the myocardium and lessen the chance of the infant developing an arrhythmia.
- In extreme cases, consider dialysis or exchange transfusion.

Hypokalemia

Hypokalemia is a serum potassium level <3.5 mEq/L. Common causes of hypokalemia are chronic diuretic use and excessive nasogastric drainage. Alkalosis accentuates hypokalemia by triggering the sequestration of potassium from the extracellular fluid to inside the cell. Electrocardiograph manifestations of hypokalemia include a flattened T wave (earliest manifestation), ST segment depression, and appearance of U waves (second recovery wave following the T wave). These changes are identical to those seen with hypomagnesemia. Hypokalemia is usually not of concern until the level drops below 3.0 mEq/L. Signs of hypokalemia include cardiac arrhythmias, ileus, and lethargy. Treatment is with Slow-K and can be intravenous or oral. Rapid administration of potassium is associated with possible life-threatening cardiac dysfunction.

Parenteral Infusion

Many inpatient infants require intravenous fluids, and there are a number of different types of access for **parenteral infusions**:

- **Umbilical cord catheterization (arterial, venous)**: This is limited to a few days only.
- **PICC line:** This allows for long-term use without repeated IV insertions. It is particularly useful for ELBW babies although they pose the danger of thrombosis, infection, and infiltration. Percutaneous insertion sites include the saphenous, antecubital, axillary, basilic, cephalic, and external jugular veins.
- **Peripheral venous access**: This is used for short-term access. Extremely small catheters and introducers (Quick-cath) may extend use to 5-7 days. There is increased risk of infiltration and skin necrosis, especially in the foot.

The catheter or needle should be secured, but must allow visualization, and the site should be checked at least every hour during administration of fluids.

Infusion Techniques and Equipment

Umbilical Artery Catheterization

Umbilical catheters may be arterial or venous, depending on primary need. Arterial catheterization indications include ABG monitoring, continuous arterial BP monitoring, and infusion of parenteral fluids.

Umbilical artery catheter placement: A sterile field must be maintained, so the infant's arms and legs are restrained to prevent contamination. The infant's temperature must be monitored and maintained at 36-37 °C (by placing on a radiant heater or in a heated incubator). The child is placed in supine position and the umbilical cord and surrounding skin cleansed with povidone iodine and then alcohol or sterile water. For infants <1250 g, a 3.5 Fr. catheter is used, and for those >1250 g, a 5 Fr. catheter. After sterile draping, iris forceps are used to dilate one of the arteries and the catheter inserted. If resistance is felt at the umbilical cord tie, it may need to be loosened. The inserted length correlates to the infant's length (using chart), traveling inferiorly and then superiorly (leg loop). Blood should be aspirated and extremities observed for circulatory compromise. Radiograph verifies correct placement.

Umbilical Vein Catheterization

Umbilical catheters may be inserted into the umbilical vein. This is easy to identify as there is only one, it is larger than the arteries, and it is usually open and does not require dilation. Indications for using the umbilical vein include exchange transfusions, CVP monitoring, and emergency administration of fluids.

Umbilical vein catheter placement: Catheter size is 3.5 Fr. for ELBW infants or 5 Fr. (most common). Length of placement is estimated by measuring the length from the umbilicus to the sternal notch and multiplying this number by 0.6. The procedure for insertion is similar to that for the umbilical artery, but insertion is usually easier. The catheter should be in the inferior vena cava, above the diaphragm but below the right atrium. Placement should be verified by echocardiography, as radiograph may not provide adequate visualization.

PICC Lines

Percutaneously inserted central catheters (PICC) are used for extended intravenous access or those with limited access and as a transition from umbilical catheters. Insertion sites include the scalp, axilla, and brachial cephalic saphenous veins. The catheter insertion length is measured:

- **Hand/arm***:* insertion site to axilla and to 1 cm above nipple line
- **Scalp**: insertion site to 1 cm above nipple line
- **Leg**: insertion site to 1 cm above umbilicus

Topical (EMLA) or local anesthetic is used and the infant's temperature maintained at 36-37 °C. Limbs are restrained to prevent contamination of sterile field. If the catheter is inserted in the hand or arm, the infant's head is turned toward insertion site to partially occlude the jugular vein and reduce risk of catheter entering the jugular. After insertion above the waist, the catheter should be in the superior vena cava above the right atrium. PICC lines in lower extremities should lie in the inferior vena cava below the right atrium. AP and lateral radiographs, ultrasound, or echocardiogram verify correct placement.

Broviac Catheters

Broviac catheters are large-bore silastic indwelling catheters that may be surgically (cutdown) or needle inserted if percutaneous insertion is not possible. The most common sites for insertion are the internal or external jugular vein and the common facial vein. **Broviac catheters** are most commonly used if long-term access (months, years) is required, such as for parenteral nutrition or medications. A Broviac catheter is tunneled subcutaneously and exits through the anterior chest. Placement is confirmed with radiograph. The Broviac catheter is cuffed at the exit point to decrease infection, but the catheter still poses a high risk of infection, especially with frequent administration of parenteral nutrition. Complications include pneumothorax, hemothorax, air embolism, misplacement or occlusion of catheter. The catheter must be secured as it is easily dislodged, so length and positioning should be carefully documented and the catheter checked frequently. The catheter is flushed with heparin to maintain patency and prevent thrombus formation.

Chapter Quiz

Ready to see how well you retained what you just read? Scan the QR code to go directly to the chapter quiz interface for this study guide. If you're using a computer, simply visit the online resources page at **mometrix.com/resources719/ccrnneonatal** and click the Chapter Quizzes link.

Professional Caring and Ethical Practice

AACN Synergy Model

AACN Synergy Model

The AACN Synergy model of nursing practice, developed by the AACN for nursing certification, places the needs of the patient as a central focus and defines the relationship between eight patient characteristics and eight nurse competencies. These competencies and characteristics are evaluated on a scale (1-5). Patient characteristics include resiliency, vulnerability, stability, complexity, resource availability, participation in care, participation in decision-making, and predictability.

Nurse competencies include clinical judgment, advocacy, caring practices, collaboration, systems thinking, response to diversity, clinical inquiry, and facilitation of learning.

The system or healthcare environment is the third element of the model. It provides support for the needs of the patients and empowers and nurtures the practice of nursing, caring, and ethical practice. All three of these systems are essential for Synergy. The needs of the patient are the driving force for nurse competencies and both are dependent on the healthcare system. When the needs, competencies, and system complement each other, Synergy is achieved, and outcomes for the nurse, the patient, and the system are optimized.

Three Levels of Outcomes

The AACN Synergy model is based on three levels of **quality outcomes** (patient, nurse, and system). Six general **indicators** of quality outcomes include:

- Satisfaction of patient and family
- Adverse incidents rates
- Rate of complications
- Adherence to discharge plans
- Mortality rate
- Length of stay in hospital

These general outcomes are based on outcomes derived from the patient, the nurse, and the system:

- **Patient outcomes** include functional change, behavioral change, trust, ratings, satisfaction, comfort, and quality of life.
- **Nurse outcomes** include physiological changes, presence or absence of complications, and the extent to which care of treatment objectives were attained.
- **System outcomes** include recidivism, costs, and resource utilization.

Advocacy and Moral Agency

Nurse competencies under the AACN Synergy model include advocacy/moral agency:

- **Advocacy** is working for the best interests of the patient despite personal values in conflict and assisting patients to have access to appropriate resources.
- **Agency** is openness and recognition of issues and a willingness to act.
- **Moral agency** is the ability to recognize needs and take action to influence the outcome of a conflict or decision.

The **levels of advocacy/moral agency** include:

- Level 1: This nurse works on behalf of the patient, assesses personal values, has awareness of the patient's rights and ethical conflicts, and advocates for the patient when consistent with the nurse's personal values.
- Level 3: This nurse advocates for the patient/family, incorporates their values into the care plan even when they differ from the nurse's, and can utilize internal resources to assist patient/family with complex decisions.
- Level 5: This nurse advocates for the patient/family despite differences in values and is able to utilize both internal and external resources to help to empower the patient/family to make decisions.

Caring Practices

In the AACN Synergy model, caring practices encompass all nursing activities that respond to the individual patient's and family's needs in a caring, compassionate, and therapeutic environment to promote patient comfort and prevent unnecessary suffering. Caring practices recognize inner strength and its relation to healing and seek to enhance the dignity of the individual through vigilance, nurturing, and skilled technical and basic nursing practices. **Levels of caring practices** include:

- Level 1: This nurse provides a safe environment and cares for the present basic needs of the patient without focus on future needs and considers death a potential outcome.
- Level 3: This nurse provides compassionate care, responding to changes in the patient, and shows acts of kindness while accepting death as a possible outcome and providing measures to ensure good end-of-life care and a peaceful death.
- Level 5: This nurse is fully engaged in patient care and understands and interprets patient/family dynamics and needs, ensuring comfort, dignity, and safety while respecting the individual and family.

Problem-Solving Steps

Problem-solving to anticipate or prevent recurrences of family dissatisfaction involves arriving at a hypothesis, testing, and assessing data to determine if the hypothesis holds true. If a problem has arisen, taking steps to resolve the immediate problem is only the first step if recurrence is to be avoided:

1. **Define the issue**: Talk with the family and staff to determine if the problem is related to a failure of communication or other issues, such as culture or religion.
2. **Collect data**: This may mean interviewing additional staff or reviewing documentation in order to gain a variety of perspectives.
3. **Identify important concepts**: Determine if there are issues related to values or beliefs.

4. **Consider reasons for actions**: Distinguish between motivation and intention on the part of all parties to determine the reason for the problem.
5. **Make a decision**: A decision on how to prevent a recurrence of a problem should be based on advocacy and moral agency, reaching the best solution possible for the infant and family.

Medication Errors Safety

There are about 7,000 deaths yearly in the United States attributed to **medication errors**. Studies indicate that there are errors in 1 in 5 doses of medication given to patients in hospitals. A caring environment is one in which patient safety is ensured with proper handling and administering of medications:

- Avoiding error-prone abbreviations or symbols. The Joint Commission has established a list of abbreviations to avoid, but mistakes are frequent with other abbreviations as well. In many cases, abbreviations and symbols should be avoided altogether or restricted to a limited approved list.
- Preventing errors from illegible handwriting. Handwritten orders should be block printed to reduce the change of error.
- Instituting bar coding and scanners that allow the patient's wristband and medications to be scanned for verification.
- Providing lists of similarly-named medications to educate staff.
- Establishing an institutional policy for administering of medications that includes protocols for verification of drug, dosage, and patient as well as educating the patient about the medications.

Facilitating Safe Passage

Facilitating safe passage is part of the caring practice that ensures patient safety, in a broad sense, from a variety of perspectives:

- Giving appropriate medications and treatment without errors that endanger the infant's health is essential.
- Providing information to the family about treatments, changes, conditions, and other aspects related to care helps them to cope with the situations as they arise.
- Preventing infection is central to infant safety and includes staff using proper infection control methods, such as hand washing.
- Knowing the person requires the nurse to take the time and effort to understand the needs and wishes of the family.
- Assisting with transitions involves not only helping the family cope with moving from one form of treatment, or one unit to another but also with transitions in health, such as from illness to health or from illness to death.

Response to Diversity

In the AACN Synergy model, response to diversity is the ability to recognize a wide range of differences (social, cultural, ethnic, racial, economic, language, and religious), to appreciate these differences, and to incorporate consideration for them into the plan of care. Diverse groups also include the disabled, gay and lesbian people, and marginal groups, such as the homeless. **Levels of response to diversity** include:

- Level 1: This nurse can assess diversity with standardized questionnaires and provide care based on his or her personal belief system and past experience, but doesn't seek assistance in dealing adequately with diversity.

- Level 3: This nurse takes a much more active role in asking about diversity issues and incorporates needs into the plan of care, teaching the family about the healthcare system.
- Level 5: This nurse considers issues of diversity in all aspects of care and presents families with alternatives, responding to, anticipating, and integrating consideration of cultural and other differences.

Facilitation of Learning

According to the AACN Synergy model, facilitation of learning is the ability to facilitate learning by family/caregivers as well as other health and allied professionals and community members. Facilitation of learning requires a needs assessment and preparation of content that is suited for the receiver in terms of delivery and content. **Levels of facilitation of learning** include:

- Level 1: This nurse is able to deliver planned educational content that is disease-specific but does not have the ability to assess family readiness to learn or abilities. The family is considered a passive recipient of knowledge.
- Level 3: This nurse is able to individualize treatment according to family needs and has an understanding of different methods of teaching and learning styles. The infants' and families' needs are considered in planning.
- Level 5: This nurse has an excellent understanding of teaching methods, learning styles, and assessment for learning readiness and develops an educational plan in cooperation and collaboration with others, including families, as well as other health and allied professionals.

Systems Thinking

The promotion of organizational values and commitment requires that the organization embody **systems thinking** and the associated concepts. Systems thinking focuses on how systems interrelate, with each part affecting the entire system. **Concepts** include:

- **Individual responsibility**: Individuals are encouraged to establish their own goals within the organization and to work toward a purpose.
- **Learning process**: The internalized beliefs of the staff are respected while building upon these beliefs to establish a mindset based on continuous learning and improvement.
- **Vision**: A sharing of organizational vision helps staff to understand the purpose of change and builds commitment.
- **Team process**: Teams are assisted to develop good listening and collaborative skills so that there is an increase in dialogue and an ability to reach consensus.
- **Systems thinking**: Staff members are encouraged to understand the interrelationship of all members of the organization and to appreciate how any change affects the whole.

Steps to Systems Thinking

An approach to systems thinking is especially valuable in organizations in which there is a lack of consensus, effective change is stalemated, and standards are inconsistent. Systems thinking is a critical thinking approach to problem-solving that takes an organization-wide perspective. **Steps** include:

1. **Define the issue**: Describe the problem in detail without judgment or solutions.
2. **Describe behavior patterns**: This includes listing factors related to the problem and using graphs to outline possible trends.
3. **Establish cause-effect relationships**: This may include using the Five Whys or other root cause analyses or feedback loops.

4. **Define patterns of performance/behavior**: Determine how variables affect outcomes and the types of patterns of behavior currently taking place.
5. **Find solutions**: Discuss possible solutions and outcomes.
6. **Institute performance improvement activities**: Make changes and then monitor for changes in behavior.

Clinical Inquiry

According to the AACN Synergy model, clinical inquiry is a continual process of questioning and evaluating practice in order to provide innovative and outstanding care through application of the results of research and experience. Clinical inquiry requires a desire to acquire new knowledge, openness to accepting advice from mentors and other health and allied professionals, competency in identifying clinical problems, the ability to search the literature for research, critical skills to interpret research findings, and the willingness and ability to design and participate in research. **Levels of clinical inquiry** include:

- Level 1: This nurse recognizes problems and seeks advice, follows industry standards and guidelines, and seeks further knowledge.
- Level 3: This nurse questions industry standards and guidelines as well as current practice and utilizes research and education to improve patient care.
- Level 5: This nurse is able to deviate from industry standards and guidelines when necessary for the individual patients and utilizes literature review and clinical research to gain knowledge, establish new practices, and improve patient care.

Patient Safety

Importance of Communication to Patient Safety

Many adverse incidents related to **patient safety** result from errors or failures in **communication**. In fact, over 30% of malpractice claims result from communication failures. Communication is especially a concern during hand-off procedures. Critical information about the patient may be undocumented, forgotten, overlooked, or misplaced. For this reason, standardized hand-off procedures, such as SBAR (**s**ituation, **b**ackground, **a**ssessment, **r**ecommendation) or I-PASS (**i**llness severity, **p**atient summary, **a**ction list, **s**ituation awareness/contingency planning, **s**ynthesis by receiver) should be utilized. While an initial error in communication may not directly harm a patient, the decisions made by subsequent healthcare providers may cause harm because the healthcare providers lacked essential information. Additionally, communication failures may occur because healthcare providers don't take the time to talk with patients or family or to listen attentively and gather their input. Problems may arise if healthcare providers fail to document medications, treatments, or observations in a timely manner. Many electronic health records utilize limited narration in favor of checklists, and checking all the boxes may become a rote activity, leading to errors.

Interprofessional Practice and Patient Safety

Interprofessional practice often begins with interprofessional education in which members of two or more professions study and learn together in order to build relationships and to have a better understanding of the contributions of each profession and the role of the profession in ensuring **patient safety**. For example, in obstetrics, an interprofessional group may include a nurse, midwife, ultrasonographer, and breastfeeding specialist. Each has a different but equally important role in patient care. A better understanding of roles and responsibilities leads to better collaboration and fewer patient safety issues. Additionally, collaboration promotes cross training and awareness of patient needs. Key elements in interprofessional practice include leadership (definitions, who leads and how leadership is determined), monitoring (continually assessing processes and outcomes), communication (methods and styles of effective communication), and support (mutual and organizational). Studies indicate that interprofessional education and practice especially improves communication among participants, a critical element in patient safety.

Perinatal Patient Safety Nurse

Large birthing facilities may designate a nurse as a **perinatal patient safety nurse**. This is usually an advanced practice nurse who focuses on mother/baby safety during care. This nurse monitors nursing care for adherence to safety procedures and provides education as needed. The overall coordination of efforts to evaluate and improve care to result in a safe, optimal outcome for both mother and baby is a major part of this role. This complies with the Joint Commission's recommendations and with the goals of Healthy People 2030 that seek to improve the nursing and medical care that is given to all persons. The unit manager and staff of smaller birthing units must take this responsibility on themselves to ensure the safety of care given in their unit.

The Joint Commission's Perinatal Care Core Measures

The Joint Commission's Perinatal Care Core Measures are those measures that require data collection for accredited hospitals that have at least 300 live births each year and any hospital that wants Perinatal Care certification. From January 2021 onward, there are 4 core measures:

- **PC-01 Elective delivery**: Elective vaginal or cesarean delivery at ≥37 weeks and <39 weeks of gestation
- **PC-02 Cesarean birth**: Nulliparous patient with term singleton in vertex position
- **PC-05 Exclusive Breast Milk Feeding**: Only breast milk feeding during entire hospital stay
- **PC-06 Unexpected Complications in Term Newborns**: Percentage with unexpected complications among full-term neonates with no pre-existing conditions (such as prematurity, congenital malformations, genetic disorders, exposure to maternal drug use, poor fetal growth, and genetic disorders)

Maternal Safety Bundles Presented by the AIM

The **Alliance for Innovation on Maternal Health** (AIM), a maternal safety and quality improvement initiative, has developed a series of **Patient Safety Bundles and Tools** to improve maternal outcomes and prevent complications:

- **Perinatal Mental Health Conditions**: Identify tools, establish screening, provide education, support, and follow-up.
- **Care for Pregnant and Postpartum People with Substance Use Disorder**: Assess and provide education (patient, staff), utilize community resources, emphasize available therapies, and establish clinical pathways.
- **Obstetric Hemorrhage**: Maintain hemorrhage cart, establish protocols, create a response team, and utilize massive transfusion protocols.
- **Safe Reduction of Primary Cesarean Birth**: Educate and train providers, offer standardized pain management and fetal assessment, and develop protocols for problems.
- **Severe Hypertension in Pregnancy**: Use standardized screening and assessment and provide triage and rapid access to medications.
- **Cardiac Conditions in Obstetric Care**: Perform a basic Cardiac Conditions screening, provide appropriate patient education, establish a multidisciplinary Pregnancy Heart Team to coordinate clinical pathways, utilize appropriate consultation, and provide specific referrals and resources.
- **Sepsis in Obstetric Care**: Create and enforce protocols and pathways for treating confirmed or suspected obstetric sepsis across the hospital, provide and train staff, establish evidence-based criteria for the identification of sepsis/suspected sepsis, and empower staff to communicate concerns regardless of position.

Patient-Centered Care in the NICU

Decreasing Family Stress If Neonate Requires Intensive Care

Having a neonate admitted to the neonatal intensive care unit is a very stressful event for a family. It interrupts family interactions and the bonding process that occurs when a neonate goes home to spend time with family members. Interventions to decrease **family stress** and encourage bonding between the neonate, mother, and family include:

- Have facilities available for families to stay close to their infant to encourage bonding.
- Maintain a play area for siblings so they are not isolated from parents.

- Permit liberal visiting times for family members.
- If it is known before birth that the infant will require critical care, let the family visit the unit and ask questions.
- Give the family contact information for support groups comprised of other parents who have children with similar illnesses.
- Encourage hands-on parental care, including kangaroo care, by both parents.

Counseling Techniques for Families with Neonates in NICU

Counseling techniques for families and extended families with a neonate in the NICU include:

- **Talk with families and listen:** Assess the family members' understanding of the neonate's condition and the situation to determine if it is realistic or distorted. If distorted, try to ascertain the reason and provide useful information in a non-threatening manner to help them more fully understand. Avoid overwhelming family members with too much information, especially initially. Listen attentively and show respect at all times. Acknowledge family members feeling of guilt and explain that these feelings are normal. Pay attention to body language when delivering information.
- **Assess coping strategies/grief:** Determine how the family members cope with stress and handle grief. Provide support and information about resources and support groups that are available and may be appropriate.
- **Encourage expression of feelings:** Remain supportive of family members' feelings and responses, even if negative, and encourage them to interact and share feelings with others. Suggest keeping a journal, diary, or blog to write about their feelings and experiences.

Shared Decision-Making and Parent-Staff Disagreements

Shared decision making requires that staff members treat the parents with respect, listen to their opinions and feelings, provide full information about treatments and the neonate's condition, encourage the parents to participate in care, and encourage parents to collaborate and share in decision-making at every step in the NICU provision of care.

When **disagreements occur between parents and staff members**, it is important to respond with patience and empathy. The nurse should try to determine why the parents disagree or are angry. For example, are they afraid a treatment is harmful? Do they not understand what the treatment consists of? Have they been reading advice on the internet or getting advice from others? Have they developed a dislike or distrust for staff members? Do they feel left out of decision-making process? Do they resent lack of control? Is a treatment at odds with their cultural or religious beliefs? The staff members should ask parents what they want and why, and provide as complete information as possible, including pros and cons.

Family Education

Educational Needs of New Mothers

The educational needs of the new mother and family vary depending on age, background, education, experience, and expectations. The needs of the adolescent mother with no experience may be quite different from those of the multiparous mother. Assessing individual needs can be difficult in the short time women are usually hospitalized, so education should cover a wide range of topics. A checklist of topics may be a helpful starting point for the mother to indicate her needs. Because mothers are usually fatigued for the first 24-48 hours, teaching after that time is most effective, but many mothers leave the hospital on the second day. Demonstration with return demonstration is an effective method to ensure that a mother can carry out tasks, but education should anticipate other needs and concerns that may arise. Mothers often have concerns about a variety of issues, such as childcare, contraception, and resuming sexual relations. Pamphlets, website information, or videos that can be sent home with the mother are very helpful.

Safe Positioning for Infants

Infants should be placed on their **backs** for sleeping. Sleeping on the stomach increases the risk of **sudden infant death syndrome (SIDS)**.

- Position the infant on the back when unattended or sleeping, but alternate the direction the head faces to prevent one side of the head from flattening (**positional molding**).
- Provide supervised time each day with the infant lying on the abdomen (only on firm surfaces) to strengthen head and neck muscles and to prevent positional molding.
- Hold the infant, rather than leaving them in a carrier.
- Position baby in side-lying position, alternating from one side to the other, using specially designed supports to maintain the position.

Infant Car Seat

All infants, regardless of age, must be placed properly in an infant car seat during transit. Holding an infant while the car is in motion is not safe. Car seats should be new or in very good condition and fastened according to the manufacturer's guidelines to ensure safety.

- Place the car seat in the back seat and away from any side airbags.
- Always securely buckle the child into the seat.
- Face the infant seat toward the rear of the car.
- Recline the seat so the infant's head does not fall forward.
- Place padding around (not under) the infant if the infant slouches to one side.
- Place blankets over the straps and buckles, not under.

Umbilical Cord Care

Education surrounding the umbilical cord should include the following information:

- Protect the cord from moisture, with top of diaper folded under the cord instead of covering it.
- If the cord becomes soiled, wash with mild soap and water, rinse, and dry. Swabbing with alcohol is no longer recommended and may increase skin irritation.
- Avoid covering the cord stump with clothing, which may cause irritation.
- Give the infant only sponge baths until the cord falls off in about 10-14 days.
- Report signs of infection, such as erythema, swelling, or purulent discharge.

Note: The umbilical cord changes color from grayish-brown to black as it dries and finally falls off.

Fecal Elimination

The first stool (**meconium**) is usually passed within 24 hours and is black and tarry looking. The stool then transitions to greenish as the baby nurses or takes formula, and by the third day, the stool is usually yellow or yellow-green for breastfed babies and yellow or light brown for formula-fed babies. Typically, babies have 2-3 stools daily by day 3 and ≥4 daily by day 5, but this may vary.

- Report abnormalities, such as bloody stools, watery stools, very hard stools, clay-colored or whitish stools, black stools (after meconium has passed), and "currant jelly" stools.

- Cleanse skin thoroughly after defecation with mild soap and water, plain water, or unscented baby wipes.
- Examine skin carefully for irritation.

Urinary Elimination

Urination is estimated according to the number of **wet diapers** in a 24-hour period. Typically, the infant has 1 wet diaper the first day, 2 the next, and so on until urination stabilizes at 6-8 wet diapers by about day 6.

- Check diaper frequently. Infants often urinate during or after feeding.
- Change diapers when wet, gently cleansing skin with mild soap and water, plain water, or unscented baby wipes.

Cradle Cap

Cradle cap may appear as scaly, crusted, or flaky skin on the scalp and other parts of the face. It is not contagious and usually clears by 1 or 2 months. It is not usually a sign of poor hygiene.

- Cleanse scalp or affected areas thoroughly, gently rubbing the area with a terry cloth or brushing to loosen crust or flakes.
- If persistent, try softening the crusts with olive oil. Leave it in for 15 minutes, and then brush or gently comb to loosen crusts or flakes. Finally, wash with baby shampoo.

Diaper Rash

Diaper rash usually results from leaving the infant in soiled/wet diapers and/or not adequately cleansing the skin, although breastfed infants sometimes react to foods the mother has eaten. A rash may also indicate an allergic response to baby wipes or other products, such as lotions or creams. Antibiotics may cause diaper rash. In some cases, a **fungal infection** may occur, usually characterized by red, weepy open areas. Purulent discharge may indicate infection.

- Change diapers as soon as possible when wet or soiled.
- Cleanse skin gently with water.
- Remove diaper and expose skin to air whenever possible.
- Apply barrier cream or ointment especially formulated for diaper rash to prevent or treat diaper rash.
- Contact physician if rash worsens and does not respond to treatment, as antifungals, cortisone, or topical antibiotics may be indicated.

Choking or Gagging in Infant

Education regarding chocking/gagging should include the following:

- Ensure small hazardous items, such as pins and cotton balls or materials, such as baby powder are out of reach.
- DO NOT prop bottle for feeding.
- Burp infant regularly during feedings, whether breast or bottle.
- Keep baby in upright position with head elevated during feedings.
- Check nipple of bottle to ensure it is dripping and not running freely.
- If the infant is choking, secure face down on forearm, tilted downward, and use the heel of the hand to thump on the mid-back. Repeat as necessary. If choking does not resolve with evidence of breathing immediately, call 911 and begin CPR.

Note: Prevention is important, as most **choking and gagging episodes** can be avoided.

Burping the Infant

Both breastfed and bottle-fed babies require **burping** because they swallow air when feeding, although bottle-fed babies tend to require more burping. Infants often show indications (grimacing, squirming, spitting up, and crying) that they are uncomfortable and need to burp.

- Burp the infant routinely after 2 or 3 ounces of formula or after nursing on one breast.
- Position the infant on the shoulder with a burp cloth under the infant's head and gently pat or rub the infant's back.
- Change to a different position if the baby doesn't burp. Try on the opposite shoulder or with the infant sitting on the lap supported by one hand while the other hand pats or rubs the infant's back.

Bathing the Infant

The infant should receive **sponge baths** until the umbilical cord falls off at 10-14 days, and then a bath in an **infant tub** (NOT in an adult tub). Mild soap/shampoo intended for babies or water alone may be used for the bath.

- Make sure the environmental temperature is warm.
- Fill tub with 2-3 inches of water.
- ALWAYS check water temperature to make sure it is warm and NOT hot.
- Set water heaters ≤120 °F to prevent inadvertent scalding.
- Support the baby during the bath with one arm under upper back to support the neck and head while holding the infant under the axillae.
- Pour water over the child with the free hand and use that hand to wash the hair and the body.
- Lift the baby from the tub and wrap in a towel to dry.
- Dry thoroughly, making sure all skin folds and crevices are dry to prevent irritation and rashes.
- Avoid use of lotions or creams.

Fontanels

The infant's fontanels (anterior and posterior) are covered by thick membranous tissue and should feel flat but firm.

- Do not be afraid to touch the fontanels or cleanse the scalp.
- Report **bulging** above the level of the skull, as this may indicate increased intracranial pressure.
- Report a **soft fontanel** that sinks below the level of the skull, as this may indicate dehydration.

Circumcision

Circumcision rates have dropped by 10% over the last 30 years, with about 58% of male infants now being **circumcised** in the United States. The American Academy of Pediatrics has confirmed that the benefits outweigh the risks, though they do not have a formal recommendation for circumcision and instead leave that decision up to the parents. Benefits including decreased risk of prostate cancer, urinary tract infections, and sexually transmitted infections such as HIV. Most parents make their decision based on cultural or religious beliefs or the factor of cost, as some insurance companies and many Medicaid programs do not cover the cost of circumcision. While at one time infants were not thought to experience pain, it is now clear that they do, so circumcision should be done using a local anesthesia or topical EMLA cream.

Post-Circumcision Care

After circumcision, the end of the foreskin is typically swollen and red, and a small amount of bleeding may persist for 24 hours.

- Change the diaper immediately, because urine may cause pain to the open tissue.
- Cleanse the area gently with water and pat dry.
- Apply petroleum jelly gauze to the incision area as directed by the individual physician.
- Avoid using soap or commercial cleansing products, such as baby wipes, until the circumcision heals.
- Report any change, such as increased swelling, redness, temperature, or purulent discharge.

Care of the Uncircumcised Penis

The infant's foreskin is different from that of the adult male. It does not **separate and retract** until the child is around 5 years old.

- Do NOT attempt to retract the foreskin.
- Do NOT use cotton swabs to clean.
- Wash the penis with soap and water or just water during the routine bath.

Shaken Baby Syndrome

Shaken baby syndrome is believed to be the result of vigorous shaking of a neonate, causing acute subdural hematoma with subarachnoid, and retinal hemorrhages. The shaking of the brain may damage vessels and nerves with resultant cerebral edema. Parents should be advised of the importance of always supporting and protecting the neonate's head and avoiding activities that may injure the child, such as throwing and catching a neonate or small child. Parents should be advised that sometimes children may not exhibit obvious neurological symptoms immediately after trauma but have learning disabilities and behavioral disorders that appear in school.

Neonatal CPR

Most cardiac arrests in newborns are associated with respiratory arrest rather than cardiac arrest, so **cardiopulmonary resuscitation** of newborns follows the ABC protocol rather than the compressions only protocol used for adults. The parent should be advised to take a CPR course, especially if the neonate is at risk and if arrest occurs, immediately call 911 for help or ask someone else to call and begin CPR:

- **Airway:** Tilt the head slightly back and lift the chin to open the airway.
- **Breathing:** If the neonate does not begin breathing, administer 2 puffs to ventilate the lungs. For small neonates, place the mouth to cover the neonate's nose and mouth and ventilate each time for approximately one second, observing the chest to ensure it is rising. For the infant with a heart rate ≥60/minute without normal breathing, administer one breath every 2-3 seconds (20-30 breaths per minute).
- **Compressions:** Infants that require chest compressions should receive two breaths per 30 compressions (30:2) for a single rescuer, and two breaths per 15 compressions for two rescuers (15:2). The chest should be depressed approximately 1.5 inches, using two fingers or two thumbs while encircling the hands around the baby's body. The optimum rate of compressions is approximately 100-120 per minute.

Discharge Planning and Follow-Up Screening

Discharge Planning for Patients with Special Needs

Discharge Requirements for Preterm Infant

In the past, discharge requirements for preterm infants were based on factors such as weight and post-conceptual age. Current requirements are instead based on physiological and functional readiness. Hospitals vary, but requirements generally include:

- All medical or surgical problems that require hospitalization are resolved.
- The infant is feeding appropriately, as evidenced by:
  - Primary caregiver feeding the infant with the prescribed method (gavage, gastrostomy, or special positioning)
  - Weight gain of 15-30 grams per day over several days
  - Feeds accomplished without respiratory difficulty
- Temperature stability is maintained between 36.5 to 37.4 °C in an open crib.
- The infant has passed at least one stool.
- Cardiac and respiratory vital signs are stable: heart rate between 100 and 160 beats per minute, and respiratory rate <60 breaths per minute.
- Parents are trained appropriately concerning the administration of medications, CPR, and the proper use of a car seat.
- The infant has passed all pre-discharge tests:
  - Hearing screening
  - Other tests as needed (anemia, ROP exams, sleep study, head ultrasound)
- Age-appropriate immunizations were administered.
- The discharge environment has been evaluated.
- Appropriate post-discharge follow-up appointments are scheduled with specialists and the primary care physician.

Discharge Education for the Special-Needs Neonate

Family involvement and education are vital for the successful discharge of a **special-needs neonate** to ensure proper care. Bringing home a premature infant or one who has special needs is a daunting task for any parent, so preparation is essential.

- Educate the parents or guardians about appropriate care methods.
- Explain how to interpret the infant's cues concerning his or her needs and how to respond appropriately.
- Point out the different states of alertness during their infant's sleep and wake cycles. Identify the appropriate times and methods for infant interaction.
- Coach the parents to ensure that they perform each skill correctly and retain it. Observe interactions between the infant and parents in the nursery to help ensure continued wellness of the infant after discharge.
- Encourage kangaroo care immediately after birth for stable newborns as it is an excellent method to foster bonding between the neonate and the mother. For neonates who require resuscitation and medical intervention, delay kangaroo care until the neonate is stable.
- If the parents are not ready, contact a social worker for follow-up.

Cerebral Palsy and Cognitive/Language Delays

Important elements of discharge planning and parent teaching for patients with cerebral palsy and cognitive/language delays include:

- **Motor delays (especially with cerebral palsy)**: Parents need realistic information about what to expect and how to cope with motor delays and prevent further complications. The nurse should review the child's life care plan, including the need for follow-up therapy and the availability of resources. Instructions and education may vary according to the cause or type of CP. For example, sudden stimuli may increase spastic muscle contractions with spastic CP. Parents need information about specific feeding and positioning needs.
- **Cognitive/language delays**: Assessment of cognition and language delays often occurs over a period of time and cannot always be accurately predicted at birth. Parents should be educated about the levels of cognitive ability common to infants and methods to stimulate cognition. Additionally, parents should understand normal language development, including milestones, and interactions that promote language development.

Follow Up Screening from Neonate to Childhood

Many screening procedures are available, including extensive laboratory testing that may be indicated if there is cause for concern that an infant may have a disorder. However, some basic screening should be done for all infants and children:

- **Genetic disorders**: Screening is usually done at birth according to state guidelines, and then may be indicated if there is concern that a child has a disorder that requires treatment.
- **Hearing**: Testing is usually done with newborns and then every 2-3 years until age 18.
- **Height and weight**: These are monitored monthly during the first year and then at least yearly until age 18 to determine if the child's development is within the normal range.
- **Vision**: This is screened at birth, at 3-4 years, and periodically between 5-18. Vision problems may become obvious when the child enters school and can't see the board or has trouble reading.
- **Fasting blood sugar**: Done every 2 years for those at risk.
- **Head circumference**: Measurement is done at birth, 1 year, and 2 years.
- **Blood pressure**: This is usually checked during infancy (6-12 months) and then periodically throughout childhood.
- **Dental screening**: Bottle-fed babies may require earlier screening as they often fall asleep with the bottle in their mouths, leading to infant caries. Dental screening is done periodically throughout childhood, especially after the new teeth come in, to evaluate for malocclusion or other problems.
- **Alcohol/drug use**: Neonates are screened for parental abuse. Screening of use may be done periodically for children between 11-18 years, especially if they are at risk.
- **Developmental screening**: There are a number of screening tests that are available and can be used if a child appears to have a developmental delay or abnormality. Screening tests must be age-appropriate. The tests are not diagnostic but can help to confirm developmental abnormalities. Tests may assess motor skills, language, and cognitive ability.

Legal Principles

Informed Consent for Neonates

Parents/guardians of neonates must provide **informed consent** for all treatment the infant receives. This includes providing the parents/guardians with a thorough explanation of all procedures, treatments, and associated risks. Parents/guardians should be apprised of all options and allowed input on the type of treatments. Parents/guardians should also be apprised of all reasonable risks and any complications that might be life-threatening or might increase morbidity. The American Medical Association has established guidelines for informed consent:

- Explanation of diagnosis
- Nature of and reason for treatment or procedure
- Risks and benefits
- Alternative options (regardless of cost or insurance coverage)
- Risks and benefits of alternative options
- Risks and benefits of not having a treatment or procedure

Providing informed consent is a requirement of all states.

Advance Directives and Do-Not-Resuscitate Orders for Infants

In accordance with federal and state laws, individuals have the right to self-determination in health care, including making decisions about end-of-life care through **advance directives,** such as living wills and the right to assign a surrogate person to make decisions through a durable power of attorney. Parents/guardians have the right to make these decisions for minors. Parents/guardians should routinely be questioned about an advance directive, as they may present at a healthcare organization without the document.

If parents/guardians indicate the desire for a **do-not-resuscitate (DNR) order** for a seriously ill child, that child should not receive resuscitative treatments for terminal illness or conditions in which meaningful recovery cannot occur. For those with DNR requests or those withdrawing life support, staff should provide the child palliative rather than curative measures, such as pain control and/or oxygen, and emotional support to the child and family. Religious traditions and beliefs about death should be treated with respect.

Nurse-Patient Ratios

Nurse-patient ratios refer to the number of patients assigned to a nurse. For example, if one nurse is assigned responsibility for 4 patients, the ratio is 1:4. Ratios are an area of concern because studies have consistently shown better outcomes for patients with lower nurse-patient ratios. However, the lower the ratio, the higher the costs. California and most recently Oregon currently have mandated nurse-patient ratios. The California law, often cited as a model, requires a 1:1 ratio in the operating room and for trauma patients in the ER, and a 1:2 ratio for patients in ICU, NICU, post-anesthesia recovery, and labor and delivery, as well as ICU patients in the ER. Ratios in other areas range from 1:3 to 1:6 (the maximum). Massachusetts and New York have a mandate for ICU only: 1:1 or 1:2. A number of other states require staffing committees to establish staffing policies, and some states require public reporting of nurse-patient ratios even though they do not mandate the ratios.

Medical Record Documentation

Proper **documentation** is a cornerstone in nursing care. It is a way to communicate patient status to other caregivers. It provides a snapshot of the patient's condition during that moment in time. It documents care given, responses to that care, and further interventions taken. Documentation should be streamlined as much as possible to make efficient use of nursing time. Documentation should be thorough and provide enough information for a subsequent reviewer to reach the same conclusions as the nurse did when giving care. Proper documentation is also the best defense against litigation. Information charted in real time may need to be reviewed by the one who charted it several years later, so it is imperative that the nurse document all of the information required to defend their actions.

Sentinel Events in Perinatal Services

A sentinel event is one that requires specific actions by a Joint Commission–accredited institution. These events are so serious that they require immediate investigation and response. The **criteria** for these events in perinatal services are any event that results in:

- Unexpected death or loss of function
- Harm due to a medication error or suicide
- Maternal death during the intrapartum period
- Death of a full-term infant
- Infant abduction
- Release of the infant to the wrong family
- Blood group incompatibility causing a hemolytic transfusion reaction
- Wrong surgery
- Retention of the foreign body after surgery
- Hyperbilirubinemia above 30 mg/dL

Areas of Obstetrical Nursing Prone to Litigation

Certain areas of care are more highly scrutinized during litigation. The policies and procedures guiding care in these areas should be reviewed continually to be sure they are in line with national standards. **Litigation** is common in the areas of FHR interpretation, documentation, and communication; telephone triage; labor induction; the use of misoprostol or oxytocin; hyperstimulation interventions; response to pain; nursing role during regional anesthesia; use of fundal pressure; interventions for shoulder dystocia; management of the second stage of labor; use of forceps and vacuum extraction; expedited cesarean births; vaginal birth after cesarean birth (VBAC); care of multiple gestations; unintended prematurity; neonatal resuscitation; and prevention of Group B streptococcal infection in the newborn.

Malpractice and Negligence Risks for the Neonatal Nurse Practitioner

Neonatal nurse practitioners, as all advance practice nurses, are usually insured for **malpractice** at a higher rate than registered nurses because their scope of practice is much wider. An NNP may be sued individually or as part of a medical group to which the NNP is associated. Because a suit is a civil matter, loss of judgment may not be reported to the state board of nursing. If a charge of negligence is brought to the attention of the board, the board may initiate an investigation and disciplinary action. Negligence may involve a number of failures, such as not referring a patient when needed, incorrect diagnosis, incorrect treatment, and not providing the patient/family with adequate or essential information. Once an NNP has established a duty to a patient—by direct examination or even a casual in-person or over-the-phone conversation that involves professional advice—the NNP may be liable for malpractice if he or she does not follow up with adequate care.

TYPES OF NEGLIGENCE

Risk management must attempt to determine the burden of proof for acts of **negligence**, including compliance with duty, breaches in procedures, degree of harm, and cause. Negligence indicates that *proper care* has not been provided, based on established standards. *Reasonable care* uses rationales for decision-making in relation to providing care. State regulations regarding negligence may vary, but all have some statutes of limitations. There are a number of different types of negligence:

- **Negligent conduct**, meaning that an individual failed to provide reasonable care or to protect/assist another, based on standards and expertise.
- **Gross negligence**, or willfully providing inadequate care while disregarding the safety and security of another.
- **Contributory negligence**, in which the injured party has contributed to his/her own harm.
- **Comparative negligence**, which attributes a percentage of negligence to each individual involved.

Review Video: Medical Negligence
Visit mometrix.com/academy and enter code: 928405

Ethics

ETHICAL PRINCIPLES ENDORSED BY NANN AND ANA

Both the National Association of Neonatal Nurses (NANN) and the American Nurses Association (ANA) have **codes of ethics** that outline the responsibilities of the neonatal nurse. General concepts emphasized include:

- Respect the human rights of patients and families regardless of race, gender, etc.
- Use nursing skills for the advancement of human welfare.
- Remember, the nurse's primary responsibility is to the patient.
- Respect family autonomy and provide accurate information.
- Ensure that patient's and family's rights and privacy are maintained in accordance with HIPAA regulations.
- Ensure that colleagues are competent; report incompetents, impaired colleagues, or those with questionable behavior.
- Maintain competence through accountability, responsibility, and continuing education.
- Enhance the nursing environment through participation in policy development and participation in professional organizations.

ETHICAL PRINCIPLES

Autonomy is the ethical principle that the individual has the right to make decisions about his or her own care. In the case of children or patients with dementia who cannot make autonomous decisions, parents or family members may serve as the legal decision maker. The nurse must keep the patient and/or family fully informed so that they can exercise their autonomy in informed decision-making.

Justice is the ethical principle that relates to the distribution of the limited resources of healthcare benefits to the members of society. These resources must be distributed fairly. This issue may arise if there is only one bed left and two sick patients. Justice comes into play in deciding which patient should stay and which should be transported or otherwise cared for. The decision should be made according to what is best or most just for the patients and not colored by personal bias.

Beneficence is an ethical principle that involves performing actions that are for the purpose of benefitting another person. In the care of a patient, any procedure or treatment should be done with the ultimate goal of benefitting the patient, and any actions that are not beneficial should be reconsidered. As conditions change, procedures need to be continually reevaluated to determine if they are still of benefit.

Nonmaleficence is an ethical principle that means healthcare workers should provide care in a manner that does not cause direct intentional harm to the patient:

- The actual act must be good or morally neutral.
- The intent must be only for a good effect.
- A bad effect cannot serve as the means to get to a good effect.
- A good effect must have more benefit than a bad effect has harm.

Nursing Code of Ethics

There is more interest in the **ethics** involved in healthcare due to technological advances that have made the prolongation of life, organ transplants, prenatal manipulation, and saving of premature infants possible, sometimes with poor outcomes. Couple these with healthcare's limited resources, and **ethical dilemmas** abound. Ethics is the study of **morality** as the value that controls actions. The American Nurses Association Code of Ethics contains nine statements defining **principles** the nurse can use when faced with moral and ethical problems. Nurses must be knowledgeable about the many ethical issues in healthcare and about the field of ethics in general. The nurse must help a patient to reveal their values and morals to the health care team so that the patient, family, and team can resolve moral issues pertaining to the patient's care. As part of the healthcare team, the nurse has a right to express personal values and moral concerns about medical issues.

Bioethics

Bioethics is a branch of ethics that involves making sure that the medical treatment given is the most morally correct choice given the different options that might be available and the differences inherent in the varied levels of treatment. In the health care unit, if the patients, family members, and the staff are in agreement when it comes to values and decision-making, then no ethical dilemma exists; however, when there is a difference in value beliefs between the patients/family members and the staff, there is a bioethical dilemma that must be resolved. Sometimes, discussion and explanation can resolve differences, but at times the institution's ethics committee must be brought in to resolve the conflict. The primary goal of bioethics is to determine the most morally correct action using the set of circumstances given.

Ethical Decision-Making Model

There are many ethical decision-making models. Some general guidelines to apply in using ethical decision-making models could be the following:

- Gather information about the identified problem
- State reasonable alternatives and solutions to the problem
- Utilize ethical resources (for example, clergy or ethics committees) to help determine the ethically important elements of each solution or alternative
- Suggest and attempt possible solutions
- Choose a solution to the problem

It is important to always consider the **ethical principles** of autonomy, beneficence, nonmaleficence, justice, and fidelity when attempting to facilitate ethical decision-making with family members, caregivers, and the healthcare team.

Ethical Assessment

While the terms *ethics* and *morals* are sometimes used interchangeably, ethics is a study of morals and encompasses concepts of right and wrong. When making **ethical assessments,** one must consider not only what people should do but also what they actually do, as these two things are sometimes at odds. Ethical issues can be difficult to assess because of personal bias, which is one of the reasons that sharing concerns with other internal sources and reaching consensus is so valuable. Issues of concern might include options for care, refusal of care, rights to privacy, adequate relief of suffering, and the right to self-determination. Internal sources might include the ethics committee, whose role is to make decisions regarding ethical issues. Risk management can provide guidance related to personal and institutional liability. External agencies might include government agencies, such as the public health department.

Ethical Analysis of a Situation

Assessment of the situation is done to reveal the ethical, legal, and professional **conflicts** that are present. Those who are involved are identified, including the patient, family, and healthcare personnel. The decision maker is determined if it is not the patient. Information about the situation is collected to determine medical facts about the disease and condition of the patient, options for treatment, and nursing diagnoses. Any pertinent legal information is included. The patient and family's cultural, religious, and moral values are determined. Possible courses of action are listed and compared in terms of outcomes for the patient using the utilitarian or deontological theory of ethics. Professional codes of ethics are also applied. A decision is made and evaluated as to whether it is the most morally correct action. Ethical arguments for and against the decision are given and responded to by the decision maker.

Professional Boundaries

Gifts

Over time, patients may develop a bond with nurses they trust and may feel grateful to the nurse for the care provided and want to express thanks, but the nurse must make sure to maintain professional boundaries. Patients often offer **gifts** to nurses to show their appreciation, but some adults, especially those who are weak and ill or have cognitive impairment, may be taken advantage of easily. Patients may offer valuables and may sometimes be easily manipulated into giving large sums of money. Small tokens of appreciation that can be shared with other staff, such as a box of chocolates, are usually acceptable (depending upon the policy of the institution), but almost any other gifts (jewelry, money, clothes) should be declined: "I'm sorry, that's so kind of you, but nurses are not allowed to accept gifts from patients." Declining may relieve the patient of the feeling of obligation.

Sexual Relations

When the boundary between the role of the professional nurse and the vulnerability of the patient is breached, a boundary violation occurs. Because the nurse is in the position of authority, the responsibility to maintain the boundary rests with the nurse; however, the line separating them is a continuum and sometimes not easily defined. It is inappropriate for nurses to engage in **sexual relations** with patients, and if the sexual behavior is coerced or the patient is cognitively impaired, it is **illegal**. However, more common violations with adults, particularly elderly patients, include exposing a patient unnecessarily, using sexually demeaning gestures or language (including off-color jokes), harassment, or inappropriate touching. Touching should be used with care, such as touching a hand or shoulder. Hugging may be misconstrued.

Attention

Nursing is a giving profession, but the nurse must temper giving with recognition of professional boundaries. Patients have many needs. As acts of kindness, nurses (especially those involved in home care) often give certain patients extra attention and may offer to do **favors**, such as cooking or shopping. They may become overly invested in the patients' lives. While this may benefit a patient in the short term, it can establish a relationship of increasing **dependency** and **obligation** that does not resolve the long-term needs of the patient. Making referrals to the appropriate agencies or collaborating with family to find ways to provide services is more effective. Becoming overly invested may be evident by the nurse showing favoritism or spending too much time with the patient while neglecting other duties. On the other end of the spectrum are nurses who are disinterested and fail to provide adequate attention to the patient's detriment. Lack of adequate attention may lead to outright neglect.

Coercion

Power issues are inherent in matters associated with professional boundaries. Physical abuse is both unprofessional and illegal, but behavior can easily border on abusive without the patient being physically injured. Nurses can easily **intimidate** older adults and sick patients into having procedures or treatments they do not want. Regardless of age, patients have the right to choose and the right to refuse treatment. Difficulties arise with cognitive impairment, and in that case, another responsible adult (often the patient's child or spouse) is designated to make decisions, but every effort should be made to gain patient cooperation. Forcing the patient to do something against his or her will borders on abuse and can sometimes degenerate into actual abuse if physical coercion is involved.

Personal Information

When pre-existing personal or business relationships exist, other nurses should be assigned care of the patient whenever possible, but this may be difficult in small communities. However, the nurse should strive to maintain a professional role separate from the personal role and respect professional boundaries. The nurse must respect and maintain the confidentiality of the patient and family members, but the nurse must also be very careful about **disclosing personal information** about him or herself because this establishes a social relationship that interferes with the professional role of the nurse and the boundary between the patient and the nurse. The nurse and patient should never share secrets. When the nurse divulges personal information, he or she may become vulnerable to the patient, a reversal of roles.

Professional Organizations and Roles

Professional Organizations

Many **professional neonatal and pediatric nursing organizations** are available for neonatal nurses to join. A professional organization is a group of practitioners who share a common interest. They are able to form a collective voice that can influence standards of practice, institutional policies, and governing regulations and laws. They may have admission standards for those wishing to join and provide ethical guidelines for members. Other benefits often include educational opportunities in a chosen area of specialty, newsletters concerning healthcare trends and issues that affect their specialty area, and gatherings where peers meet for discussions. Some organizations available for neonatal nurses include:

- The Academy of Neonatal Nurses (ANN)
- The Association of Women's Health, Obstetric, and Neonatal Nurses (AWHONN)
- The National Association of Neonatal Nurses (NANN)
- The National Association of Pediatric Nurse Practitioners (NAPNP)

Board of Nursing

Each state has its own Nurse Practice Act, which is governed by the state **Board of Nursing**. The Nurse Practice Act outlines requirements for licensure and certification and delineates the scope of practice of nurses, including duties and delegation. Typically, licensure is granted to those who complete an accredited LVN/LPN or RN program and pass the nursing exam (NCLEX) or receive endorsement because of licensure in another state. The neonatal nurse practitioner (NNP) must practice within the standards of advanced practice under the Nurse Practice Act in the state in which the person works and the individual's scope of practice, which is directly related to the individual's educational preparation and certification. In some cases, NNP certification in one state is automatically recognized in other states through the Compact agreement. Educational experience and scope of practice must relate to patient population in terms of age, disease, diagnosis, and treatment.

Organizations Regulating the Philosophy of Care in Birthing Facility

The philosophy of care in a birthing unit must be an agreement that all care given be based on evidence and national standards and guidelines. All policies and procedures should be written with the guidance of these materials. They should be reviewed as needed in the light of additional evidence and changes in guidelines by major professional organizations. These organizations include the Association of Women's Health, Obstetric and Neonatal Nurses (AWHONN), the American College of Obstetricians and Gynecologists (ACOG), the American College of Nurse Midwives (ACNM), the American Academy of Pediatrics (AAP), the American Society of Anesthesiologists (ASA), the Joint Commission (TJC), the Centers for Disease Control (CDC), the American Heart Association (AHA), and the Food and Drug Administration (FDA).

Neonatal Nurse Practitioner

A neonatal nurse practitioner (NNP) is a registered nurse who also has a graduate degree in nursing with a concentration in advanced care of the neonate. The NNP manages daily care of several neonates in the Intensive Care Unit. The NNP assesses physical signs, evaluates laboratory results and clinical data, consults with specialists, writes orders, and interacts with parents to provide support and updates on the clinical status of their neonate. The NNP is responsible for delivery room management of the high risk neonate, intubation, placement of umbilical lines, lumbar punctures, percutaneous placement of arterial and central lines, and insertion of chest tubes. These activities are performed under the direction and supervision of an attending neonatologist.

Prerequisites for RN to Become NNP and Expansion in Scope from RN to NNP

Prerequisites for an RN to become a Neonatal Nurse Practitioner include a current state nursing license demonstrating successful completion of a nursing program and completion of a post-baccalaureate accredited graduate program at the doctorate or master's level in neonatal nursing. In order to receive NNP certification from the National Certification Corporation (NCC), the graduate program must have been at least one academic year in duration with at least 200 hours didactic and 600 clinical. The certification exam must be taken within 8 years of graduation. While both the RN and NNP monitor patients and provide direct nursing care, the NNP has a broader **scope of practice** and prescriptive authority and can order medications and treatments while the RN cannot. Additionally, the NNP can establish an independent practice (supervisory requirements may vary from state to state) and work directly with patients and family to establish plans of care. The NNP may bill Medicare, Medicaid, and insurance companies directly for services provided while the RN may not.

Evidence-Based Practice

Classes of Evidence-Based Practice

Evidence-based practice is treatment based on the best possible evidence, including a study of current research. Literature is searched to find evidence of the most effective treatments for specific diseases or injuries, and those treatments are then utilized to create clinical pathways that outline specific multi-departmental treatment protocols, including medications, treatments, and timelines. Evidence-based guidelines are often produced by specialty organizations that undertake the task of searching and analyzing literature to produce policies, procedures, and guidelines that become the standard of care for the disease. These guidelines are then used when a patient fits the disease criteria for that guideline. **Evidence-based nursing** aims to improve the quality of nursing care by integrating evidence-based research into nursing practice. This can be done on the individual level or the systems level, in which facilities incorporate evidence-based research into the development of clinical pathways and guidelines.

Evidence-Based Practice Guidelines

The creation of evidence-based practice guidelines is usually facility-driven as a means of ensuring these practices are implemented across the system. The process of guideline creation usually includes the following components:

- **Focus on the topic/methodology:** This includes outlining possible interventions and treatments for review, choosing patient populations and settings, and determining significant outcomes. Search boundaries (such as types of databases, types of studies, dates of studies) should be determined.
- **Evidence review:** This includes review of literature, critical analysis of studies, and summarizing of results, including pooled meta-analysis.
- **Expert judgment:** Recommendations based on personal experience from a number of experts may be utilized, especially if there is inadequate evidence based on review, but this subjective evidence should be explicitly acknowledged.
- **Engage stakeholders and patients:** Survey relevant key stakeholders (physicians, nurses, etc.) and patients who would be implementing or subjected to the care outlined in the guideline for feedback.
- **Policy considerations:** This includes cost-effectiveness, access to care, insurance coverage, availability of qualified staff, and legal implications.

- **Policy:** A written policy must be completed with recommendations. Common practice is to utilize letter guidelines, with "A" being the most highly recommended, usually based on the quality of supporting evidence.
- **Review:** The completed policy should be submitted to peers for review and comments before instituting the policy.

Clinical Pathways

Clinical pathway development is done by those involved in direct patient care. The pathway should cover the entire scope of an illness. Steps include:

1. Selection of patient group and diagnosis, procedures, or conditions, based on analysis of data and observations of wide variance in approach to treatment and prioritizing organization and patient needs; consider inclusion/exclusion criteria
2. Creation of interdisciplinary team of those involved in the process of care, including physicians to develop pathway
3. Analysis of data including literature review and study of best practices to identify opportunities for quality improvement
4. Identification of all categories of care, such as nutrition, medications, and nursing
5. Discussion and reaching consensus
6. Identifying the levels of care and number of days to be covered by the pathway (with flexibility to accommodate various possible lengths of stay)
7. Pilot testing and redesigning steps as indicated
8. Educating staff about standards
9. Monitoring and tracking variances in order to improve pathways

HICPAC Categories of Evidence-Based Practice

Levels of evidence are categorized according to the scientific evidence available to support the recommendations, as well as existing state and federal laws. While recommendations are voluntary, they are often used as a basis for state and federal regulations.

- **Category IA** is well supported by evidence from experimental, clinical, or epidemiologic studies and is strongly recommended for implementation.
- **Category IB** has supporting evidence from some studies, has a good theoretical basis, and is strongly recommended for implementation.
- **Category IC** is currently required by state or federal regulations.
- **Category II** is supported by suggestive clinical or epidemiologic studies, has a theoretical basis, and is suggested for implementation.
- **Unresolved** means there is no recommendation because of a lack of consensus or evidence.

Process Monitoring and Outcome Evaluation

Process monitoring and outcome evaluation are important components of evidence-based practice, which incorporate both internal and external research with subject matter expert opinion and patient preferences. All treatments are subjected to review to determine if they produce positive outcomes, and policies and protocols for outcome evaluation should be in place. **Process monitoring** over the course of treatment involves careful observation and record-keeping that notes progress, with supporting laboratory and radiographic evidence as indicated by condition and treatment **Outcome evaluation** includes the following:

- **Evaluating** results includes reviewing records as well as current research to determine if outcomes are within acceptable parameters.
- **Sustaining** involves maintaining treatment that has proven effective and continuing to monitor and evaluate.
- **Improving** means to continue the treatment but with additions or modifications in order to improve outcomes.
- **Replacing** the treatment with a different treatment must be done if outcome evaluation indicates that current treatment is ineffective.

Evidence-Based Nursing Interventions

Evidence-based nursing interventions enable nurses to provide high-quality patient care that is based upon research and knowledge, as opposed to giving care that is based upon tradition or information that is out of date. An evidence-based nursing approach is based on the integration of practical clinical experience with medical and clinical research; it utilizes proven clinical guidelines and assessment practices. Evidence-based nursing interventions allow nurses to make patient care decisions based on the most current research that has been scientifically validated. Studies show that evidence-based nursing practice yields improved patient outcomes, enables nurses to practice up-to-date methods, improves nurse confidence and decision-making skills, and supports compliance with Joint Commission standards.

Resources

There are numerous information resources for evidence-based nursing interventions. These resources include evidence-based textbooks; databases such as CINAHL Plus, COCHRANE library, PubMed/MEDLINE, TRIP Database, and ClinicalKey for Nursing; evidence-based nursing metasites such as the Academic Center for EBN, Joanna Briggs Institute, McGill University, ONS-EBN section, and EBN-University of Minnesota; online evidence-based nursing journals such as Clinical Nurse Specialist, Clinical Nursing Research, Evidence-Based Nursing, Journal of Nursing Care Quality, Journal of Advanced Nursing, Journal of Nursing Scholarship, Nurse Researcher, Nursing Research, Western Journal of Nursing Research, and Worldviews on Evidence-Based Nursing; and various online tutorials.

Obtaining Results of Research to Use in Evidence-Based Practice

When searching for **current evidence** in print and online literature, the nurse should look for **systematic reviews, analyses, and reports**. PUBMED is a large database of biomedicine and life sciences and can be searched for all published articles on a particular subject. These articles can be analyzed to determine treatments that have the best evidence of efficacy. Subject and methodological terms and clinical filters can be used to find necessary information, including a specific medical subject heading (MH), subheading (SH), publication type (PT), and text word (TW). The nurse should also search the Cochrane Databases, Agency for Healthcare Research and Quality, and US Preventive Services Task Force Recommendations for evidence and guidelines. When trials of a treatment provide evidence of effectiveness, the evidence is weighed for strength and confidence. Those that provide the strongest evidence become recommendations and guidelines for use in the field. Research is also done on a smaller scale by specialists who publish in peer-reviewed journals their research results related to the use of a particular intervention.

Nursing Research

Elements of Research

The following are elements of research:

- **Variable**: An entity that can be different within a population
- **Independent variable**: The variable that the researchers hypothesize will impact the outcome and therefore is controlled by the researchers to evaluate its effect
- **Dependent variable**: The variable that is measured based on the impact of the independent variable
- **Hypothesis**: The proposed explanation to describe an expected outcome in a study
- **Sample**: The selected group to be studied that is meant to represent the larger population to which the study will be applied
- **Experimental group**: The subset within the sample that undergoes the treatment or intervention
- **Control group**: The subset within the sample that is not exposed to the treatment or intervention being evaluated (placebo)

The nurse must be taught and must understand the process of critical analysis and know how to conduct a survey of the literature. **Basic research concepts** include:

- **Survey of valid sources**: Information from a juried journal and an anonymous website or personal website are very different sources, and evaluating what constitutes a valid source of data is critical.
- **Evaluation of internal and external validity**: Internal validity shows a cause-and-effect relationship between two variables, with the cause occurring before the effect and no intervening variable. External validity occurs when results hold true in different environments and circumstances with different populations.
- **Sample selection and sample size**: Selection and size can have a large impact on the results, but a sample that is too small may lack both internal and external validity, depending on the population it is meant to represent. Selection may be so narrowly focused that the results can't be generalized to other groups.

Validity, Generalizability, and Replicability

Many research studies are most concerned with **internal validity** (adequate unbiased data properly collected and analyzed within the population studied), but studies that determine the efficacy of procedures or treatments, for example, should have **external validity** as well; that is, the results should be **generalizable** (applicable) for the population that was targeted by the study. **Replication** of the study under different circumstances and with different subjects and researchers should produce similar results. For various reasons, some people may be excluded from a study so that instead of randomized subjects, the subjects may be highly selected (a non-probability sample) so when data is compared with another population in which there is less or more selection, results may be different. The selection of subjects, in this case, would interfere with external validity. Part of the design of a study should include considerations of whether or not it should have external validity or whether there is value for the institution based solely on internal validation, which would then determine the sampling technique utilized.

Hypothesis

A hypothesis should be generated about the probable cause of the disease/infection based on the information available in laboratory and medical records, epidemiologic study, literature review, and expert opinion. For example, a hypothesis should include the infective agent, the likely source, and the mode of transmission: "Wound infections with *Staphylococcus aureus* were caused by the reuse of single-use irrigation syringes used during wound care in the ICU." Population, setting, and time frame may also be added.

Hypothesis testing includes data analysis, laboratory findings, and outcomes of environmental testing. It usually includes case-control studies, with 2-4 controls picked for each case of infection. They may be matched according to age, sex, or other characteristics, but they are not infected at the time they are picked for the study. Cohort studies, whose particpants are defined by exposure rather than utilizing controls, may also be instituted. If the hypothesis cannot be supported, then a new hypothesis or different testing methods may be necessary.

Critical Reading

There are several steps to critical reading to evaluate research:

- **Consider the source** of the material. If it is in the popular press, it may have less validity compared to something published in a peer-reviewed journal.
- **Review the author's credentials** to determine if a person is an expert in the field of study.
- **Determine the hypothesis**, or the central claim of the research. It should be clearly stated.
- **Examine the organization** of the article, whether it is based on a particular theory, and the type of methodology used.
- **Review the evidence** to determine how it is used to support the main points. Look for statistical evidence and sample size to determine if the findings have wide applicability.
- **Evaluate** the overall article to determine if the information seems credible and useful and should be communicated to administration and/or staff.

Major Study Types Utilized in Statistical Analysis

When conducting research, the nurse should be aware of the **types of studies** available and when each type of study is appropriate and most reliable:

- **Case-control studies** are simple. They review pre-existing cases of individuals with the disorder of interest and controls (individuals without the disorder) to assess prior exposures that may have contributed to the disorder. For example, case-control studies may be done with mesothelioma and exposure to possible pleural irritants. These are good for rare diseases to determine possible association.
- **Cross-sectional studies** utilize a cross-section of data from the population and analyze variables at one time point. They are not good for determining cause and effect, but they are useful for estimating exposure prevalence and disease burden.
- **Cohort studies** follow a cohort of a population for a period of time and attempt to make a link with diseases. As in the previous example, researchers could follow a group exposed to asbestos and study the incidence of mesothelioma.
- **Randomized controlled trial** is the gold standard, with patients assigned to the control or experimental group. This is a difficult type of test to design and implement but very useful, as the data is often well-controlled. It is the most expensive type of study.

Bias in Research

Selection bias occurs when the method of selecting subjects results in a cohort that is not representative of the target population because of inherent error in design. For example, if all patients who develop urinary infections are supposed to be evaluated with urine culture and sensitivities for microbial resistance, but only those patients with clinically-evident infections are included, a number of patients with sub-clinical infections or no symptoms may be missed, skewing the results. Selection bias can occur in a variety of study designs.

Information bias occurs when there are errors in classification, so an estimate of association is incorrect. Non-differential misclassification occurs unrelated to the disease or exposure status (often related to equipment/instruments or random error). Differential misclassification occurs when there is a misclassification of disease or exposure that is dependent on outcome or exposure (often related to recall bias).

Qualitative and Quantitative Data

Both qualitative and quantitative data are used for analysis, but the focus is quite different:

- **Qualitative data**: Data are described verbally or graphically, and the results require reporting or observation. Interviews may be used as a tool to gather information, and the researcher's interpretation of data is important. Gathering this type of data can be time-intensive, and is not intended for generalization to a larger population.
- **Quantitative data**: Data are described in terms of numbers within a statistical format. This type of information gathering is done after the design of data collection is outlined. Tools may include surveys, questionnaires, or other methods of obtaining numerical data.

Quality Improvement and Risk Assessment

Continuous Quality Improvement

Continuous quality improvement is a multidisciplinary management philosophy that can be applied to all aspects of an organization, whether related to such varied areas as the cardiac unit, purchasing, or human resources. The skills used for epidemiologic research (data collection, analysis, outcomes, action plans) are all applicable to the analysis of multiple types of events, because they are based on solid scientific methods. Multi-disciplinary planning can bring valuable insights from various perspectives, and strategies used in one context can often be applied to another. All staff, from housekeeping to supervising, must be alert to not only problems but also opportunities for improvement. Increasingly, departments must be concerned with cost-effectiveness as the costs of medical care continue to rise, so the quality professional in the cardiovascular unit is not in an isolated position in an institution but is just one part of the whole, facing similar concerns as those in other disciplines. Disciplines are often interrelated in their functions.

Juran's Quality Improvement Process

Joseph Juran's quality improvement process (QIP) is a 4-step method of change (focusing on quality control) which is based on a trilogy of concepts that includes quality planning, control, and improvement. The steps to the QIP process include the following:

1. **Defining** the project and organizing includes listing and prioritizing problems and identifying a team.
2. **Diagnosing** includes analyzing problems and then formulating theories related to cause by root cause analysis and test theories.
3. **Remediating** includes considering various alternative solutions and then designing and implementing specific solutions and controls while addressing institutional resistance to change. As causes of problems are identified and remediation instituted to remove the problems, the processes should improve.
4. **Holding** involves evaluating performance and monitoring the control system in order to maintain gains.

FOCUS Performance Improvement Model

Find, organize, clarify, uncover, start (FOCUS) is a performance improvement model used to facilitate change:

- **Find**: Identifying a problem by looking at the organization and attempting to determine what isn't working well or what is wrong.
- **Organize**: Identifying those people who have an understanding of the problem or process and creating a team to work on improving performance.
- **Clarify**: Determining what is involved in solving the problem by utilizing brainstorming techniques, such as the Ishikawa diagram.
- **Uncover**: Analyzing the situation to determine the reason the problem has arisen or that a process is unsuccessful.
- **Start**: Determining where to begin in the change process.

FOCUS, by itself, is an incomplete process and is primarily used as a means to identify a problem rather than a means to find the solution. FOCUS is usually combined with PDCA (FOCUS-PDCA), so it becomes a 9-step process; however, beginning with FOCUS helps to narrow the focus, resulting in better outcomes.

Nurse's Involvement in Quality Improvement

The following are ways in which nurses can be involved in quality improvement in their facility:

- **Identify situations** in the nursing unit that require improvement and might benefit patient outcomes (cost containment, incident reporting, etc.) if changed.
- **Identify potential items** that can be measured to be able to test the problem or to be able to monitor patient outcomes.
- **Collect data** on those measurements and determine current patient outcomes.
- **Analyze the data** and identify procedures, methods, etc., that can be utilized to potentially make positive changes in patient outcomes, doing research if necessary.
- **Make recommendations for changes** to be implemented to determine the effect on patient outcomes.
- **Implement recommendations** after approval from administrative personnel.
- **Collect data** using the same measurements and determine if the changes improved patient outcomes or not.

Risk Management

Risk management attempts to prevent harm and legal liability by being proactive and by identifying a patient's **risk factors**. The patient is educated about these factors and ways that they can modify their behavior to decrease their risk. Treatments and interventions must be considered in terms of risk to the patient, and the patient must always know these risks in order to make healthcare decisions. Much can be done to avoid mistakes that put patients at risk. Patients should note medications and other aspects of their care so that they can help prevent mistakes. They should feel free to question care and to have their concerns heard and addressed. When mistakes are made, the actions taken to remedy the situation are very important. The physician should be made aware of the error immediately, and the patient notified according to hospital policy. Errors must be evaluated to determine how the process failed. Honesty and caring can help mitigate many errors.

Nursing Malpractice, Negligence, Unintentional Torts, and Intentional Torts

- **Malpractice** is unethical or improper actions or lack of proper action by the nurse that may or may not be related to a lack of skills that nurses should possess.
- **Negligence** is the failure to act as any other diligent nurse would have acted in the same situation.
- Negligence can lead to an **unintentional tort**. In this case, the patient must prove that the nurse had a duty to act, a duty proven via standards of care, and that the nurse failed in this duty and harm occurred to the patient as a result of this failure.
- **Intentional torts** differ in that the duty is assumed and the nurse breached this duty via assault and battery, invasion of privacy, slander, or false imprisonment of the patient.

Review Video: Medical Negligence
Visit mometrix.com/academy and enter code: 928405

Chapter Quiz

Ready to see how well you retained what you just read? Scan the QR code to go directly to the chapter quiz interface for this study guide. If you're using a computer, simply visit the online resources page at **mometrix.com/resources719/ccrnneonatal** and click the Chapter Quizzes link.

CCRN Practice Test

1. A newborn with a congenital heart defect causing systemic to pulmonary shunting develops signs of cardiogenic shock. Which of the following are characteristics of cardiogenic shock?

a. Decreased cardiac output, increased systemic vascular resistance, pulmonary edema, and right ventricular failure.
b. Decreased cardiac output, peripheral edema, decreased systemic vascular resistance, and left ventricular failure.
c. Decreased cardiac output, decreased systemic vascular resistance, pulmonary edema, and left ventricular failure.
d. Increased cardiac output, increased systemic vascular resistance, peripheral edema, and right ventricular failure.

2. A neonate on mechanical ventilation develops a left pneumothorax with obvious tachypnea, displaced apical heartbeat, and unequal air exchange, requiring needle aspiration. What is the correct insertion site for the needle?

a. Left anterior axillary line, second or third intercostal space.
b. Left midsternal line, second or third intercostal space.
c. Left midclavicular line, third or fourth intercostal space.
d. Left midclavicular line, second or third intercostal space.

3. The nursing staff is preparing posters to explain handwashing and gowning procedures for family members to reduce the chance of cross-contamination in the NICU. Which of the following is the best type of poster?

a. A poster with detailed text at 9th grade level and small sketches.
b. A poster with large pictures and minimal text written at 6th grade level.
c. A poster with pictures only.
d. A poster with text only at adult reading level.

4. After insertion of an endotracheal tube (ETT), the nurse auscultates the infant for breath sounds and notes that the right lung is better ventilated than the left. What does this suggest?

a. The ETT is positioned too high.
b. The ETT is positioned too low.
c. The ETT is in the stomach.
d. The ETT is correctly positioned.

5. A premature neonate was maintained on mechanical ventilation for 3 weeks. Extubation was done with some difficulty, and the infant subsequently developed stridor, recurrent pneumonitis, and frequent choking. What complication of long-term intubation most likely explains these symptoms?

a. Tracheal stenosis.
b. *Staphylococcus aureus* infection.
c. Pulmonic stenosis.
d. Tracheobronchial fistula.

6. If a newborn's stroke volume is about 5 mL, what is the average pulse required to ensure adequate cardiac output?

a. 100 bpm.
b. 145 bpm.
c. 180 bpm.
d. 195 bpm.

7. A neonate suffered perinatal asphyxia and developed moderate hypoxic-ischemic encephalopathy (HIE) with neurological dysfunction, including seizures. Which treatment may be used to increase cerebral blood flow?

a. Phenobarbital.
b. Calcium channel blocker.
c. Allopurinol.
d. Heparin.

8. Evidence-based guidelines are being developed for insertion and care of peripherally inserted central catheters (PICCs) to reduce infection rates. The most reliable information derives from which of the following?

a. Opinion of the medical director.
b. Staff observations.
c. Review of literature, focusing on research studies with critical analysis.
d. Reports of best practices at another hospital.

9. After emergent treatment for a pneumothorax, a neonate has a chest tube inserted and attached to a 3-chamber Pleur-Evac system. Which chamber or chambers control the vacuum necessary to create suction?

a. Chambers 1 and 3.
b. Chamber 1.
c. Chamber 2.
d. Chamber 3.

10. A woman with placenta previa delivers a neonate at near term. Which of the following neonatal conditions is an increased risk with placenta previa?

a. Asphyxia.
b. Congenital anomalies.
c. Cerebral hemorrhage.
d. Neural tube defects.

11. A postoperative neonate is assessed for pain using the CRIES tool. This tool requires supplemental oxygen as needed to maintain oxygen saturation at which of the following levels?

a. > 94%.
b. > 95%.
c. > 96%.
d. > 97%.

12. A neonate has had frequent blood draws to monitor electrolyte and glucose levels. Phlebotomy has caused anemia of prematurity (AOP), although the infant is not acutely hypoxemic. Which initial treatment is indicated?

a. Recombinant human erythropoietin (rHuEPO).
b. Fresh frozen plasma (FFP)
c. Packed red blood cells (PRBC).
d. Platelets.

13. What is the best approach to ensure collaboration between the parents of a seriously ill neonate and the medical staff?

a. Provide printed guidelines outlining parents' rights and responsibilities.
b. Tell the family what their rights are in relation to care.
c. Advise the family that they should devise a list of concerns.
d. Sit down with the family and ask what they want.

14. A neonate with hypoxia is receiving noninvasive positive pressure ventilation. Which of the following provides a steady stream of pressurized air with increased pressure during inspiration?

a. Bilevel positive airway pressure (BiPAP).
b. Continuous positive airway pressure (CPAP).
c. Free flow (blow-by) oxygen.
d. Oxygen per high-flow nasal cannula.

15. A premature neonate is receiving enteral feedings. Which of the following is most important in reducing the risk of necrotizing enterocolitis (NEC)?

a. Increasing feeding volume rapidly to goal to maximize benefits.
b. Using breast milk in enteral feedings.
c. Using hyperosmolar feedings.
d. Administering immunoglobulins.

16. A neonate develops a stable tachyarrhythmia. Which first action is most appropriate?

a. Give a synchronized electrical cardioversion at 0.5-2.0 Joules/kg.
b. Give asynchronous cardioversion.
c. Try esophageal pacing.
d. Apply ice to the neonate's face to trigger the diving response.

17. New policies are being instituted in the NICU, based on evidence-based research. Some of the staff members are vocally resistant to the changes. What is the most appropriate action for the unit supervisor?

a. Advise staff that complaining is counterproductive.
b. Provide honest information about the reasons for the changes and how the changes will affect the staff, including positives.
c. Suggest that staff vote on whether to implement the changes.
d. File a report with Human Resources about those complaining.

18. An infant has been treated with a CoolCap® for brain cooling (hypothermia) for 70 hours and is being rewarmed. What is the correct rate of rewarming?

a. 0.5°C/hr.
b. 1°C/hr
c. 1.5°C/hr.
d. 2°C/hr.

19. A neonate with bronchopulmonary dysplasia is receiving high-frequency jet ventilation (HFJV). Which assessment is best used to determine airway patency and effectiveness of ventilation?

a. Auscultation of the lungs.
b. Heart and respiratory rate.
c. Chest wall vibration.
d. Oxygen saturation level.

20. A premature neonate has developed acute renal failure (ARF). There is a proportionate rise in the BUN/creatinine ratio with creatinine concentration 1.8 mg/dL. What finding in the urinalysis suggests an intrinsic cause for the ARF rather than prerenal or postrenal?

a. White blood cells.
b. Red blood cells.
c. Protein, tubular cells, and casts.
d. Mucous and red blood cells.

21. A mother brings her term infant (and first child) for an exam at 2 weeks after birth. The baby has poor skin turgor, face drawn, appears listless, and has not regained birth weight. The mother is breast-feeding. Which of the following first actions is most appropriate?

a. Question mother about breast-feeding technique and frequency and observe the infant breast-feeding.
b. Report the mother to Child Protective Services for neglect.
c. Order laboratory tests for electrolytes.
d. Advise the mother to stop breast-feeding and switch to formula.

22. A mother developed abruptio placentae during pregnancy. Which of the following conditions in the neonate is commonly associated with abruptio placentae?

a. Congenital anomalies.
b. Neurological deficits.
c. Cerebral hemorrhage.
d. Microcephaly.

23. A neonate receiving mechanical ventilation has a $PaCO_2$ rate of 33 with pH of 7.5 from a blood sample obtained from the umbilical artery. These values indicate:

a. Metabolic acidosis from decreased tissue perfusion.
b. Metabolic alkalosis from loss of acid.
c. Respiratory acidosis from hypoventilation.
d. Respiratory alkalosis from hyperventilation.

24. A term neonate is diagnosed with osteogenesis imperfecta (OI) type 1 at birth based on a rib fracture, blue sclera, and short limbs. What information must the parents receive before taking the child home?

a. Correct methods of handling, bathing, and placing their child in the crib.
b. Instructions for tube feedings.
c. Printed guide for genetic testing.
d. Schedule for grief counseling.

25. The parents of a neonate are considering genetic testing for their son because the father was recently diagnosed with Huntington disease. They ask the nurse's opinion. Which is the most appropriate response?

a. "Testing the infant now can help relieve your anxiety."
b. "You should not have the infant tested until his teen years."
c. "The information cannot be used for health purposes now, and your child may want to make this decision himself when he is older."
d. "You should ask the doctor."

26. A 6-day-old newborn develops signs of congestive heart failure with tachypnea, heart rate 175 at rest, fine pulmonary rales, and difficulty feeding. Which of the following is the most likely underlying cause?

a. Hypoplastic left heart syndrome.
b. Coarctation of the aorta.
c. Patent ductus arteriosus.
d. Pulmonary stenosis.

27. A premature neonate born at 33 weeks' gestation is 2 days old and exhibiting episodes of apnea that range from 15-25 seconds, associated with cyanosis, bradycardia, oxygen saturation less than 85%, and swallowing during apneic periods. The most likely diagnosis is:

a. Periodic breathing.
b. Pulmonic stenosis.
c. Apnea of prematurity.
d. Pneumothorax.

28. A neonate is being treated in the NICU. A woman calls and identifies herself as the child's mother and asks for information about the infant's condition. What is the appropriate action?

a. Provide the information.
b. State that no information can be given over the phone
c. State that a return call must be made to the home before information can be given.
d. Ask for identifying information, such as an agreed-upon password, to ensure that the person has a right to confidential information.

29. A term neonate in apparent good health develops seizures on day 2 but appears healthy between seizures. After a CT scan, which test is indicated to confirm subarachnoid hemorrhage?

a. Ultrasound.
b. Hemoglobin and hematocrit.
c. Lumbar puncture.
d. MRI.

30. A neonate born 11 weeks before due date and weighing less than 2500 g exhibited respiratory distress syndrome at birth and has been maintained on HFJV with supplementary oxygen for more than 28 days. What medications are used to prevent/treat bronchopulmonary dysplasia and allow the lungs to mature?

a. Surfactant, furosemide, and theophylline/albuterol.
b. Surfactant, dexamethasone, and theophylline/albuterol.
c. Dexamethasone and indomethacin.
d. Prostaglandin and theophylline/albuterol.

31. A full-term neonate fails to pass meconium in the first 48 hours of life. The infant exhibits abdominal distension, poor feeding, and bilious vomiting. An x-ray of the abdomen shows dilated loops of bowel. Which diagnostic procedure is used both to confirm a diagnosis of meconium plug syndrome and to treat?

a. MRI.
b. Colonoscopy.
c. Contrast enema.
d. Saline enema.

32. A neonate with severe sepsis has developed indications of multiorgan dysfunction syndrome (MODS). Cardiac function is depressed, and acute respiratory distress syndrome develops with renal failure related to acute tubular necrosis. The neonate's platelet count is falling, suggesting the onset of which complication?

a. Anemia.
b. Apnea.
c. Pulmonary edema.
d. Disseminated intravascular coagulation.

33. A neonate who is breast-feeding has onset of jaundice 5 days after birth associated with a decrease in stools. Serum bilirubin is 20 mg/dL. The mother is producing adequate breast milk and the infant's intake has also been adequate. Which initial treatment is appropriate?

a. Breast-feeding more frequently with caloric supplements and phototherapy.
b. Discontinuation of breast-feeding for 24 hours, substituting formula, and providing phototherapy.
c. Providing phototherapy only
d. No treatment is indicated.

34. In the ACCN Synergy Model, the three levels of quality outcomes include:

a. Nurse, patient, and system.
b. Resiliency, vulnerability, and stability.
c. Recidivism, cost, and resource utilization.
d. Trust, ratings, and satisfaction.

35. A neonate with congestive heart failure (CHF) is very agitated and crying, with a decrease in oxygen saturation (PaO_2). Which treatment is most appropriate?

a. Increased flow of supplemental oxygen to improve oxygenation.
b. Furosemide to reduce excess intravascular fluid.
c. Morphine or fentanyl to produce sedation.
d. Digoxin therapy to improve cardiac output.

36. A neonate born at 38 weeks' gestation is severely compromised and exhibits tachypnea, nasal flaring, and retractions; nail beds are yellow-green; crackles are noted on auscultation of the lungs; arterial blood gases (ABGs) show pH of 7.28 with hypoxemia and hypercapnia; and radiograph shows infiltrates, atelectasis, and both hypoinflated and hyperinflated areas. The most likely diagnosis is:

a. Apnea of prematurity.
b. Bronchopulmonary dysplasia.
c. Transient tachypnea of newborn.
d. Meconium aspiration syndrome (MAS).

37. A neonate has been taking oral fluids well but has been agitated and crying during feedings. He develops dyspnea, respiratory distress, and cyanosis. The most likely diagnosis is:

a. Pneumonitis.
b. Aspiration pneumonia.
c. Atrial septal defect.
d. Congestive heart failure.

38. A neonate is severely ill and may die. The parents are Hmong and ask that a traditional healer be allowed into the NICU to treat the child. Generally, only family members are allowed into the NICU. What is the most appropriate action?

a. Explain that only family members are allowed into the NICU.
b. Arrange a viewing so that the healer can see the child through a window.
c. Make an exception and allow the healer to attend the child.
d. Refer the matter to risk management.

39. A neonate at 28 weeks' gestation and weighing 1400 g has a fall in hematocrit at 24 hours and gradual neurological deterioration, although motor function is symmetric. Oxygen saturation decreases, and the infant is hyperglycemic with metabolic acidosis. The anterior fontanelle is tense but not bulging. The most likely cause of these symptoms is:

a. Intraventricular hemorrhage.
b. Subarachnoid hemorrhage.
c. Subdural hemorrhage.
d. Congenital hydrocephalus.

40. A neonate at 37 weeks' gestation is born to a mother who has abused cocaine throughout pregnancy. The neonate exhibits persistent hypertonia, startles easily, and shows signs of distress at any disturbance. Which is the most appropriate treatment?

a. Anticonvulsant.
b. Opioid.
c. Sedative.
d. Swaddling and reduction in external stimuli.

41. Which of the following metabolic abnormalities is associated with acute renal failure (ARF)?

a. Hypokalemia.
b. Hypophosphatemia.
c. Hypercalcemia.
d. Hypernatremia.

42. A neonate has a venous umbilical catheter inserted to receive exchange transfusions. Placement is best verified by which of the following procedures?

a. Proper estimation of length by measuring the distance from the shoulder to the umbilicus, multiplying the number by 0.75.
b. An echocardiogram or ultrasound.
c. A radiograph.
d. Auscultation with a stethoscope.

43. A 40-year-old mother with a history of binge drinking delivers a term neonate by breech presentation. Which of the following indicate fetal alcohol syndrome (FAS)?

a. Facial abnormalities and neurological deficits.
b. Growth retardation.
c. Congenital cardiac anomalies.
d. All of the above.

44. A premature neonate born at 34 weeks' gestation has a low birth weight (less than 2500 g) and develops respiratory distress syndrome (RDS) with increasing hypoxemia because of inadequate surfactant. Which of the following results from lack of surfactant?

a. Alveolar collapse.
b. Alveolar obstruction.
c. Alveolar dilation.
d. Alveolar necrosis.

45. A neonate whose parents are Jehovah's Witnesses has a life-threatening hypovolemic anemia and requires blood products. The parents have indicated that they oppose transfusions of whole blood or blood cells. Which of the following is the most appropriate first action?

a. Ask that a hospital attorney to speak with the parents.
b. Explain the child's condition and need for blood products.
c. Refer the issue to Child Protective Services.
d. Refer the issue to risk management.

46. Onset of drug withdrawal symptoms for a neonate whose mother used heroin during pregnancy is usually:

a. 12-24 hours postnatal.
b. At least 48 hours (up to 1 month) postnatal.
c. ≥48 hours (up to 1 month) postnatal.
d. 4-7 days (up to 14 days) postnatal.

47. A neonate has a large exposed myelomeningocele. She has been feeding poorly and her skin turgor is decreased. Symptoms include tachycardia, tachypnea, decreasing systolic blood pressure, capillary refill greater than 3 seconds, cyanosis, cold extremities, and markedly decreased urinary output with increased specific gravity. She is most likely exhibiting indications of:

a. Hypovolemic shock.
b. Obstructive shock.
c. Renal failure.
d. Sepsis.

48. A neonate exhibits severe respiratory distress and cyanosis with a left hemithorax, right mediastinal shift, and right pulmonary hypoplasia. What would auscultation of the chest and abdomen likely show?

a. Lack of bowel sounds.
b. Hyperactive abdominal bowel sounds.
c. Bowel sounds across the chest.
d. Bowel sounds in the right abdomen only.

49. A female neonate is found to have an imperforate anus with no external opening or dimple on initial physical exam. The abdomen is slightly distended, but the neonate passes some meconium at 24 hours. What type of anomaly does this suggest?

a. Low anomaly with rectourethral fistula.
b. Intermediate anomaly with a perineal fistula.
c. Intermediate anomaly with rectovaginal fistula.
d. High anomaly with rectovaginal fistula.

50. In the care of a patient, any procedure or treatment should be done with the ultimate goal of benefitting the patient, and any actions that are not beneficial should be reconsidered. This is an example of which ethical principle?

a. Justice
b. Autonomy
c. Nonmaleficence.
d. Beneficence

51. A neonate is 40 weeks' gestation and breast-feeding well but has onset of jaundice at 36 hours. Total serum bilirubin is 12 mg/dL. Which treatment is indicated at this time?

a. Increasing frequency of breast-feeding.
b. Phototherapy.
c. Continued observation and jaundice assessment.
d. Exchange transfusion.

52. A neonate exhibits an enlarged head with widened sutures, dilated vessels, bulging fontanelles and increasing frontooccipital circumference (FOC). Which of the following signs may indicate damage to brain tissue associated with congenital hydrocephalus?

a. Frontal release signs.
b. Babinski sign.
c. Setting sun eyes.
d. Pyramidal tract signs.

53. An infant of a diabetic mother (IDM) is large for gestational age (LGA) and is at risk for developing hypoglycemia because of hyperinsulinism. Blood glucose level has fallen to 45 mg/dL. The infant is breast-feeding poorly. Which first preventive treatment is indicated?

a. Glucagon.
b. IV glucose administration at 4-6 mg/kg/min.
c. Diazoxide.
d. Somatostatin.

54. Which of the following neonatal symptoms at birth is associated with maternal cocaine use?

a. Tremors, hypertonicity, hyperirritability.
b. Congenital malformations.
c. Pronounced lethargy.
d. Seizures.

55. A neonate exhibits respiratory distress and cyanosis that is alleviated by crying. The nurse is unable to pass a suctioning tube through the nares on either side. What first action should the nurse take?

a. Insert a small-gauge nasogastric (NG) tube.
b. Place infant with upper body elevated.
c. Administer free-flow (blow-by) oxygen at 5 L/min.
d. Stimulate the infant to cry.

56. During the initial physical examination, the neonate's chest circumference is 34 cm. What is the expected head circumference?

a. 32 cm.
b. 34 cm.
c. 36 cm.
d. 38 cm.

57. The best determinant of the effectiveness of teaching is:

a. Observable/Measurable behavioral modification.
b. Parent's report of compliance.
c. Parent satisfaction based on surveys.
d. Instructor's knowledge base.

58. A neonate has received a transfusion and fluids for treatment of hypovolemic shock and is being treated with a dopamine infusion to increase cardiac output and improve blood pressure. He is receiving 10 mcg/kg/min. Possible side effects include:

a. Bradycardia and pulmonary edema.
b. Hypertension and peripheral edema.
c. Tachypnea and hypotension.
d. Tachycardia, ectopic beats, and dysrhythmias.

59. A 3-day old neonate with tracheomalacia has respiratory stridor, reflex periods of apnea, and cough during feeding. Which initial treatment is probably indicated?

a. Insertion of endotracheal tube.
b. Nasogastric feeding.
c. PICC for parenteral nutrition.
d. Careful feeding with infant's upper body elevated and administration of humidified air.

60. When doing clinical research, which of the following sources is NOT valid?

a. Popular press report.
b. Juried medical journal.
c. Professional physician's association.
d. Chief of medical staff.

61. A neonate is receiving supplemental oxygen per a medium-sized oxygen hood and develops signs of hypercapnia from rebreathing CO_2 retained within the hood. The most likely cause is:

a. Rate of oxygen flow is too high for the size of the hood.
b. Rate of oxygen flow is too low for the size of the hood.
c. Size of hood is too small for the infant.
d. Size of hood is too large for the infant.

62. The nurse is obtaining blood from the heel of a neonate for a potassium level. Because the infant is crying and moving his limbs, she grasps the heel very tightly during the procedure. How can squeezing the heel too hard affect the laboratory results?

a. It may give an artificially high reading.
b. It may give an artificially low reading.
c. It has no effect on the laboratory reading.
d. It may have a varied effect (high or low) on the laboratory reading.

63. A term female neonate has a large occipital encephalocele, which is covered by skin. The neonate is to be sent home prior to surgical repair to place the herniated mass inside the skull and repair the bony defect. What instruction is most important for the parents to prevent complications?

a. Feeding instructions to ensure adequate nutrition.
b. Measuring head for signs of hydrocephalus.
c. Observing for signs of infection.
d. Positioning and care of encephalocele.

64. A premature neonate with respiratory distress maintained on positive pressure mechanical ventilation exhibits sudden swelling of the scrotal area. This is most likely an indication of:

a. Impaired circulation resulting in edema.
b. Improper positioning of infant.
c. Alveolar damage resulting in pneumoperitoneum.
d. Testicular torsion.

65. Placing the neonate above the level of the mother's placenta during delivery while the cord is clamped can result in:

a. Hypoxia.
b. Apnea.
c. Anemia.
d. No untoward effects.

66. Which of the following is an indication of stress in an extremely low birth weight (ELBW) neonate?

a. Hypertonicity.
b. Increased startle response.
c. Jitteriness.
d. Decreased activity, nonreactive.

67. A newly hired nurse is assisting her team leader, who is preparing to insert an IV peripheral catheter. The team leader drops the sterile catheter onto the bed linens and then picks up the contaminated catheter and continues to prepare for insertion. Which is the best response?

a. Wait until the team leader finishes the procedure and ask why she used the contaminated catheter.
b. Report the team leader's behavior to a supervisor after the catheter is inserted.
c. Say nothing to anyone because the linens were clean.
d. Immediately say, "The catheter was contaminated when it fell. Would you like me to get another setup or stay with the patient while you get it?"

68. A 20-day-old male neonate returns to the hospital because of poor feeding, vomiting of bile, and bouts of crying with evidence of abdominal pain, although his abdomen is not distended. He has passed only small amounts of liquid stool in the past 48 hours and stool guaiac is positive for blood. A slight abdominal mass is palpable. The radiograph is positive for the "double bubble" sign. What diagnosis do these findings suggest?

a. Malrotation defect with volvulus.
b. Renal calculus with ileus.
c. Gastroenteritis.
d. Fecal impaction with overflow diarrhea.

69. A 5-day-old neonate has been diagnosed with patent ductus arteriosus (PDA). Her heart rate is 185 bpm with a 4+ bounding pulse and respiratory rate is 76 per minute. Hepatomegaly is 4 cm below costal margin. The most likely treatment for the PDA is:

a. Surgical repair
b. Indomethacin or ibuprofen lysine.
c. Prostaglandin.
d. No specific treatment is necessary because the PDA will close.

70. An immigrant mother delivered her second child at home with no prenatal care. The mother is Rh- and the child Rh+. The mother brings her newborn to the hospital because the infant is swollen, cyanotic, and jaundiced with enlarged liver and spleen. Testing indicates immune hydrops fetalis with severe anemia. Which type of transfusion is most commonly prescribed?

a. Complete exchange transfusion with whole blood.
b. Fresh frozen plasma.
c. Partial exchange transfusion with PRBCs.
d. Platelets.

71. A neonate with esophageal atresia (EA) and tracheoesophageal fistula (TEF) (distal communication with trachea) accumulates white, frothy oral secretions and exhibits drooling, coughing, and choking. The correct positioning to decrease incidence of reflux and aspiration prior to surgical repair is:

a. Prone or side-lying with head elevated 30-45 degrees.
b. Supine position with head elevated 30 degrees.
c. Prone position with head below chest.
d. Normal supine or side-lying position.

72. The best method to evaluate a parent's educational outcomes related to being taught a procedure is to:

a. Ask the parent for feedback.
b. Give the parent a verbal test.
c. Ask the parent to do a demonstration.
d. Give the parent a written test.

73. A near-term neonate shows indications of persistent pulmonary hypertension of newborn (PPHN) 6 hours after birth:

- Cyanosis with poor cardiac perfusion, tachycardia. Hypoxemia, persisting even with supplemental oxygen.
- Systolic murmur with regurgitation of the tricuspid valve.
- Tachypnea and general respiratory distress.

Which of the following treatments are initially indicated?

a. Intubation and conventional mechanical ventilation, surfactant, sedation, and inhaled nitrous oxide.
b. Extracorporeal membrane oxygenation (ECMO) and induced paralysis (pancuronium or vecuronium).
c. Albuterol, surfactant, and sedation.
d. High-frequency oscillatory ventilation (HFOV), surfactant, and theophylline.

74. A neonate had vacuum-assisted delivery and exhibits a collection of fluid beneath the skin of the scalp but superficial to the periosteum. The swelling crosses suture lines. The symptoms are consistent with:

a. Cephalohematoma.
b. Caput succedaneum.
c. Craniotabes.
d. Abusive head trauma.

75. A neonate with apnea of prematurity is treated with a maintenance dose of theophylline 2 mg/kg every 12 hours to stimulate the central nervous system and dilate the bronchi. Which of the following is the correct IV administration?

a. Rapid IV push.
b. IV push over 5 minutes.
c. Slow infusion of at least 10 minutes.
d. Slow infusion of at least 20 minutes

76. The mother of a healthy preterm neonate born at 36 weeks' gestation asks if her child will likely be developmentally delayed. Which is the correct response?

a. Developmental delay usually subsides by age 2.
b. Development is usually normal.
c. Development is usually markedly delayed for 3 years.
d. Developmental delay usually persists throughout childhood.

77. A 40-year-old multiparous mother is 36 weeks' gestation and exhibits hypertension and general flu-like symptoms, including nausea and vomiting. She complains of pain in the right upper quadrant. Laboratory testing shows hemolysis, elevated liver enzymes, and low platelets (30,000), consistent with HELLP syndrome. Which treatment approach is most critical?

a. Deliver the infant as soon as possible.
b. Provide IV steroids.
c. Give platelet transfusion.
d. Give fresh frozen plasma (FFP) transfusion.

78. A 14-day-old neonate is showing marked cyanosis and decreased cardiac output with increasing signs of congestive heart failure and cardiovascular collapse. The most likely diagnosis is:

a. Hypoplastic left heart syndrome.
b. Ventricular septal defect.
c. Aortic stenosis.
d. Pulmonic stenosis.

79. A nursing team leader delegates a task to unlicensed assistive personnel. Who is responsible for patient outcomes?

a. The unlicensed person who completes the task.
b. Both the team leader and the unlicensed person who completes the task.
c. The team leader who delegates the task.
d. The administrative staff.

80. A post-term neonate born at 43 weeks' gestation and weighing 4100 g with postmaturity syndrome will most likely exhibit which of the following?

a. Lack of creases in plantar area of feet.
b. Long body with extra layers of fat and moist, resilient skin.
c. Long, thin body with loose, parchment-like skin.
d. Large head in proportion to the rest of the body.

81. A neonate is delivered per cesarean. The infant exhibits tachypnea with slight sternal retraction, grunting exhalations, and perioral cyanosis at birth, with mild symptoms still evident but much improved with no cyanosis by 8 hours. The most likely treatment at this point is:

a. Oxygen administration through mask or hood.
b. CPAP.
c. Careful monitoring only.
d. Intubation and mechanical ventilation.

82. A 2-day-old infant of a diabetic mother (IDM) exhibits jitteriness, irritability, stridor, tetany, high-pitched cry, seizures, and decreased myocardial contractility with decreased cardiac output. An electrocardiogram shows a prolonged QT interval and a flattened T wave. What electrolyte imbalance is consistent with these symptoms?

a. Hypercalcemia.
b. Hypocalcemia.
c. Hyperkalemia.
d. Hypokalemia.

83. A 5-day-old neonate with a PICC in place and an endotracheal tube for ventilation develops respiratory distress with tachypnea, hypoglycemia, sternal retractions, grunting respirations, hypoxemia, hypercapnia, and cyanosis. Breath sounds are diminished over the left lower lung and audible rales are present. Radiograph shows unilateral alveolar infiltrates. Which further laboratory tests are indicated to verify a diagnosis of pneumonia?

a. WBC count and ESR.
b. ESR, blood culture, and urinalysis.
c. ABGs and culture from about PICC insertion site.
d. CBC, blood culture, ABGs, and cultures of tracheal aspirate and cerebral spinal fluid.

84. The Health Insurance Portability and Accountability Act (HIPAA) regulates:

a. Rights of the individual related to privacy of health information.
b. Transfer of patients from one facility to another.
c. Medical trials.
d. Workplace safety.

85. Which of the following is an indication that a neonate has an intussusception?

a. Very bloody liquid stools.
b. "Current jelly" stools.
c. Tarry stools.
d. Liquid brown stools.

86. Two weeks after delivery, a mother brings her baby to the hospital because the child has "colic" and cries almost constantly. The mother expresses anger at the infant. The infant has a severe excoriating diaper rash, numerous bruises, and appears dehydrated. Which of the following is most appropriate?

a. Make a referral for the mother for counselling.
b. Make a referral for the mother for child-care classes.
c. Make a referral to Child Protective Services for suspected abuse/neglect.
d. Make a referral to a support group for new parents.

87. A neonate with severe intracranial pressure develops herniation of the brain into the brainstem area at 7 days' postnatal. Criteria for declaring brain death include:

a. Possible diagnosis that excludes reversible causes, clinical observation, and two examinations separated by at least 24 hours.
b. Unclear diagnosis, clinical observation, and two examinations separated by at least 12 hours.
c. Diagnosis that explains condition and excludes reversible causes, testing for higher brain function, and two examinations separated by at least 48 hours.
d. Diagnosis that explains condition and excludes reversible causes, testing for higher brain function, and clinical observation.

88. A pregnant woman at 36 weeks' gestation complains of menstrual-like cramps, diarrhea, and low dull backache with painless contractions of the uterus. The most likely cause is:

a. Gastroenteritis.
b. Preterm labor.
c. Renal infection.
d. Preeclampsia.

89. Tetralogy of Fallot is a combination of which 4 congenital heart defects?

a. Aortic stenosis, atrial septal defect, aorta overriding atrial septal defect (ASD), and left ventricular hypertrophy.
b. Patent ductus arteriosus, pulmonic stenosis, aortic stenosis, and left ventricular hypertrophy.
c. Coarctation of the aorta, aortic stenosis, patent ductus arteriosus, and right ventricular hypertrophy.
d. Pulmonic stenosis, ventricular septal defect, aorta overriding ventricular septal defect (VSD), and right ventricular hypertrophy.

90. A term neonate develops a *Staphylococcus aureus* infection 5 days after birth with sepsis and subsequent symptoms that include hypoxemia; hypercapnia; tachypnea with wheezing, sternal retractions, and expiratory grunting; CNS depression with lethargy and tachycardia. These symptoms are consistent with which of the following?

a. Meningitis.
b. Acute respiratory failure.
c. Congestive heart failure.
d. Pulmonary abscess.

91. Which of the following infants exhibiting indications of acute respiratory failure meets the criteria for treatment with extracorporeal membrane oxygenation (ECMO)?

a. Gestational age 33 weeks, weight 1900 g, and received conventional mechanical ventilation for 5 days.
b. Gestation age 34 weeks, weight 2000 g, intracranial hemorrhage grade 3.
c. Gestational age 35 weeks, weight 2200 g, coarctation of the aorta, and received conventional mechanical ventilation for 10 days.
d. Gestational age 35 weeks, weight 2200 g, intracranial hemorrhage grade 2, and received conventional mechanical ventilation for 12 days.

92. A neonate with ABO incompatibility develops hyperbilirubinemia, which is treated with phototherapy. The infant is not anemic. What follow-up is advised for the next few weeks?

a. Total serum bilirubin levels.
b. Blood cell counts (Hgb and Hct).
c. Electrolyte levels.
d. White blood counts.

93. A neonate at 37 weeks' gestation is born with gastroschisis with intestines exposed through an opening near the umbilicus on the right side, but the abdomen is normal in size, the opening is small, and the bowel tissue appears healthy. The child receives IV nutrition and antibiotics to prevent infection prior to surgery. Which of the following is a primary concern prior to surgery?

a. Hypothermia/Hypovolemia.
b. Hemorrhage.
c. Respiratory distress.
d. Hypotension.

94. Which of the following is an example of therapeutic communication?

a. "Don't worry. Everything will be fine."
b. "You should listen to your baby's doctor."
c. "Why are you upset?"
d. "Is there anything you'd like to discuss?"

95. Which of the following is a disadvantage of flow-inflating bag and mask ventilation?

a. It cannot be used to deliver positive end-expiratory pressure (PEEP).
b. It must be connected to a gas source to function.
c. It cannot attain high pressures necessary for noncompliant lungs.
d. It requires attachment of a reservoir to deliver high concentrations of oxygen.

96. A newborn was born with tricuspid atresia, but testing indicates there are no septal defects. What is the purpose of administering prostaglandin to the infant?

a. To ensure the ductus arteriosus closes.
b. To lower blood pressure through vasodilation.
c. To ensure the ductus arteriosus and foramen ovale remain open.
d. To regulate cardiac contractions.

97. A neonate large for gestational age (LGA) has delivery complicated by shoulder dystocia. The neonate exhibits weak right arm muscles and holds the arm adducted and internally rotated. The startle reflex is abnormal on the affected side but grasp reflex is normal. The symptoms indicate which of the following conditions?

a. Shoulder dislocation.
b. Erb palsy.
c. Klumpke paralysis.
d. Congenital muscular torticollis.

98. A 14-day-old term neonate develops croup with severe cough. Which of the following is the most common risk associated with croup?

a. Pulmonary hemorrhage from strain of coughing.
b. Dehydration.
c. Respiratory obstruction from inflammation.
d. Seizures from high fever.

99. A mother at 33 weeks' gestation has preeclampsia and undergoes a number of fetal function tests. Which test is indicated to determine fetal lung maturity?

a. Ultrasound.
b. Umbilical artery Doppler studies.
c. Contraction stress tests.
d. Amniocentesis.

100. A neonate with respiratory distress syndrome and acute respiratory failure has been receiving conventional mechanical ventilation and is being weaned off ventilation. His pulmonary status is stabilizing, but ABGs show he is becoming hypocapnic. What adjustments are necessary to increase his $PaCO_2$?

a. Decrease peak inspiratory pressure (PIP), inspiratory to expiratory ratio (I:E), or positive end-expiratory pressure (PEEP).
b. Increase PIP, I:E, or PEEP.
c. Decrease respiratory rate (RR) or tidal volume (Vt).
d. Increase RR or Vt.

101. A neonate with abdominal distention, vomiting, and failure to pass meconium in 48 hours is diagnosed with meconium ileus. Based on this diagnosis, for which of the following congenital disorders should the infant be tested?

a. Cystic fibrosis.
b. Hirschsprung disease.
c. Congenital malrotation.
d. Congenital megacolon.

102. The best time to initiate conflict resolution is:

a. When those in conflict have had time to resolve their differences.
b. When conflict first emerges.
c. When conflict interferes with function.
d. When those involved ask for conflict resolution.

103. A premature neonate is 24 hours' postnatal and her potassium level is 6.2 mEq/L. What does this laboratory value indicate?

a. A normal rise from a shift in potassium from intracellular to extracellular space.
b. A normal value for potassium.
c. Hypokalemia.
d. Hyperkalemia.

104. In the first postnatal exam, the neonate exhibits a respiratory rate of 50 per minute with prolonged expiratory phase and slight substernal retraction. Coarse rales are heard throughout the lung fields. Skin appears slightly mottled, and heart rate is 160. These findings indicate:

a. Respiratory distress syndrome.
b. Normal postnatal transitional findings.
c. Acute respiratory infection.
d. Aspiration pneumonia.

105. On physical exam, the neonate exhibits wrist flexion to 0°, arm recoil past 90°, and hips, knees, and arms all flexed past 90°. This is consistent with the neuromuscular characteristics of which of the following:

a. Small for gestational age.
b. Very small for gestational age.
c. Postterm infant.
d. Normal full-term infant.

106. When considering the use of a translator for a parent who does not speak English, which consideration is most important?

a. The translator speaks both languages well.
b. The translator knows the patient's history.
c. The translator has training in medical vocabulary for both languages.
d. The translator is available onsite.

107. A neonate with asymmetric intrauterine growth restriction (IUGR) has a head that is normal in size for gestational age but a body that is growth restricted. A common cause for this type of IUGR includes:

a. Chromosomal abnormalities.
b. Infection.
c. Genetic abnormalities.
d. Preeclampsia.

108. Which of the following are subtle clinical signs of seizures?

a. Eye blinking and horizontal ocular deviation.
b. Jitteriness without ocular deviation.
c. 10-15 seconds of fast tremors occurring up to 100 times daily.
d. Jitteriness upon stimulation and fast and slow clonic jerking.

109. After 6 days of enteral feedings, a premature neonate is switched to parenteral nutrition (PN). What change in daily caloric content is required?

a. Increase caloric intake for PN by about 25% over those needed for enteral nutrition.
b. Maintain the same caloric intake.
c. Decrease caloric intake for PN by about 30% from those needed for enteral nutrition.
d. Decrease caloric intake for PN by about 20% from those needed for enteral nutrition.

110. A neonate with respiratory distress syndrome has developed bleeding from the umbilicus and trachea with bloody diarrhea, as well as hypotension, petechiae, and purpura, indicating disseminated intravascular coagulation. Blood volume is still adequate. Which treatment is indicated to control active bleeding?

a. Platelets only.
b. Platelets and fresh frozen plasma.
c. Packed red blood cells.
d. IV glucose.

111. According to Knowles' principles of adult learning, adult learners tend to be:

a. Unmotivated.
b. Lacking in self-direction.
c. Practical and goal-oriented.
d. Insecure.

112. A neonate that is small for gestational age (SGA) and unable to take adequate oral fluids has an umbilical artery catheter in place and is receiving glucose but begins to show indications of hypoglycemia with increased glucose utilization. Which procedure is advised initially:

a. Do an ultrasound to check position of tip of umbilical artery catheter.
b. Stop IV glucose immediately.
c. Do a repeat blood glucose level in an hour.
d. Increase IV glucose.

113. A neonate recovering from cardiovascular surgery has been receiving heparin, but a blood cell count shows a drop in platelet count of 50%, indicative of heparin-induced thrombocytopenia (HIT), with no active bleeding. Which initial action is indicated:

a. Stop all forms of anticoagulation.
b. Stop all forms of heparin and give platelet transfusion.
c. Continue heparin at lower dose and give platelet transfusion.
d. Stop all forms of heparin and begin treatment with direct thrombin inhibitor, such as lepirudin, danaparoid, or argatroban.

114. Working for the best interests of the patient, despite personal values in conflict, and assisting patients to have access to appropriate resources comprise:

a. Moral agency.
b. Advocacy.
c. Agency.
d. Collaboration.

115. A neonate is recovering from thoracic surgery and is receiving oxygen. Which of the following is a major principle of neonatal oxygen administration?

a. Concentration should be individually titrated to maintain the arterial oxygen level at 50-80 mmHg.
b. Oxygen should be humidified to 20%.
c. Oxygen should be warmed to 28°C.
d. Oxygen levels should be monitored every 2 hours.

116. A neonate with congenital heart disease and congestive heart failure is receiving both a loop diuretic (furosemide) and digoxin. Which electrolyte imbalances are of primary concern with loop diuretics?

a. Hyperkalemia, hypocalcemia, and hypernatremia.
b. Hypokalemia, hyponatremia, and hypocalcemia.
c. Hypokalemia, hyponatremia, and hypomagnesemia.
d. Hyperkalemia, hypernatremia, and hypermagnesemia.

117. The nurse inserts a nasogastric tube into a premature infant for feeding. Prior to administering feedings per the NG tube, the nurse should confirm correct placement of the tube. The nurse injects air through the NG tube while auscultating the gastric area and hears air flow. Which is of the following is correct?

a. The NG tube is placed correctly and feedings can begin.
b. The NG tube is placed incorrectly and should be removed and reinserted.
c. NG placement must be verified by other methods.
d. The NG tube is in the distal esophagus and should be advanced.

118. A neonate is born to an HIV-positive mother by elective cesarean. The mother had been receiving antiretroviral medications and the neonate is to receive them for the first 6 weeks. The infant has a low birth weight but otherwise appears healthy. Which of the following should the mother avoid?

a. Breast-feeding.
b. Kissing the infant.
c. Exposing the infant to other HIV-negative family members during the 6 weeks of treatment.
d. Changing the infant's diapers.

119. A premature neonate experienced fetal distress during delivery and fails to breathe well or cry after birth, with an Apgar score of 2 at one minute, indicating neonatal asphyxia. Which symptoms are indicative of increasing hypoxia?

a. Tachycardia and peripheral cyanosis.
b. Hypertonia and central cyanosis.
c. Bradycardia and central cyanosis.
d. Cardiac arrhythmias and peripheral cyanosis.

120. In instituting continuous quality improvement (CQI), which members of the health care institution are responsible for identifying quality performance improvement projects?

a. Administrative staff.
b. Nursing team leaders.
c. Physicians
d. All staff.

121. With mechanical ventilation, settings are carefully adjusted to meet the neonate's needs and to maintain the pH, PaO_2, and PO_2 at target levels. The fraction of inspired oxygen (FiO_2) must be carefully monitored to prevent oxygen toxicity. What FiO_2 level is usually maintained to prevent toxicity?

a. $\leq$80%.
b. <60%.
c. $\leq$50%.
d. <40%.

122. A mother received magnesium as a treatment for eclampsia prior to delivery, and this is reflected in an increased magnesium level in the neonate. Which of the following are signs of hypermagnesemia in a neonate?

a. Hypertonia and hyperreflexia.
b. Hypotonia and hypertension.
c. Hypotension and flushing secondary to vasodilation.
d. Constipation and hypertension.

123. During mechanical ventilation, excessive pressure settings may result in which of the following ventilation-induced lung injuries (VILI)?

a. Barotrauma.
b. Volutrauma.
c. Atelectrauma.
d. Biotrauma.

124. If all patients who develop infections around catheter-insertion sites are evaluated with culture and sensitivities for microbial resistance, but only those with clinically evident infections are included, those with subclinical infections may be missed, skewing results. This is an example of:

a. Selection bias.
b. Information bias.
c. Hypothesis testing.
d. Generalizability.

125. When auscultating a neonate's heart sounds, the nurse notes that there is no split in the S2 sound, a grade IV harsh systolic murmur in the upper right sternal border, and a thrill in the suprasternal notch. Which condition could account for these abnormalities?

a. Aortic stenosis.
b. Atrial septal defect.
c. Pulmonary stenosis.
d. Ebstein anomaly.

126. End-tidal CO_2 monitoring is most useful in the following circumstances:

a. Full-term neonate with mild to moderate lung disease.
b. Full-term neonate with normal lung function or premature neonate with mild to moderate lung disease.
c. Neonate with abnormal ventilation to perfusion ratio.
d. Full-term or premature neonate with severe lung disease.

127. The "5 rights of delegation" include:

a. Right time, right place, right person, right direction, and right evaluation.
b. Right person, right place, right time, right assignment, and right supervision.
c. Right task, right time, right circumstance, right place, and right supervision.
d. Right task, right circumstance, right person, right direction, and right supervision.

128. A mother with an unremarkable pregnancy delivers a neonate that exhibits retinochoroiditis. On questioning, the mother states that she has 6 cats that she cares for in her home. The most likely cause of the child's condition is:

a. Toxoplasmosis.
b. Rubella.
c. Cytomegalovirus.
d. Guillain-Barré.

129. A neonate is receiving perioperative IV fentanyl. Which of the following complications can result from fentanyl?

a. Obstruction of the biliary tract.
b. Chest wall rigidity.
c. Hypotonia.
d. Diarrhea.

130. A full-term neonate born to a mother with idiopathic thrombocytopenic purpura has a platelet count of 40,000/mcL and is stable with no signs of bleeding. Which of the following is recommended?

a. Platelet transfusion.
b. Observation only.
c. Immunosuppressant therapy.
d. Continued serial platelet counts and sonogram, CT, or MRI to rule out intracerebral hemorrhage.

131. When using transcutaneous CO_2 monitoring, how long should the electrode(s) be left in place after calibration before measurements are taken?

a. Measurements can be taken immediately.
b. 5 minutes.
c. 15 minutes.
d. 30 minutes.

132. A 21-day-old neonate develops green-bronze jaundice, dark urine, clay-colored stools, abdominal distention with distended abdominal veins, and hepatosplenomegaly with firm liver. Liver biopsy and test shows extrahepatic biliary atresia, and a hepatoportoenterostomy (Kasai procedure) is done to create a conduit between the liver and small intestine. Which added vitamin(s) or minerals should the baby receive postoperatively?

a. Water-soluble vitamins (B-complex, C).
b. Fat-soluble vitamins (A, D, E, K).
c. Calcium.
d. Potassium.

133. During the interdisciplinary team meeting, the leader stresses the importance of following the rules of the organization exactly. What type of leadership style is this?

a. Bureaucratic.
b. Autocratic.
c. Consultative.
d. Participatory.

134. The nurse is inserting a PICC for an infant who requires extended IV therapy because of very low birth weight. During the procedure, the infant must be monitored for which of the following?

a. Tachycardia and tachypnea.
b. Bradycardia and hypoxia.
c. Atrial fibrillation
d. Blood pressure.

135. A neonate requires an endotracheal tube (ETT). The infant has a gestational age of 33 weeks and weighs 1900 g. Which internal diameter (ID) is correct for the ETT?

a. 2.5 mm.
b. 3 mm.
c. 3.5
d. 3.5-4 mm.

136. Normal weight loss after full-term birth is:

a. 5-7%.
b. 7-9%.
c. 9-11%.
d. 11-13%.

137. A neonate had an atrioventricular shunt for treatment of hydrocephalus. Twenty-four hours postoperatively, the shunt becomes obstructed. Which of the following symptoms indicate early signs of increasing intracranial pressure in a neonate?

a. Vomiting, lethargy, bulging fontanelles, and increased head circumference.
b. Decerebrate or decorticate posturing.
c. Respiratory depression with Cheyne-Stokes, bulging fontanelles, and increased head circumference.
d. High-pitched cries, poor feeding, irritability, bulging fontanelles, increasing head circumference, and distended scalp veins.

138. Which neuromuscular assessment measures the resistance to stretching of extensor muscles in the infant's forearm to help determine gestational age?

a. Arm recoil test.
b. Scarf sign test.
c. Square window test.
d. Heel to ear test.

139. A mixed venous oxygen saturation (SvO_2) level of less than 60% can indicate which of the following?

a. Increased hemoglobin, PaO_2, and/or cardiac output.
b. Decreased hemoglobin, PaO_2, and/or cardiac output.
c. Decreased oxygen consumption.
d. Sepsis.

140. What is the initial IV dose of naloxone to reverse opioid-induced depression in a neonate?

a. 1 mg/kg.
b. 0.2 mg/kg.
c. 0.1 mg/kg.
d. 2 mg/kg.

141. A neonate has been diagnosed with physiologic gastroesophageal reflux (GER). What symptom is associated with this condition?

a. Respiratory distress and regurgitation.
b. Esophagitis and regurgitation.
c. Regurgitation-related malnutrition.
d. Regurgitation only.

142. A neonate has a differential diagnosis of congenital muscular dystrophy (CMD) (laminin alpha-2 deficiency) and exhibits hypotonia at birth with poor feeding and mild respiratory distress. Which tests are necessary to establish the diagnosis?

a. Creatinine kinase.
b. Electromyogram, nerve conduction studies, and muscle biopsy.
c. Muscle biopsy only.
d. MRI only.

143. The nurse should identify learner outcomes as part of the plan for teaching parents to care for their neonate. The most appropriate learner outcome for teaching parents to do NG feedings is:

a. Demonstrate skill in preparing and administering NG feeding.
b. List and describe different types of NG tubes.
c. Explain the nutritional composition of the tube feeding solution.
d. Explain the benefits of giving the infant a pacifier during feedings.

144. The correct incremental volume for administration of transfusions to neonates receiving PRBCs to prevent overhydration is:

a. 5-10 mL/kg at rate of 5 mL/kg/hr.
b. 15-20 mL/kg at rate of 5 mL/kg/hr.
c. 20-30 mL/kg at rate of 10-20 mL/kg/hr.
d. 30-40 mL/kg at rate of 10-20 mL/kg/hr.

145. A neonate develops herpetic lesions at 6 days after birth and is diagnosed with herpes simplex encephalitis (HSE) although the mother has no history of herpes virus infection. The infant is extremely lethargic, breast-feeding poorly, and exhibits tremors. Liver function tests are abnormal. Which medication is indicated to treat the infection?

a. Immunoglobulin.
b. Zidovudine.
c. Acyclovir.
d. Oseltamivir.

146. A neonate with anoxic encephalopathy develops seizures. Which of the following anticonvulsants is the treatment of choice for seizures in neonates?

a. Fosphenytoin (*Cerebyx*)
b. Lorazepam (*Ativan*).
c. Phenobarbital (*Luminal*).
d. Phenytoin (*Dilantin*).

147. The purpose of administration of heliox during mechanical ventilation is to:

a. Promote vasodilation and decrease pulmonary hypertension.
b. Decrease airway resistance to reduce respiratory effort and improve oxygenation.
c. Reduce pulmonary blood flow and increase peripheral vascular resistance.
d. To stabilize the fraction of inspired oxygen (FiO_2) level.

148. A preeclamptic mother at 35 weeks' gestation has an amniocentesis and lecithin to sphingomyelin (L:S) ratio to determine if the fetal lungs are mature enough for early delivery. Which ratio demonstrates adequate lung maturity to make respiratory distress syndrome (RDS) unlikely?

a. 0.5:1
b. 1:1
c. 1:2
d. 2:1

149. A male neonate has a left abdominal mass, low urinary output, and poor urinary stream. His serum creatinine and BUN are elevated and renal function is compromised. Ultrasound shows hydronephrosis secondary to ureteropelvic junction (UPJ) obstruction. What treatment is indicated?

a. Pyeloplasty to remove obstruction.
b. Antibiotics to prevent infection.
c. Monitoring only unless symptoms worsen.
d. Kidney dialysis.

150. A neonate is extremely low birth weight (less than 1000 g). In providing skin care, which is the most appropriate for cleansing the skin and preventing irritation that my lead to infection?

a. Sterile water.
b. Mild soap.
c. Mild povidone-iodine solution.
d. Isopropyl alcohol.

Answer Key and Explanations

1. A: Cardiogenic shock causes increased preload and afterload and decreased contractibility. Together, these result in decreased cardiac output and increased systemic vascular resistance to compensate. This increases afterload in the left ventricle, which fails to adequately pump blood as cardiac output and coronary and peripheral perfusion continue to decrease. Fluid builds up, causing pulmonary edema and right ventricular failure.

2. D: The correct needle insertion point for a needle aspiration to treat pneumothorax in a neonate is on the left midclavicular line at the second or third intercostal space. The infant should be given oral sucrose, placed in supine position, given IV fentanyl 250 mcg over 2-3 minutes, and given a local anesthetic with 1% lidocaine. The needle is inserted directly into the intercostal space until air is aspirated in a syringe. The air is expelled through a stopcock. A chest tube may be inserted in the same space or at the anterior axillary line, fourth, fifth, or sixth intercostal space.

3. B: The best poster is one with large pictures so that family members can see what they need to do and minimal text at 6th-grade reading level. Readability (the grade level of material) is a concern because many patients and families may have limited English skills or low literacy, so pictures are important. The average American reads effectively at the 6th- to 8th-grade level (regardless of education achieved). Additionally, research indicates that even people with much higher reading skills learn medical and health information most effectively when the material is presented at the 6th- to 8th-grade readability level.

4. B: If the right lung is better ventilated than the left after insertion of an ETT, this suggests that the ETT is positioned too low. ETT placement should immediately be verified by auscultation and radiograph, ultrasound, or disposable end-tidal carbon dioxide detectors. Esophageal intubation is indicated if no air exchange is detected bilaterally or if there is air sound over left upper abdomen. The tube may be too high if air sounds are diminished. An ETT may be inserted nasally or orally.

5. A: The difficulty extubating the infant and subsequent development of strider, recurrent pneumonitis, and frequent choking are often associated with tracheal stenosis caused by pressure necrosis of the tissues from the intubation tube. Incidence of tracheal stenosis increases if the infant's mucosa becomes infected, so pathogens may have a role in the disorder. Treatment with balloon dilatation per endoscopy is often successful, although some infants require surgical repair.

6. B: A newborn requires a cardiac output of about 800 mL/min, but the stroke volume is usually only about 5 mL because of the small size, so a heart rate of about 145 bpm is needed to ensure adequate output. A period of apnea is usually followed by decreased heart rate and oxygen saturation. Heart rates will vary depending on whether the neonate is awake, sleeping, or active.

- <1 week: At rest, 100-180; asleep, 80-160; active/sick, ≤220
- 1-2 weeks: At rest, 100-220; asleep, 80-200; active/sick, ≤220

7. B: Calcium channel blockers may increase cerebral blood flow with ischemia caused by HIE. Other treatments include phenobarbital for seizures. Allopurinol (40 mg/kg) 4 hours after birth reduces mortality rates. HIE results when oxygen supply to the brain is impaired. HIE is classified as mild, moderate, or severe, depending on the degree of ischemia and symptoms. Mild HIE usually resolves in 3-4 days and moderate HIE in 1-2 weeks, but permanent brain damage can occur with severe HIE.

8. C: The most reliable information derives from an evidence review that includes review of literature, critical analysis of studies, and summarizing of results, including pooled meta-analysis. Recommendations based on personal experience from a number of experts may be utilized, especially if there is inadequate evidence based on review, but this subjective evidence should be acknowledged because people may be biased. Considering best practices may be helpful but does not take the place of evidence review.

9. C: Chamber 2 creates a vacuum to allow suction. The first chamber is the collection chamber where the air and/or fluid are drained from the pleural space. Bubbling in this chamber is the result of air being pumped out of the pleural space and is expected. The second chamber is the water seal chamber where the water, in an amount prescribed by the physician, is placed to create the vacuum necessary to pull the fluid and/or air out of the pleural space. The level of water affects the amount of pressure and should be carefully monitored to make sure it remains at the ordered level. The third chamber is the suction chamber, which is responsible for the suction that creates the pressure, removing the air from the pleural space.

10. B: Placenta previa puts the neonate at increased risk for congenital anomalies of the CNS and cardiac, respiratory, and gastrointestinal systems. Placenta previa is also associated with poor growth and anemia. Implantation of the placenta is over or near the internal cervical os. Placenta previa may also cause premature birth with associated neonatal complications of prematurity. Women with placenta previa have increased incidences of hemorrhage in the third trimester.

11. B: CRIES is an effective tool for evaluation postoperative pain in neonates and requires maintaining oxygen saturation greater than 95%. A score of at least 4 indicates pain:

	Characteristic	0	1	2
C	Crying	No cry, or normal cry	High-pitched crying but can be consoled.	High-pitched crying and cannot be consoled.
R	Requires O_2 (To keep O_2 saturation at 95%)	No oxygen required.	Oxygen required. (< 30% below baseline)	Oxygen required. (> 30% below baseline)
I	Increased VS (HR, BP)	HR and BP unchanged or below baseline.	HR and BP increase < 20%.	HR and BP increase > 20%.
E	Expression	No grimace.	Grimace.	Grimace and non-audible grunt
S	Sleeplessness	Continuously sleeping.	Awakens frequently.	Constantly awake.

12. A: rHuEPO is indicated to stimulate erythropoiesis in phlebotomy-related AOP. Infants with signs of hypoxemia (poor feeding, tachypnea, tachycardia, pallor) may require transfusions. AOP represents a pathologic exaggeration of the normal decrease in hematocrit that occurs in every newborn. Other causes include:

- Decreased RBC production because the premature neonate's response to erythropoietin (EPO), the main stimulus for RBC production, has not matured. Lowest hemoglobin (Hgb) levels are usually at 2-3 months of age.
- Premature RBCs have a shortened lifespan when compared with the full-term neonate's because of decreased levels of intracellular ATP and enzyme activity.

13. D: Including parents in planning for an infant takes time initially, but sitting down and asking the parents, "What do you want?" and using the Synergy Model to evaluate the infant's (and parents') characteristics can provide valuable information that saves time in the long run and facilitates planning and expenditure of resources. Nurses and others on the health care team must always remember that the point of collaborating is to improve patient care, so the patient and patient's family must remain central to all planning.

14. A: BiPAP (similar to CPAP) provides a steady stream of pressurized air but senses inspiratory effort and increases pressure during inspiration. CPAP provides a steady stream of pressurized air throughout both inspiration and expiration. Free-flow oxygen is administered to the neonate by the use of either a mask hooked up to an oxygen source or by the use of the oxygen tubing to direct and concentrate the oxygen at the infant's airway. Free-flow oxygen should be administered at a rate of 5 L/min. Oxygen per high-flow nasal cannula (1.5-2.0 L/min) can result in positive pressure, depending on the size of catheter and the flow rate.

15. B: Recent studies have supported the use of breast milk for feedings as the most preventive strategy for NEC in preterm infants due to the many protective qualities the breast milk provides. Risk for NEC increases if volume of feedings is increased more than 20 mL/kg/day, so feeding tolerance should be carefully monitored with a slow increase to goal. Other risk factors include intestinal ischemia and bacterial colonization. NEC is also associated with the use of hyperosmolar feedings. Administering immunoglobulins and Bifidobacterium may give some protective effect.

16. D: Apply ice to the neonate's face to trigger the diving response to slow the heart rate. The vagal maneuver increases parasympathetic input to the heart and slows the rate. If unsuccessful, try adenosine, digoxin, or propranolol. Use synchronized cardioversion at 0.5-2.0 Joules/kg for unstable arrhythmia with narrow QRS complex. Treat a stable arrhythmia with wide QRS complex initially with esophageal pacing. If unresponsive, try procainamide and lidocaine, flecainide, and asynchronous cardioversion if necessary.

17. B: When instituting changes, the best approach is to provide honest information about the reasons for changes and how staff will be affected. Resistance to change is common for many people, so coordinating collaborative processes requires anticipating resistance and taking steps to achieve cooperation. Resistance often relates to concerns about job loss, increased responsibilities, and general denial or lack of understanding and frustration. The nurse should be empathetic and patient, allowing people to express their opinions and encouraging their participation.

18. A: Both the *CoolCap* and body cooling devices used for cooling therapy require rewarming at the rate of 0.5 °C/hr. Duration of cooling for both types of devices is usually 72 hours. The *CoolCap* requires 2 hours to reach target core temperature while the body cooling device requires 1.5 hours.

The target core site for the *CoolCap* is the rectum while the target core site for body cooling is the esophagus.

19. C: Assessment of chest wall vibrations is the best indicator that the airway is patent and HFJV settings are appropriate for effective ventilation. Chest wall vibrations may decrease if the ETT is not patent or a pneumothorax occurs. The vibrations may cause interference with monitoring devices for heart rate and respirations. HFJV directs a high velocity stream of air into the lungs in a long spiraling spike that forces carbon dioxide against the walls, penetrating dead space and providing gas exchange by using small tidal volumes of 1-3 ml/kg, much smaller than with conventional mechanical ventilation. Inspiration is controlled while expiration is passive, but the rate of respiration is up to 11 per second ("panting" respirations).

20. C: Protein, tubular cells, and casts are usually found in the urine with intrinsic acute renal failure. This occurs when the kidneys themselves have an abnormality and may be the result of a "prerenal" insult. A common condition is acute tubular necrosis precipitated by shock, perinatal asphyxia, drugs, or a prolonged prerenal state. Prerenal or functional renal failure (accounting for 50% of ARF in neonates) is usually caused by renal hypoperfusion, also called prerenal azotemia, from shock, dehydration, myocardial failure, or severe hypoxia. The kidneys themselves are normal. Postrenal or obstructive renal failure occurs when an obstruction exists in the urinary system distal to the kidneys.

21. A: The mother should be questioned about her breast-feeding technique and frequency, and should be observed while breast-feeding the child. Since this is her first child, she may need further assistance in breast-feeding properly to ensure the infant receives adequate nutrition. While further tests may be indicated, these signs are indicative of dehydration and poor nutrition, so that should be dealt with first. As there are no other indications of neglect, referral to Child Protective Services is not appropriate at this time. Switching from breast milk to formula is rarely necessary if mothers receive adequate support and instruction.

22. B: With abruptio placentae, irreversible brain damage may occur with fetal hypoxia, and neurological deficits occur in about 14% of survivors.

Abruptio placentae are related to maternal hypertension, and incidence increases with cocaine abuse, causing the placenta to prematurely detach partially or completely from the uterine. Partial detachment interferes with the functioning of the placenta, causing intrauterine growth retardation. Severe bleeding occurs with total detachment. Common fetal complications are preterm labor, hypoxia, and anemia. Fetal mortality is about 25% with partial detachment and 100% with complete.

23. D: These values indicate respiratory alkalosis from hyperventilation associated with excessive mechanical ventilation, which decreases the level of carbon dioxide. Respiratory alkalosis occurs with $PaCO_2$ less than 35 and pH greater than 7.45. Normal $PaCO_2$ is 35-45 mmHg and normal pH 7.35-7.45. Arterial blood gas (ABG) is the most informative measurement of blood gas status. Venous blood gas (VBG) is easier to obtain if an arterial catheter is not in place. To compare the values in the VBG with an ABG, add 0.05 to the pH of the VBG. Subtract 5-10 mmHg from the PCO_2 of the VBG. Capillary blood gas (CBG) can be obtained with a heel stick, but the values obtained are the least accurate and rarely useful.

24. A: The parents of an infant with OI should receive information about methods of handling, bathing, and placing their child in the crib to minimize trauma and avoid fractures. OI is genetic disorder of collagen synthesis that results in brittle, easily fractured bones. Common features of OI include brittle bones, bowing of long bones, shortened limbs, blue sclera, skeletal deformities (including scoliosis), respiratory difficulties, and weak muscles. Infants do not generally require feeding tubes. OI is usually inherited in a dominant fashion, but a new mutation may cause the disorder in approximately 25% of cases. Parents of children should receive genetic advice from a health care professional rather than a brochure. Type 1 is nonlethal and the mildest of 4 types of OI.

25. C: The information derived from testing for Huntington disease cannot be used for health promotion or disease prevention, so the parents should be counseled to wait until the child is at least in the teen years and can make an informed decision about whether to have testing. Avoid using "should" statements or deferring a discussion to others. This type of information can be devastating to young people who are not provided adequate support and counseling prior to testing. Some people with adult-onset diseases choose not to be tested, and childhood testing robs them of this choice.

26. C: Onset of symptoms varies with different structural defects, and symptoms of congestive heart failure within the first week may be caused by patent ductus arteriosus, as well as transposition of the great vessels and total anomalous pulmonary return with pulmonary venous obstruction. Hypoplastic left heart syndrome is evident at birth. Coarctation of the aorta and pulmonary stenosis are usually evident between one and four weeks after birth.

27. C: Apnea of prematurity occurs in premature infants (less than 34 weeks) and is believed caused by immaturity of the nervous system, improving as the brain matures. It may persist for a 4-8 weeks. There are 3 types of apnea:

- Central: no airflow or effort to breathe
- Obstructive: no airflow, but effort to breathe
- Mixed: both central and obstructive elements (75% of AOP)

AOP symptoms include swallowing during apneic periods, apnea greater than 20 seconds, apnea less than 20 seconds with bradycardia 30 beats below normal, oxygen saturation less than 85% persisting at least 5 seconds, and cyanosis.

28. D: Confidentiality is ensured through the use of required passwords when parents call for information about their children and through the limitation of who is allowed to visit a child (usually restricted to only those who accompany parents). Confidentiality is the obligation that is present in a professional-patient relationship. Nurses are under an obligation to protect the information they possess concerning the family and/or infant. Care should be taken in the unit to safeguard information and provide the privacy that the family deserves.

29. C: A lumbar puncture should show bloodstained cerebral spinal fluid, consistent with a subarachnoid hemorrhage. Subarachnoid hemorrhage may result from the trauma of childbirth (one of the most common causes) or from shaken impact syndrome. The presenting symptom may be seizures, usually at about day 2, although many neonates are asymptomatic. If seizures occur, the neonate typically appears healthy between seizures. The condition is usually self-limiting and does not require treatment.

30. A: Bronchopulmonary dysplasia, a chronic lung disease characterized by alveolar damage resulting from abnormal development with inflammation and development of scar tissue, may require surfactant rescue treatment, diuretics (furosemide) to reduce pulmonary edema, and bronchodilators (theophylline/albuterol) to increase airflow. Respiratory syncytial virus (RSV) prophylaxis (such as *RespiGam*) is also commonly given because of increased risk of infection.

Steroids, such as dexamethasone, are no longer advised because of significant risks associated with the drugs.

31. C: A contrast enema is used to confirm a diagnosis of meconium plug syndrome and helps differentiate that from other causes of intestinal obstruction. The contrast enema also is often therapeutic and helps the plug to pass. Meconium plug syndrome usually occurs in full-term infants, infants of diabetic mothers, or infants with hypermagnesemia. A small percentage of infants initially identified as having meconium plug syndrome (5-10%) have Hirschsprung disease. The cause of meconium plug syndrome is thought to be immaturity of the ganglion cells of the colon.

32. D: Thrombocytopenia appears in about 30% of those affected with MODS and may result in disseminated intravascular coagulation (DIC). Liver damage and bowel necrosis may occur. MODS is the most common cause of sepsis-related death. Cardiac function becomes depressed, acute respiratory distress syndrome (ARDS) may develop, and renal failure may follow acute tubular necrosis or cortical necrosis.

33. C: Breast milk jaundice may result from breast milk breaking down bilirubin and its being reabsorbed in the gut. Treatment for bilirubin level of 20 mg/dL or higher involves discontinuing breast-feeding for 24 hours and substituting formula. Phototherapy is usually indicated for total serum bilirubin of at least 18 mg/dL for infants at medium risk. This type of pathological hyperbilirubinemia is characterized by less frequent stools and onset in the fourth to seventh day, peaking in 10-15 days, but jaundice may persist for up to 12 weeks.

34. A: The ACCN Synergy Model is based on three levels of quality outcomes. These general outcomes are based on outcomes derived from the patient, the nurse, and the system:

- Patient outcomes include functional change, behavioral change, trust, ratings, satisfaction, comfort, and quality of life.
- Nurse outcomes include physiological changes, presence or absence of complications, and extent to which care of treatment objectives were attained.
- System outcomes include recidivism, costs, and resource utilization.

35. C: An agitated infant with CHF should receive morphine or fentanyl, as agitation increases oxygen consumption and can lower the PaO_2. Once the infant has calmed, the necessary flow of supplemental oxygen can be determined more effectively. Furosemide is indicated for fluid retention. Digoxin is used to improve cardiac output, but this may not be necessary if the child is resting.

36. D: Meconium aspiration syndrome (MAS) occurs when meconium expelled in the amniotic fluid is aspirated by the fetus *in utero* or by the neonate at first breath. Infants may present with symptoms at birth or within a few hours. Typical symptoms include tachypnea, lethargy, depressed state, hypoxemia and hypercapnia, metabolic acidosis, yellow-green staining of nail beds, and hyperventilation in early stages and hypoventilation later. Symptoms are similar to transient tachypnea of the newborn (TTN) but more severe. Chest x-rays may show infiltrates, atelectasis, or hypoinflated areas as well as hyperinflated areas.

37. B: Crying during feeding puts the neonate at risk for aspiration pneumonia. Aspiration pneumonia may occur as the result of any type of aspiration, including foreign objects. The aspirated material creates an inflammatory response, with the irritated mucous membrane at high risk for bacterial infection secondary to the aspiration. With infants who are weak, have paralysis or congenital anomalies, or lack adequate cough reflex, the most common causes of aspiration pneumonia are oral fluids. Infants with respiratory stress or crying during feeding can easily aspirate.

38. C: An exception should be made to allow the healer to attend the child. The Hmong believe that illness occurs when the spirit, soul, and body are out of balance and may want a traditional healer, a shaman, to treat the spiritual cause of the disease. Hmong believe that both spiritual and physical worlds exist and that a person has a number of souls. Sickness occurs when one or more souls are lost or taken by other spirits. These souls must be reclaimed for healing to occur.

39. A: These symptoms are consistent with intraventricular hemorrhage (IVH), which is common in premature neonates less than 32 weeks' gestational age. Fifty percent of IVH occur in the first 24 hours and 90 percent within 72 hours.

Grade	Extent of Hemorrhage	Degree
I	Limited to the germinal matrix (subependymal region).	Mild (5% death rate; 5% motor or cognitive impairment).
II	Extends 10-40% into the lateral ventricles on sagittal view, but minimal ventricular dilation.	Moderate (10% death rate; 30% to 40% motor or cognitive impairment).
III	Extends 50% or more into the lateral ventricles with significant ventricular dilation.	Severe (27-50% death rate; 35% motor or cognitive impairment).
IV	Extends into brain tissue with periventricular hemorrhagic infarction.	Catastrophic (80% death rate; 90% motor or cognitive impairment).

40. D: Swaddling a neonate exposed to cocaine and eliminating as much environmental noise and excessive light as possible can reduce stimulation and relieve symptoms. Medications are rarely required to control symptoms. Hypertonia may last 2 years or less. Head circumference may be smaller for the first 2 years as well, although the infant usually attains normal weight and height by the end of the first year.

41. D: Hypernatremia is associated with ARF. Typical ARF metabolic abnormalities that should be monitored include:

- Hypernatremia: > 146 mEq/L (critical value > 160).
- Hyperkalemia: > 6 mEq/L (critical value > 7 mEq/L).
- Hypocalcemia: < 7.6 mg/dL (critical value < 7 mg/dL).
- Hyperphosphatemia: > 8 mg/dL (increases when serum calcium decreases).

42. B: An echocardiogram or ultrasound is necessary to verify placement of a venous umbilical catheter; a radiograph may not provide adequate visualization. Measuring from the shoulder to the umbilicus and multiplying by 0.75 only estimates the proper length for insertion, but this does not ensure that the tip is actually situated correctly in the inferior vena cava above the diaphragm but below the right atrium. Auscultation with a stethoscope cannot be used to verify placement, although misplaced catheters may cause arrhythmias.

43. D: Facial abnormalities, neurological deficits, growth retardation, and congenital abnormalities, including cardiac, skeletal, renal, ocular, and auditory, may all be signs of FAS. Facial abnormalities can include hypoplastic (underdeveloped) maxilla, micrognathia (undersized jaw), hypoplastic philtrum (groove beneath the nose), and short palpebral fissures (eye slits between upper and lower lids). Neurological deficits may include microcephaly, intellectual disabilities, motor delay, and hearing deficits.

44. A: Lack of surfactant produces alveolar collapse (atelectasis) and less compliant lungs, resulting in laborious breathing. Collapsed areas of lung may still receive blood flow, but no exchange of gases occurs (ventilation perfusion mismatch). RDS is caused by the absence or deficiency of surfactant. Surfactant is a lipoprotein that reduces surface tension in the alveoli. Surfactant causes the lungs to be more compliant (alveoli expand with less effort), and the alveoli do not collapse on end expiration. Surfactant production begins at 22 weeks of gestation, but levels are inadequate until 36 weeks of gestation

45. B: It is important to approach the family with full information and reasons for the transfusion or blood components without being judgmental. Allow the parents to express their feelings. In fact, studies show that while adults often refuse transfusions for themselves, they frequently allow their children to receive blood products, so one should never assume that an individual would refuse blood products based on the religion alone. Jehovah's Witnesses can receive fractionated blood cells, thus allowing hemoglobin-based blood substitutes.

Basic Blood Standards for Jehovah Witnesses

Not acceptable	Whole blood: red cells, white cells, platelets, plasma
Acceptable	Fractions from red cells, white cells, platelets, and plasma

46. A: The onset of withdrawal symptoms in a neonate varies depending on the mother's type of drug use, but the onset of symptoms of heroin is generally within 12 to 24 hours. Rarely, symptoms may present up to 7 days after birth, in which case the neonate may already have been discharged home. Mothers should be carefully screened to try to identify infants at risk.

47. A: The infant is showing indications of uncompensated hypovolemic shock, a risk associated with myelomeningocele, which increases fluid loss because of impaired skin integrity. Perfusion of tissue and organs is inadequate, so fluid moves from the intravascular compartment to the interstitial spaces, further decreasing volume. Hypovolemic shock occurs when intravascular volume decreases by 15-25%.

48. C: Bowel sounds are heard over the chest area with left-sided congenital diaphragmatic hernia, which includes herniation of the large and small intestines and intraabdominal organs into the thoracic cavity. Hypoplasia of the right lung results from pressure exerted from displaced organs. Infants exhibit severe respiratory distress and cyanosis and may develop pulmonary hypertension and cardiopulmonary failure. Immediate surgical repair is indicated with high-frequency oscillatory ventilation (HFOV) and nitric oxide for pulmonary hypoplasia and extracorporeal membrane oxygenation (ECMO) for cardiopulmonary dysfunction.

49. D: In a high anomaly, the rectum ends above the puborectalis muscles, and internal sphincter is absent; frequently, there is a rectourethral fistula in males or a rectovaginal fistula in females, allowing passage of some meconium. There may be fistulas to the bladder or perineum. Low anomalies have no external opening, but rectum is otherwise in normal position through the puborectalis muscle, with normal function, and no connection to the genitourinary tract. Intermediate anomalies have rectum at or below the level of puborectalis muscle and an anal dimple. The external sphincter is in normal position.

50. D: Beneficence is ensuring that procedures and treatments are done to benefit the patient. Nonmaleficence is providing care in a manner that does not cause direct intentional harm to the patient. Autonomy is the individual's right to make decisions about his or her own care. In the case of children, the child cannot make autonomous decisions, so the parents serve as the legal decision maker. The nurse must keep the parents fully informed so that they can exercise their autonomy in informed decision-making. Justice relates to the distribution of the limited resources of health care benefits to the members of society. These resources must be distributed fairly.

51. C: While the neonate's bilirubin is elevated (normal range, 3.4-11.5 mg/dL at 1-2 days), only continued observation and jaundice assessment is indicated at this time. Physiologic hyperbilirubinemia is common in newborns and usually benign, resulting from immature hepatic function and increased RBC hemolysis. Infants have larger red blood cells with a shorter life than adults, leading to more RBC destruction and resulting in an increased load of serum bilirubin, which the liver of the newborn cannot handle. Onset is usually within 24-48 hours, peaking in 72 hours for full-term or 5 days for preterm infants and declining within a week. Phototherapy is the indicated treatment for total serum bilirubin at least 18 mg/dL for those at medium risk.

52. C: The setting sun sign occurs when the upper eyelids retract and the eyes turn downwards because of pressure on the mesencephalic tegmentum and paralysis of upward gaze, indicating damage to brain tissue related to hydrocephalus. An indication of hydrocephalus is the positive Macewen sign, resonance on tapping near the frontal-temporal-parietal juncture. Congenital hydrocephalus is present at birth and can occur because of aqueductal stenosis, spina bifida, or Arnold-Chiari malformations.

53. B: Glucose administration at 4-6 mg/kg/min is advised as a preventive treatment for an IDM at risk for hyperinsulinism. Blood glucose levels must be regularly monitored with acute hypoglycemia present with blood glucose less than 40 mg/dL. Glucagon stimulates release of glycogen from the liver but can stimulate insulin production, so it must be given after initiation of glucose IV. Diazoxide is used to suppress insulin production if other treatment fails. Somatostatin suppresses both insulin and glucagon secretion but is very short acting.

54. A: A neonate whose mother abused cocaine often exhibits tremors, hyperirritability, and hypertonicity at birth. Other symptoms include hypertension with decreased cardiac output, episodes of apnea or periodic breathing, and abnormal sleep patterns. Withdrawal symptoms usually occur within 48 hours during which the hyperirritability is replaced with lethargy and drowsiness. The infant may startle easily, exhibit abnormal muscle movement, and fail to respond to comfort measures. Poor feeding may result from an abnormal suck and swallow pattern.

55. D: The infant is exhibiting signs of bilateral choanal atresia, so the nurse should stimulate the infant to cry to promote mouth breathing. The choana are the two openings in the posterior nares connecting the nasal passages with the nasopharynx. Newborns are obligate nasal breathers. Successful nose breathing requires air to pass through the choana, so if these openings fail to form during fetal development, the infant must become a mouth breather. If atresia occurs only on one side (unilaterally), the infant may have no symptoms. The infant with bilateral choanal atresia has periods of respiratory distress and cyanosis that are alleviated by crying. Bilateral choanal atresia often becomes a medical emergency requiring intubation.

56. C: The head circumference is usually about 2 cm greater than the chest circumference, so the head circumference should be about 36 cm.

Head	Disproportionately large for body.
Body	Long with prominent abdomen and narrow hips.
Extremities	Short and in flexed position. (Feet usually dorsiflexed after breech birth.) Hands clenched.
Neck	Short and chin resting on chest
Weight	2500-4000 g (average about 3400 g). Physiologic weight loss is 5-10% for full-term and 15% for preterm.
Length	45-55 cm (average 50 cm).
Head circumference	32-38 cm (usually 2 cm greater than chest circumference).
Chest circumference	Chest rounded and 30-36 cm

57. A: The best determinant of teaching effectiveness is behavioral modification noted through observation and measurement. Many times, compliance rates are based on parent reports, but these are not always accurate. Satisfaction does not necessarily lead to compliance. A knowledgeable instructor is important, but knowledge does not always relate to teaching abilities.

58. D: Typical side effects of a dopamine infusion are tachycardia, ectopic beats, and dysrhythmias. Dopamine is used to improve cardiac efficiency by strengthening contractions and increasing cardiac output. Moderate doses (5-10 mcg/kg/min) increase blood pressure and improve perfusion of tissues, but hypovolemia must be treated before use of a dopamine infusion or the drug is not effective. Higher doses cause vasoconstriction, especially of the pulmonary vasculature.

59. D: Treatment for tracheomalacia includes humidified air, care in feeding with the infant's upper body elevated, and antibiotics (if needed for respiratory infection). The condition usually resolves as the infant grows, but in rare cases, surgery may be indicated. Tracheomalacia is a congenital abnormality of the trachea in which the supporting cartilage is weak and posterior membranous wall is widened. The distal third of the trachea is most commonly affected, and the condition may be associated with other congenital defects, such as cardiovascular abnormalities and/or tracheoesophageal fistula. Recurrent respiratory infections are common.

60. A: Popular press, including both print and other media (television, Internet), is not a valid source of information. Juried medical journals and professional physician's associations are valid because they present information based on research, critical analysis, and best practices. Physicians on staff, such as the chief of medical staff, may also provide valid information but should not be relied on solely as they may have bias.

61. B: CO_2 retention in an oxygen hood and rebreathing of CO_2 is usually caused by an oxygen flow rate that is too low. Small hoods usually require a flow rate of at least 4 L/min and medium and large hoods 3 L/min. An oxygen hood is appropriate for an infant who has a mild form of RDS and can maintain normal carbon dioxide levels in his blood, only needing supplemental oxygen. A hood too large will allow oxygen to escape and lower the concentration the infant is receiving. A hood too small will irritate the infant's skin at contact points. If the infant is to be held for feedings or otherwise removed from the hood, a secondary O_2 delivery tool should be available.

62. A: Squeezing the heel to hard when obtaining capillary blood can cause the sample to hemolyze and give an artificially elevated laboratory value. Prewarming the heel with a heel warmer or warm cloth may increase blood flow. The heel should be grasped firmly by placing the thumb behind the heel and the second finger near the toes while the other fingers secure the ankle. The area is swabbed with alcohol. The lancet should not enter deeper than 2-3 mm. The first drop is wiped away with a sterile swab, and then the foot is gently "milked." Hemolysis is reduced by allowing drops to form and drop into the tube rather than scraping them off the skin.

63. D: Because the stretched skin is taught over the encephalocele, pressure can cause it to easily rupture, so the parents must be taught how to position the child and protect the area with foam and sheepskin. Encephalocele is a neural defect involving a bony defect and herniation of the brain and/or cerebrospinal fluid through part of the skull in a skin-covered sac, most commonly midline in the occipital area. The encephalocele may be as large as the skull or may look like a small nasal polyp. Rupture may result in meningitis. Hydrocephalus occurs in about 50%.

64. C: Pneumoperitoneum is air in the peritoneal area, including the abdomen and occasionally the scrotal sac. This air leak syndrome results from ventilation-induced lung injury (VILI). As pressure increases inside alveoli, the alveolar wall pulls away from the perivascular sheath and subsequent alveolar rupture allows air to follow the perivascular planes and flow into adjacent areas:

- Pneumothorax: air in pleural space
- Tension pneumothorax: one-way airflow into the pleural cavity, with pressure build-up
- Pneumomediastinum: air in mediastinal area. Pneumopericardium: air in pericardial sac
- Subcutaneous emphysema: air in subcutaneous tissue planes of the chest wall
- Pulmonary interstitial emphysema (PIE): air trapped in the interstitium between the alveoli

65. C: Anemia can occur from blood loss if a neonate is held above the level of the placenta while the umbilical cord is clamped (fetoplacental transfusion). Blood can also transfer from the placenta into the mother's circulation (fetomaternal transfer). There is almost always some mixing of blood during delivery, but fetomaternal transfer can also occur with trauma (falls, injuries, assaults) to the abdominal area during pregnancy. Fetomaternal transfusion is especially a concern if the mother is Rh- and the infant Rh+ because the fetal blood can result in anti-D antibodies in the mother. These anti-D antibodies can cross the placenta and attack the fetal Rh+ red blood cells (maternal-fetal transfusion), resulting in hemolytic anemia.

66. D: Decreased activity and increasing nonreactivity are indications of stress in the ELBW neonate. Protecting the infant from stress is a critical part of nursing care and includes decreasing environmental stimuli (lowering lights, reducing noise), handling gently, using facilitated tucking to mimic fetal positioning, providing nonnutritive sucking, allowing long periods of sleep, and spacing procedures.

67. D: As an advocate for the patient, the nurse must prevent possible injury to a patient. "The catheter was contaminated when it fell," states the problem. "Would you like me to get another setup or stay with the patient?" suggests a solution without assigning blame. A contaminated catheter could cause a serious infection. Reporting the team leader's behavior to the supervisor, while appropriate, does not protect the patient. Saying nothing protects only the first nurse from possible repercussions but is unprofessional and unethical conduct.

68. A: Volvulus results from a genetic malrotation defect in which the intestines are attached to the back of the abdominal wall by one single attachment rather than a broad band of attachments across the abdomen, essentially suspending the bowels so that they can easily twist, resulting in a volvulus (twisted bowel), cutting off blood supply. It may untwist but can lead to bowel infarction. Symptoms usually present by 2 months and typically include bilious vomiting and cycles of abdominal pain. The "double bubble" sign shows air in the stomach and proximal intestine but none distally, suggesting intestinal obstruction.

69. B: Ibuprofen lysine or indomethacin (3 doses of either) is successful in causing PDA to close in 70-80% of infants. If the PDA remains open, then surgical repair may be indicated. Symptoms are usually evident at 4-7 days after birth. Mild cases may close without treatment, but clinically significant cases (HR greater than 170 bpm, respirations greater than 70/min, bounding pulses, and hepatomegaly greater than 3 cm below costal margin) require medical or surgical treatment. Prostaglandin is used to reopen a PDA.

70. C: The most common treatment for severe anemia associated with hydrops fetalis related to Rh sensitivity is a partial exchange transfusion with PRBCs to treat anemia without increasing blood volume. Rh sensitivity may occur when an Rh-negative mother's blood contacts blood of an Rh-positive fetus, resulting in antibodies that can cross the placenta and attack the fetal Rh-positive red blood cells, resulting in hemolysis. This is primarily a problem during second or subsequent pregnancies. In the fetus, hemolysis triggers increased RBC production (erythroblastosis fetalis), a form of anemia that left untreated results in severe/fatal edema (hydrops fetalis) that can cause congestive heart failure. Hyperbilirubinemia and jaundice occur from RBC destruction, leading to neurological impairment (kernicterus).

71. A: A neonate with EA and TEF should be positioned in prone or side-lying position with head elevated 30-45 degrees to prevent reflux and aspiration of gastric secretions until surgical repair, which may be done in stages, especially for premature infants. Crying increases air swallowing and risk of reflux, so comfort measures should be used to prevent crying. Medications include gastric acid blockade and antibiotics if necessary to prevent infection.

72. C: The best method to evaluate a parent's educational outcomes related to being taught a procedure is to ask the parent to do a demonstration. Parent feedback is not a reliable indicator of ability to perform. Tests, whether oral or written, can identify what a parent knows and may be appropriate for testing general knowledge about a subject (such as infant care), but knowing and doing are different skills, so demonstration is critical and allows the nurse to provide feedback or additional training if needed.

73. A: Initial treatment for PPHN includes intubation and mechanical ventilation, surfactant to reduce surface tension, sedation (fentanyl or morphine) to reduce restlessness, and inhaled nitrous oxide to promote vasodilation. Nitrous oxide is FDA-approved for use in term or near-term neonates. Other treatments may include sodium bicarbonate or tromethamine for metabolic acidosis and vasopressors (dopamine, dobutamine, nitroprusside, or epinephrine) to maintain systemic pressure above pulmonary pressure. HFOV or ECMO is indicated if conventional mechanical ventilation is ineffective.

74. B: Caput succedaneum is a collection of fluid beneath the skin, but superficial to the periosteum, with swelling that crosses suture lines. It often occurs when the head presses against the dilating cervix during the birth process or with vacuum-assisted deliveries. Cephalohematoma occurs when blood vessels between the skull and the periosteum rupture, causing a subperiosteal collection of blood. The swelling appears several hours after birth and does not cross suture lines. Craniotabes is an area of softened skull that is softer and more pliable than surrounding tissue and gives way when pressure is applied. Abusive head trauma may occur from shaking the infant.

75. D: Theophylline should always be administered slowly over at least 20 minutes. A rapid infusion or IV push can result in cardiac arrest. The infant must be observed carefully for side effects such as tachycardia, irritability, gastrointestinal irritation with vomiting, slowed gastric emptying, and seizures.

76. A: A healthy preterm infant (born at least 32 weeks of gestation) usually has little risk of long-term developmental delays and catches up with full-term infants by 2 years of age. Some types of developmentally delays or problems, such as learning disabilities, may not be evident until school age. Disabilities and developmental delays related to premature birth are more common in those born fewer than 26 weeks of gestation or with ELBW.

77. A: Delivering the infant as soon as possible, even if premature, is critical with HELLP syndrome because the mother may develop severe irreversible liver damage or hepatic hemorrhage. Platelet transfusions are generally recommended for platelet counts less than 20,000/mcL, although a transfusion may be considered with platelet counts less than 50,000/mcL for cesareans. IV steroids are sometimes administered to stabilize platelet count if the fetus is fewer than 32 weeks' gestation and the condition of the fetus and mother is stable.

78. A: Hypoplastic left heart syndrome is a cyanotic congenital heart disease characterized by underdevelopment of the left ventricle and ascending aortic atresia. This causes an inability of the heart to pump blood, so most blood flows from the left atrium through the foramen ovale to the right atrium and to the lungs, with the descending aorta receiving blood through the ductus arteriosus. Symptoms may be mild until the ductus arteriosus closes at about 2 weeks, causing a marked increase in cyanosis and decreased cardiac output, leading to cardiovascular collapse unless surgical repair is successful.

79. C: The nurse who delegates remains accountable for patient outcomes and for supervision of the person to whom the task was delegated. The scope of nursing includes delegation of tasks to unlicensed assistive personnel, provided those personnel have adequate training and knowledge. Delegation can be used to manage the workload and to provide adequate and safe care. Delegation should be done in a manner that reduces liability by providing adequate communication.

80. C: Many post-term (more than 42 weeks) neonates are normal in size and appearance but some continue to grow *in utero* and weigh more than 4000 g, and about 5% exhibit postmaturity syndrome, which may include:

- Appearance: alert (may indicate intrauterine hypoxia)
- Skin: loose, dry, cracking, parchment-like, lacking lanugo or vernix; may have meconium staining, yellow to green (indicating recent)
- Fingernails: long (sometimes with meconium staining)
- Scalp hair: long/thick
- Body: long, thin (fat layers absent), increasing risk of cold stress and hypothermia because of decreased brown fat and liver glycogen
- Complications: hypoglycemia from nutritional deprivation, meconium aspiration, polycythemia and/or seizures as response to hypoxia, and congenital anomalies

81. C: This neonate exhibits signs of transient tachypnea of newborn (TTN) ("wet lungs") and requires only careful monitoring, especially if symptoms are improving, as symptoms usually subside within 24-72 hours. TTN results from fluid remaining in the alveoli in the lungs after birth, decreasing oxygen exchange. Small or premature infants or those delivered by rapid vaginal or cesarean have increased risk because they do not receive the pressure during delivery that helps to squeeze the fluid from the lungs. TTN is also more common in infants of mothers who smoke or are diabetic.

82. B: These symptoms are consistent with hypocalcemia. Normal calcium value for a neonate (0-10 days) is 7.6-10.4 mg/dL. The critical value for hypoglycemia is less than 7 mg/dL. Early-onset hypocalcemia usually presents in the first 3 days of life, and is associated with prematurity, birth asphyxia, and infants of diabetic mothers. Late-onset hypocalcemia presents after the first week and is associated with DiGeorge syndrome, hyperphosphatemia, vitamin D deficiency, magnesium deficiency, diuretic therapy, and hypoparathyroidism. Hypocalcemia is treated with a slow infusion of calcium gluconate.

83. D: A number of tests should be done to verify a diagnosis of pneumonia and rule out other disorders with similar symptoms, such as RDS and sepsis: CBC to indicate neutropenia or shift to left; blood culture to rule out septicemia; ABGs to determine presence and degree of metabolic acidosis; culture of tracheal aspirate for presence of organisms; and culture of cerebrospinal fluid to rule-out comorbid meningitis.

84. A: HIPAA regulations are designed to protect the rights of individuals regarding the privacy of their health information. The nurse must not release any information or documentation about a child's condition or treatment without consent, as the parents have the right to determine who has access to personal information, which is considered protected health information (PHI), including health history, condition, treatments in any form, and any documentation. Personal information can be shared with parents, legal guardians, and those with durable power of attorney.

85. B: "Current jelly" stool, a mixture of blood and mucous, is typical of intussusception, which is a telescoping of one portion of the intestine into another, usually at the ileocecal valve, causing an obstruction. As the walls of the intestine come in contact, inflammation and edema cause decreased perfusion, which can result in infarction with peritonitis and death. Other symptoms include sudden acute episodes of abdominal pain, vomiting, lethargy, distended abdomen, and sausage-shaped mass in the right upper quadrant of abdomen.

86. C: While these symptoms could be attributed to other physical causes, they are consistent with child abuse, so a referral should be made to Child Protective Services. Nurses and other health care providers are mandatory reporters in all states and must report cases of suspected abuse and neglect. This mother may benefit from counseling, childcare classes, and a support group, but the primary concern is safety of the child.

87. C: The criteria for declaring that a neonate 7-60 days postnatal has suffered brain death include a diagnosis that explains the condition that caused brain death and excludes conditions that are reversible, testing of higher brain functions with EEG or cerebral blood flow testing, and two separate clinical examinations done at least 48 hours apart. Infants 60 days to 1 year must meet the same criteria except that two separate clinical examinations must be done at least 24 hours apart.

88. B: Menstrual-like cramps, diarrhea, and low dull backache with painless uterine contractions often signify preterm labor. Other indications include feelings of abdominal or pelvic pressure and increase or change in vaginal discharge, which may be thin and watery, mucoid, or blood-tinged. African-American women have double the rate of pre-term delivery as other ethnic groups, and incidence increases in multiple gestations or with a history of previous preterm labor.

89. D: Tetralogy of Fallot (TOF) is a combination of 4 different congenital defects:

- Pulmonic stenosis with decreased blood flow to the lungs
- Ventricular septal defect (VSD), usually with a large opening
- Overriding aorta with displacement to the right so that it appears to come from both ventricles, usually overriding the VSD and resulting in mixing of oxygenated and deoxygenated blood
- Right ventricular hypertrophy

Infants are often acutely cyanotic immediately after birth, but those with less severe defects may have increasing cyanosis over the first year of life. Total surgical repair during the first year of life is the preferred treatment.

90. B: Acute respiratory failure (ARF) is a possible complication of sepsis. *Staphylococcus aureus* infections are generally nosocomial infections acquired after birth from family, staff, or other infants. Other common causes of ARF are respiratory distress syndrome and meconium aspiration syndrome. Early signs of ARF include changes in the depth and pattern of respirations with flaring nares, sternal retractions, expiratory grunting, wheezing, and extended expiration as the body tries to compensate for hypoxemia and increasing levels of carbon dioxide. Cyanosis may be evident. CNS depression occurs with decreased perfusion to the brain. As the hypoxemia worsens, cardiac arrhythmias, including bradycardia, may occur with either hypotension or hypertension.

91. D: A neonate with gestational age at least 35 weeks and weight more than 2000 g meets criteria for ECMO if she has no significant blood abnormalities (bleeding, clotting), no intracranial hemorrhage greater than grade 2, and no lethal malformations or major cardiac abnormalities. Respiratory and cardiac conditions should be reversible. Conventional mechanical ventilation is usually given 10-14 days prior to ECMO. Indications include RDS, MAS, PPHN, sepsis, ARDS, and congenital diaphragmatic hernia. ECMO is also indicated as life support before or after cardiac surgery to correct defects.

92. B: Because of increased rate of RBC breakdown, the neonate should be monitored with blood cell counts to assess anemia. About 20-25% of pregnancies involve ABO incompatibility, usually with the mother type O and the fetus A or B. Anti-A and anti-B antibodies occur naturally when a woman is exposed to A and B antigens in foods or bacteria, so these antibodies can cross the placenta and result in hemolysis of fetal RBC; however, the antibodies are relatively large and do not enter the fetal circulation easily. If fetal blood leaks into maternal blood (a common occurrence), then smaller antibodies form and these can cross the placenta more easily. Serious complications for the fetus are rare.

93. A: Hypothermia and hypovolemia are a primary concern with an infant awaiting surgical repair of gastroschisis because the exposed bowels increase loss of body heat and fluid. The infant should be placed in a sterile bowel bag (feet to axilla) to protect the area and reduce heat loss. The bowel bag is better than applying dampened gauze because the wet gauze cools and can increase hypothermia. Respiratory distress can occur, especially if the abdominal cavity is small in size. IV fluids reduce danger of hypotension, and the danger of hemorrhage is reduced because the bowel tissue appears healthy.

94. D: Open-ended questions, such as "Is there anything you'd like to discuss?" encourage parents to express feelings. Nurses should avoid meaningless clichés, such as "Don't worry. Everything will be fine," as this may not be true. Providing direct advice should also be avoided, such as "You should..." or "The best thing to do is..." Instead, provide facts and encourage parents to make decisions. "Why are you upset?" questions behavior that may not directly relate to care and requires analysis of feelings.

95. B: Flow-inflating mask ventilation requires direct connection to a gas (oxygen) in order to function and does not function on room air. Flow-inflating bag and mask ventilation have the ability to deliver anywhere from 21% (room air) to 100% oxygen; any pressure desired can be set. This type of bag and mask also has the ability to maintain positive end-expiratory pressure (PEEP) and CPAP. The high pressures possible with this type of equipment make overinflation of the lungs possible, sometimes resulting in pneumothorax. A complete seal is necessary to deliver a tidal volume.

96. C: Prostaglandin is given to an infant with tricuspid atresia and no septal defects to ensure that the ductus arteriosus and foramen ovale remain open. Tricuspid atresia is lack of tricuspid valve between the right atrium and right ventricle so blood flows through the foramen ovale (or an atrial defect) to the left atrium. Blood flows to the lungs from the left ventricular outflow through the patent ductus arteriosus. If a ventricular septal defect is present, some blood shunts from the left ventricle to the right and then to the pulmonary artery.

97. B: Erb palsy results from damage to the upper part of the brachial plexus from delivery complicated by shoulder dystocia. The brachial plexus is a collection of nerve tissue located in the shoulder area that is the pathway for nerves traveling from the spine to the arm and shoulder, controlling movement. Most commonly, the upper portion of this plexus is damaged, leading to weak arm muscles (Erb palsy). When examined, the infant holds the arm adducted and internally rotated. The startle reflex is abnormal on the affected side, but the grasp reflex is normal. If the lower portion of the plexus is damaged, the hand is paralyzed also, and the grasp reflex is absent (Klumpke paralysis).

98. C: Because the larynx is very small in infants and small children, inflammation may become obstructive because of swelling of the larynx and trachea. Atelectasis may occur if the bronchioles become obstructed. Croup is not a disease in itself but rather a syndrome of disorders characterized by a distinctive, harsh, "barking" repetitive cough and hoarseness, resulting from inflammation in the area of the larynx. Croup syndromes may affect all areas of the upper respiratory tract system. Croup usually follows an upper respiratory tract infection, and only about 50% of infants develop a fever.

99. D: The amniocentesis indicates fetal lung maturity. If lungs are immature and the fetus is fewer than 34 weeks' gestation, IV corticosteroids may be administered to increase fetal lung maturity if the mother is stable enough to delay delivery for 48 hours. During treatment for preeclampsia, the fetus must have continuous fetal monitoring. The ultrasound helps to determine fetal age and to diagnose intrauterine growth restriction. Other tests include serial nonstress and contraction stress tests.

100. C: Decrease respiratory rate (RR) or tidal volume (Vt) to increase PaO_2 for an infant showing signs of hypocapnia during weaning from conventional ventilation. If hypercapnia is present, decrease the peak inspiratory pressure (PIP), inspiratory to expiratory ratio (I:E), or positive end-expiratory pressure (PEEP). ABGs are essential to monitor weaning, especially pH and PaO_2, and keep O_2 use as low as possible to avoid toxicity.

101. A: Meconium ileus is usually the first clinical sign of cystic fibrosis. Meconium ileus is obstruction of the ileum with inspissated (thick) mucilaginous meconium that clings to the side of the narrowed lumen of the intestine and forms hard pellets. The mucus interferes with absorption of fat, protein, carbohydrates, and other nutrients, leading to malabsorption syndromes.

- Uncomplicated*:* abdominal distention, vomiting, and no meconium in first 24-48 hours.
- Complicated *(*may include volvulus, gangrene, perforations, or bowel atresia)*:* pain, fever, erythema, and edema of abdominal wall consistent with peritonitis.

102. B: The best time to initiate conflict resolution is when conflict first emerges but before open conflict and hardening of positions. Steps include:

- Allowing both parties to present their sides without bias.
- Encouraging cooperation through negotiation and compromise.
- Maintaining focus and avoiding arguments.
- Evaluating the need for renegotiation, formal resolution process, or third party.
- Utilizing humor and empathy to diffuse tension.
- Summarizing and outlining key arguments.
- Avoiding forced resolution if possible.

103. D: The neonate is developing hyperkalemia (greater than 6 mEq/L). Shortly after birth (within the first 24-72 hours), serum potassium concentrations are expected to rise from a shift of potassium from the intracellular space to the extracellular space. Potassium shift is more extreme in premature infants and can result in life-threatening hyperkalemia, so preterm infants must be monitored carefully for 48 hours or until potassium levels stabilize.

104. A: During the early postnatal period, some fluid remains in the lungs, so coarse rales with prolonged expiratory phase and slight substernal or intercostal retraction are normal findings. Respiratory rate of 30-60 and heart rate of 120-160 are also within normal parameters. The neonate's skin usually appears slightly mottled.

105. D: Neuromuscular characteristics of a full-term infant include:

Test	Result
Supine resting posture	Hips, knees, and arms all flexed past 90°, indicating mature muscular tone.
Square window	The wrist flexes to 0°, reflecting very little resistance to the extensor muscles of the wrist.
Arm recoil	Arms recoil past 90°. Contact between the infant's fist and face demonstrates mature tone in the biceps muscles.
Popliteal angle	< 90° knee flexion.
Scarf sign	The arms cannot be drawn past the ipsilateral axillary line because of the mature tone of the posterior shoulder girdle flexor muscles.
Heel to ear	Resistance is felt in the knee and hip when the heel is at the femoral crease because of the tone of the posterior pelvic girdle flexor muscles.

106. C: The translator should have training in medical vocabulary for both languages because just speaking the languages well does not mean that the translator will adequately translate specialized vocabulary. It is not necessary for the translator to know the patient's history as the translator's job is only to translate what is said, not add to it or interpret it based on prior knowledge. While onsite translators are ideal, translation can be done with a speakerphone at a distance.

107. D: Preeclampsia and placental insufficiency can both cause asymmetric IUGR. IUGR is classified according to the size of the infant's head.

Symmetric IUGR	Asymmetric IUGR
Both head and body are small (growth-restricted). Occurs early in pregnancy. Common causes are chromosomal abnormalities and infections.	Large head in proportion to the body; the head is spared. The head is normal in size for gestational age, while the body is growth-restricted. Occurs late in pregnancy. Common causes include placental insufficiency and preeclampsia.

108. A: Subtle signs of seizures include eye blinking and horizontal ocular deviations, as well as peddling, rowing, or stepping movements, nonnutritive sucking, lip smacking, drooling, and periods of apnea. Jitteriness must be differentiated from seizures. Characteristics of jitteriness include lack of ocular deviations or other abnormalities and clonic jerking that has both fast and slow elements. Stimulation elicits jitteriness and gentle restraint halts it. Autonomic changes involving the heart rate, respirations, and blood pressure are not present, and EEG is normal. Jitteriness is distinct from shuddering, a 10- to 15-second period of fast tremors that may recur 100 times or less daily.

109. D: Since calories are delivered into the circulatory system with PN, the caloric needs are usually about 20% less than those needed for enteral nutrition (averaging about 90-100 kcal/kg/d). Caloric needs may vary according to the neonate's body temperature, activity, and stress, so PN should be individualized for the needs of each neonate. Fluid requirements usually range from 100-150 mL/kg/d, depending on gestational age, ambient environmental temperature, and type of heat source.

110. B: Platelets and fresh frozen plasma (FFP), which contains all the clotting factors, treat active bleeding associated with DIC. PRBCs treat hypovolemia. DIC triggers both coagulation and hemorrhage through a complex series of events that include trauma, causing tissue factor (transmembrane glycoprotein) to enter the circulation and bind with coagulation factors, triggering the coagulation cascade. This stimulates thrombin to convert fibrinogen to fibrin, causing aggregation and destruction of platelets and forming clots that can be disseminated throughout the intravascular system. Platelets adhere to the clots, increasing their size and causing blockage of both the microvascular systems and larger vessels, resulting in ischemia and necrosis. Clot formation triggers fibrinolysis and plasmin to breakdown fibrin and fibrinogen, causing destruction of clotting factors and hemorrhage.

111. C: According to Knowles, adult learners tend to be practical and goal-oriented, so they like to remain organized and keep the goal in mind while learning. Other characteristics include:

- Self-directed: Adults like active involvement and responsibility.
- Knowledgeable—adults can relate new material to information that they are familiar with from previous life experiences or education.
- Relevancy-oriented—adults like to know how they will use information.
- Motivated: Adults like to see evidence of their own achievement, such as earning a certificate.

112. A: An ultrasound to check the position of the tip of the umbilical catheter is indicated. If the tip is directly above the pancreas, the delivery of glucose directly to the pancreas can stimulate overproduction of insulin and increased glucose utilization. Other causes of increased glucose utilization can include:

- Cold stress and hypothermia
- Sepsis
- Increased work of breathing
- Perinatal asphyxia
- Rh incompatibility
- Persistent neonatal hyperinsulinism
- Maternal tocolytic drugs

113. D: Treatment for HIT includes immediately stopping all forms of heparin and beginning treatment with a direct thrombin inhibitor, such as argatroban, lepirudin, or danaparoid. The alternative anticoagulation is necessary because of the danger of thrombosis. Hemorrhage usually does not occur despite low thrombocyte count, and platelet transfusions are rarely indicated. An ultrasound of lower extremities should be done to assess for thromboses, and daily platelet counts should be done until recovery.

114. B: Advocacy is working for the best interests of the patient, despite personal values in conflict, and assisting patients/families with access to appropriate resources. Moral agency is the ability to recognize needs and take action to influence the outcome of a conflict or decision. Agency is openness and recognition of issues and a willingness to act. Collaboration is working together to achieve better results.

115. A: Oxygen administration should be titrated to the needs of the individual infant to keep the arterial oxygen level between 50 and 80 mmHg. Additionally, oxygen should be humidified to 30-40% to avoid drying nasal passages and respiratory distress. Oxygen should be warmed to 31-34 °C to prevent cold stress and should never be given without some method of monitoring the level of oxygen in the infant's blood at all times, such as with pulse oximetry or arterial blood gas studies. Adjustments to the concentration of oxygen must be done slowly to prevent sudden vasoconstriction.

116. B: Hypokalemia, hyponatremia, and increased calcium excretion resulting in hypocalcemia are the adverse reactions seen with loop diuretics. Loop diuretics (e.g., furosemide) are the most potent of the diuretics and work on the ascending limb of the loop of Henle. They disrupt the Na+/K+/2Cl- transporter and also limit K+ reabsorption. Hypokalemia and hypocalcemia may cause cardiac arrhythmias. Hyponatremia may increase fluid retention.

117. C: Hearing airflow is not sufficient to ensure that the NG tube is correctly placed as the tip may be in the distal esophagus. Placement must be confirmed by other methods, such as aspirating gastric contents and checking the pH or assessing nature of aspirant to determine if it is gastric fluid. NG tube placement should be verified by radiograph, a definitive procedure, prior to beginning tube feedings. Complications include perforation if the tube is forced during insertion and aspiration if the tube is misplaced and not in the stomach.

118. A: An HIV-positive mother should avoid breast-feeding her infant because the risk of HIV transmission with breast-feeding is 0.7% per month of breast-feeding. There is virtually no chance of passing the virus through kissing or exposing the child to other HIV-negative family members, and changing the infant's diaper poses no danger to the child. The perinatal transmission rate is

30% in untreated HIV-positive mothers, usually acquired during delivery, but drops to 1-2% with optimal treatment. Neonates are usually asymptomatic but are at risk for prematurity, low birth weight, and small for gestational age (SGA). Infants may show failure to thrive, hepatomegaly, interstitial lymphocytic pneumonia, recurrent infections, and CNS abnormalities.

119. C: Neonatal asphyxia, indicated by failure to breathe well or cry at delivery, causes increasing hypoxia with bradycardia, hypotonia, central cyanosis, and lack of response to stimuli. While a normal Apgar score is at least 7, infants with Apgar score of 3 or less are at risk of dying without immediate resuscitation to increase oxygen to tissues. Initial Apgar scores are usually taken at 1 minute after birth. Resuscitation is generally necessary for all neonates with Apgar score less than 7 at 1 minute.

120. D: All staff members are responsible for identifying quality performance improvement projects. Continuous quality improvement (CQI) is a management philosophy that emphasizes the organization and the systems and processes within that organization rather than individuals. Total quality management (TQM) is a management philosophy that espouses a commitment to meeting the needs of the customers (patients, staff) at all levels within an organization. Both management philosophies recognize that change can be made in small steps and should involve staff at all levels.

121. D: While the FiO_2 delivery may range from 21-100%, it is usually maintained less than 40% to avoid toxicity. The inspiratory to expiratory ratio (I:E) is usually 1:2 to 1:5 with the tidal volume (Vt) set in relation to the respiratory rate. The rate of flow controls the L/min speed of the Vt, and the pressure setting controls the pressure exerted in delivering the Vt. Sensitivity determines the effort needed to trigger inspiration.

122. C: Hypermagnesemia in a neonate is characterized by hypotension and marked flushing secondary to vasodilation, as well as hypotonia, hyporeflexia, and constipation. Elevated magnesium blocks neurosynaptic transmission by interfering with the release of acetylcholine. Treatment is usually supportive, as the elevated serum magnesium will be cleared by the infant's kidneys. In severe cases, the infant may require respiratory and/or blood pressure support.

- Neonate: 1.5-2.2 mg/dL
- Critical values: less than 1.2 mg/dL and greater than 3 mg/dL (neonates)

123. A: Ventilation-induced lung injury (VILI) is damage caused by mechanical ventilation. VILI comprises 4 interrelated elements:

- *Barotrauma*: Damage to the lung caused by excessive pressure
- *Volutrauma*: Alveolar damage related to high tidal volume ventilation
- *Atelectrauma*: Injury caused by repetitive forced opening and closing of alveoli
- *Biotrauma*: Inflammatory response

VILI is common in acute respiratory distress syndrome (ARDS) but can affect any ventilation patient.

124. A: Selection bias occurs when the method of selecting subjects results in a cohort that is not representative of the target population because of inherent error in design. Information bias occurs when there are errors in classification, so an estimate of association is incorrect. A hypothesis should be generated about the probable cause based on the information available in laboratory and medical records, epidemiologic study, literature review, and expert opinion. Hypothesis testing includes data analysis, laboratory findings, and outcomes of testing. Generalizability is when results of research are true for similar populations.

125. A: Aortic stenosis can result in no split in the S2 sound, a harsh systolic murmur in the upper right sternal border, and a suprasternal notch thrill. The S2 sound is normally split. A lack of split indicates that both the aortic valve and pulmonic valve are closing at the same time, or that one valve is not closing. Atrial septal defect, pulmonary stenosis, and Ebstein anomaly cause a widening of the S2 split.

126. B: End-tidal CO_2 ($ETCO_2$) is useful for neonates with normal lung function or in premature infants with mild-moderate lung disease, but results may be inaccurate if there is a large alveolar-arterial gradient. End-tidal CO_2 monitors are used to confirm correct placement of endotracheal tubes during intubation and to ensure adequate oxygenation. Both sidestream analysis with a double-lumen ETT and mainstream analysis within the ventilator circuit are used. Transcutaneous monitoring is preferred with severe lung disease.

127. D: The "5 rights of delegation" include:

- Right task: The nurse determines as appropriate task to delegate for a specific patient.
- Right circumstance: The nurse has considered all relevant information to determine the appropriateness of delegation.
- Right person: The nurse chooses the right person based on education and skills to perform the task.
- Right direction: The nurse provides a clear description of the task, purpose, limits, and expected outcomes.
- Right supervision: The nurse can supervise, intervene as needed, and evaluate performance.

128. A: Because the mother cares for 6 cats in the home, the most likely cause of the retinochoroiditis is toxoplasmosis, a protozoal infection. About 1:1000 pregnant women become infected during pregnancy, from eating undercooked meat, drinking unpasteurized goat's milk, or contacting infected cat feces. Risk to the fetus is greatest if the disease occurs during the first trimester, often causing severe fetal abnormalities, such as microcephaly and hydrocephalus, or miscarriage. However, risk of fetal transmission is greatest during the third trimester, although 70% are born without indications of infection. Mild infection may be manifest by retinochoroiditis at birth (with other symptoms delayed). Severe infection may result in convulsions and coma from CNS abnormalities.

129. B: Neonates receiving IV fentanyl must be carefully observed for chest wall rigidity. Some infants exhibit generalized rigidity and may develop laryngospasm. An opiate antagonist (naloxone) is indicated to reverse these adverse effects. Infants born to mothers who received fentanyl during labor and delivery may exhibit depressed respirations and central nervous system, impaired thermoregulation, and difficulty feeding, requiring IV naloxone to reverse the effects of the drug.

130. D: An infant with idiopathic thrombocytopenic purpura (ITP) and a platelet count less than 50,000/mcL requires serial platelet counts to monitor platelets and a sonogram, CT, or MRI to evaluate for possible hidden intracranial hemorrhage. General guidelines for transfusing platelets depend on the clinical stability of the neonate. If the infant is stable, a transfusion is considered when the count is less than 25,000/mcL. If the infant is unstable, a transfusion is considered when the count is less than 50,000/mcL.

131. C: The electrodes are calibrated (usually every 4 hours to ensure accuracy), and then heat (43-44 °C) the underlying skin, so they must be left in place for 15 minutes after calibration to ensure adequate heating of the skin. One or two leads are placed on the infant's skin over any part of the body that allows good contact. O_2 and CO_2 diffuse through the skin, and monitors provide a digital display. If right-to-left shunting is suspected, then leads are usually placed on right shoulder and lower abdomen or leg (above and below the ductus arteriosus).

132. B: As part of postoperative management of surgery to repair extrahepatic biliary atresia, the neonate should receive fat-soluble vitamins (A, D, E, K) because these nutrients were not absorbed before surgical repair. Biliary atresia prevents bile from leaving the liver, causing the liver to become inflamed and scarred. With extrahepatic biliary atresia, the ducts outside of the liver are damaged, so surgical repair may be successful if liver is not severely compromised. Intrahepatic and severe extrahepatic biliary atresia require liver transplant.

133. A: The leader who wants everyone to follow the organization's rules exactly is bureaucratic. Autocratic leaders make decision independently and enforce rules while charismatic leaders rely on personal charm to influence and persuade. Consultative leaders present a decision and welcome input but rarely change decisions while participatory leaders present potential decisions but make final decisions based on input. Democratic leaders present the problem and ask teams to arrive at a solution. Laissez-faire leaders exert little control and allow staff to make decisions with little interference.

134. B: A neonate receiving a PICC should be monitored for bradycardia and hypoxia during the procedure. PICCs are contraindicated if IV therapy is less than 6 days, if vessels are inadequate, or if abnormalities of the thoracic area or extremities may impede insertion. If the infant has active bacteremia or sepsis, the PICC line should be inserted only after administration of antibiotics for 24-48 hours. Caution must be exercised with coagulation disorders or concurrent treatment with high-frequency ventilation. PICCs should not be used for blood products or to obtain blood specimens.

135. B: The correct internal diameter (ID) for the ETT for an infant at 28-34 weeks' gestation and weight of 1000-2000 g is 3 cm. Infants less than 1000 g or less than 28 weeks' gestation require ID of 2.5 mm. Infants at 34-38 weeks' gestation and weight of 2000-3000 g require ID of 3.5 mm. Infants greater than 3000 g or greater than 38 weeks' gestation require ID of 3.5-4.0 mm.

136. A: Normal weight loss after full-term birth is 5-7%, but the infant usually regains this weight within 2 weeks; the infant should gain 4-7 ounces per week. During the first month, the infant needs to breast-feed about every 2-3 hours to ensure adequate nutrition. At birth, the infant's gastric capacity is about 5-6 mm, increasing to 1.5-2.0 ounces by 7 days. Trying to feed the infant larger amounts more frequently can result in regurgitation.

137. D: Symptoms of increasing intracranial pressure vary with age. Neonates typically exhibit bulging fontanels without normal pulsations, distention of scalp veins, and increased head circumference. Infants may be irritable with high-pitched cries and poor feeding. Infants have open fontanels that allow for some expansion; however, the ability to compensate is limited. Late signs of increase intracranial pressure include pupil size and reactivity changes, decerebrate or decorticate posturing, respiratory depression with Cheyne-Stokes, and papilledema.

138. C: The square window test measures the resistance to stretching of extensor muscles in the infant's forearm. Increased ability to flex the infant's wrist correlates with greater gestational age. Arm recoil test measures the tone of the biceps muscles. Increased amount of arm recoil (flexion by the infant after the infant's arms are extended) correlates with greater gestational age. Scarf sign test measures the tone of shoulder flexor muscles. Increased resistance to movement of the infant's arm across the chest is associated with greater gestational age. The heel to ear test measures the tone of pelvic girdle muscles. Increased resistance to movement of the infant's foot to the ear is associated with greater gestational age.

139. B: A mixed venous oxygen saturation (SvO_2) level less than 60% indicates a decrease in delivery of oxygen because of decreased hemoglobin, PaO_2, and/or cardiac output OR increased consumption of oxygen (VO_2), which can occur with fever or seizures. Increased SvO_2 level greater than 80% usually indicates the presence of sepsis.

140. C: The initial neonatal dose of the opioid antagonist naloxone is 0.1 mg/kg. Naloxone can be administered intramuscularly or subcutaneously, but IV use is recommended if rapid onset of action is needed because of severe depression. If the infant does not respond adequately to the initial dose, additional doses can be administered at 2- to 3-minute intervals, depending on the severity of the condition.

141. D: Physiologic GER is associated only with regurgitation ("spitters") and is common in about 50% of neonates. Usually, this condition subsides as the infant matures. Pathologic GER may cause esophagitis, malnutrition, and respiratory distress. While regurgitation is common, other symptoms can occur without regurgitation if the distal esophagus is irritated. Premature infants less than 1500 g have increased risk of GER. With pathologic GRE, other anomalies, such as esophageal atresia, may be present.

142. B: Tests to confirm diagnosis of congenital muscular dystrophy (laminin alpha-2 deficiency), the most common type (40%), includes electromyogram and nerve conduction studies to both confirm that the symptoms relate to myopathy and to rule out other disorders. These tests are followed by a muscle biopsy to confirm the diagnosis. Changes in the periventricular white matter are usually not evident on MRI until after 6 months. Creatinine kinase is typically elevated with CMD but this cannot establish a diagnosis.

143. A: The learner outcome for teaching a patient about NG feedings should relate directly to that goal: Demonstrate skill in preparing and administering NG feeding. While all of the other things (different types of NG tubes, nutritional composition, and pacifier use) are important, they do not relate to the specifically to the topic and should not be the learner outcome for this activity. In some cases, one class or session may cover multiple topics with multiple outcomes, but a patient may be overwhelmed by too much information.

144. B: Packed red blood cells are usually administered in volumes of 15-20 mL/kg at a rate of 5 mL/kg/hr. Platelet concentrations and fresh frozen plasma are administered in volumes of 10-20 mL/kg at a rate of 10-20 mL/kg/hr. Cryoprecipitate is administered in volume of 5-10 mL/kg at a rate of 10-20 mL/kg/hr.

145. C: Herpes simplex encephalitis (HSE) is treated with IV acyclovir 20 mg/kg every 8 hours. While HSE can be transmitted by shedding of maternal virus during delivery, in most cases the mother has no history of the disease. The most common pathogen is herpes simplex virus type 2 but type 1 can also cause HSE. HSE can be acquired after birth from someone with herpes infection. Mortality rates are high even with treatment.

146. C: Phenobarbital is the neonatal anticonvulsive of choice for seizures. Loading dose is 20 mg/kg IV in 10-15 minutes and then 5 mg/kg to maximum 40 mg/kg to control seizures. Maintenance dose is 3-4 mg/kg per 24 hours in 2 doses beginning at least 12 hours after loading dose. Fosphenytoin is used if phenobarbital is ineffective. Phenytoin is sometimes used instead of fosphenytoin if phenobarbital is ineffective. Lorazepam is used if other drugs are ineffective. Hypoglycemia may trigger seizures, which are treated with glucose 10% solution.

147. B: Heliox is administered during mechanical ventilation to decrease airway resistance in order to reduce respiratory effort and improve oxygenation. It is often used to relieve respiratory distress caused by respiratory obstruction. Helium replaces nitrogen, which is more viscous than helium, so nitrogen causes more airway resistance. Heliox may be administered in different concentrations, but a mixture of 21% oxygen and 79% helium is common.

148. D: The ratio of the phospholipids lecithin and sphingomyelin (two components of surfactant) changes during pregnancy with L:S ratio at 0.5:1 early in pregnancy, 1:1 at 30-32 weeks, and 2:1 at 35 weeks. At 2:1, RDS is unlikely, although this finding is not always accurate for infants of diabetic mothers (IDM); they may show adequate ratio but still develop RDS, so these neonates must be monitored carefully. A second test is phosphatidylglycerol (PG). This phospholipid first appears in surfactant at about week 35 in IDM with complications and week 36 in other pregnancies, indicating lung maturity.

149. A: If kidney function is compromised, then a pyeloplasty is advised to remove the UPJ obstruction and reattach ureter to renal pelvis to allow normal urinary drainage. The most common cause of UPJ is the lack of proper canalization of the renal pelvis during embryologic development. The obstruction can be mild or severe and may be asymptomatic in the newborn period. In milder cases without renal compromise, the infant may be treated with antibiotics because infection is common, and monitored to ensure condition is stable or improving. If renal deterioration occurs, then a pyeloplasty is indicated. Another congenital anomaly occurs with UPJ obstruction in approximately 50% of cases.

150. A: Sterile water should be used for skin care, as the skin is very thin and friable. Antimicrobials (such as povidone-iodine) used to prep skin for procedures should be wiped off the skin as soon as possible, and isopropyl alcohol use should be avoided because it dries the skin. Soap may alter the acidity of the skin. If sterile water is not adequate for cleansing, then only a product with a neutral pH and no preservatives is appropriate.

How to Overcome Test Anxiety

Just the thought of taking a test is enough to make most people a little nervous. A test is an important event that can have a long-term impact on your future, so it's important to take it seriously and it's natural to feel anxious about performing well. But just because anxiety is normal, that doesn't mean that it's helpful in test taking, or that you should simply accept it as part of your life. Anxiety can have a variety of effects. These effects can be mild, like making you feel slightly nervous, or severe, like blocking your ability to focus or remember even a simple detail.

If you experience test anxiety—whether severe or mild—it's important to know how to beat it. To discover this, first you need to understand what causes test anxiety.

Causes of Test Anxiety

While we often think of anxiety as an uncontrollable emotional state, it can actually be caused by simple, practical things. One of the most common causes of test anxiety is that a person does not feel adequately prepared for their test. This feeling can be the result of many different issues such as poor study habits or lack of organization, but the most common culprit is time management. Starting to study too late, failing to organize your study time to cover all of the material, or being distracted while you study will mean that you're not well prepared for the test. This may lead to cramming the night before, which will cause you to be physically and mentally exhausted for the test. Poor time management also contributes to feelings of stress, fear, and hopelessness as you realize you are not well prepared but don't know what to do about it.

Other times, test anxiety is not related to your preparation for the test but comes from unresolved fear. This may be a past failure on a test, or poor performance on tests in general. It may come from comparing yourself to others who seem to be performing better or from the stress of living up to expectations. Anxiety may be driven by fears of the future—how failure on this test would affect your educational and career goals. These fears are often completely irrational, but they can still negatively impact your test performance.

Elements of Test Anxiety

As mentioned earlier, test anxiety is considered to be an emotional state, but it has physical and mental components as well. Sometimes you may not even realize that you are suffering from test anxiety until you notice the physical symptoms. These can include trembling hands, rapid heartbeat, sweating, nausea, and tense muscles. Extreme anxiety may lead to fainting or vomiting. Obviously, any of these symptoms can have a negative impact on testing. It is important to recognize them as soon as they begin to occur so that you can address the problem before it damages your performance.

The mental components of test anxiety include trouble focusing and inability to remember learned information. During a test, your mind is on high alert, which can help you recall information and stay focused for an extended period of time. However, anxiety interferes with your mind's natural processes, causing you to blank out, even on the questions you know well. The strain of testing during anxiety makes it difficult to stay focused, especially on a test that may take several hours. Extreme anxiety can take a huge mental toll, making it difficult not only to recall test information but even to understand the test questions or pull your thoughts together.

Effects of Test Anxiety

Test anxiety is like a disease—if left untreated, it will get progressively worse. Anxiety leads to poor performance, and this reinforces the feelings of fear and failure, which in turn lead to poor performances on subsequent tests. It can grow from a mild nervousness to a crippling condition. If allowed to progress, test anxiety can have a big impact on your schooling, and consequently on your future.

Test anxiety can spread to other parts of your life. Anxiety on tests can become anxiety in any stressful situation, and blanking on a test can turn into panicking in a job situation. But fortunately, you don't have to let anxiety rule your testing and determine your grades. There are a number of relatively simple steps you can take to move past anxiety and function normally on a test and in the rest of life.

Physical Steps for Beating Test Anxiety

While test anxiety is a serious problem, the good news is that it can be overcome. It doesn't have to control your ability to think and remember information. While it may take time, you can begin taking steps today to beat anxiety.

Just as your first hint that you may be struggling with anxiety comes from the physical symptoms, the first step to treating it is also physical. Rest is crucial for having a clear, strong mind. If you are tired, it is much easier to give in to anxiety. But if you establish good sleep habits, your body and mind will be ready to perform optimally, without the strain of exhaustion. Additionally, sleeping well helps you to retain information better, so you're more likely to recall the answers when you see the test questions.

Getting good sleep means more than going to bed on time. It's important to allow your brain time to relax. Take study breaks from time to time so it doesn't get overworked, and don't study right before bed. Take time to rest your mind before trying to rest your body, or you may find it difficult to fall asleep.

Along with sleep, other aspects of physical health are important in preparing for a test. Good nutrition is vital for good brain function. Sugary foods and drinks may give a burst of energy but this burst is followed by a crash, both physically and emotionally. Instead, fuel your body with protein and vitamin-rich foods.

Also, drink plenty of water. Dehydration can lead to headaches and exhaustion, especially if your brain is already under stress from the rigors of the test. Particularly if your test is a long one, drink water during the breaks. And if possible, take an energy-boosting snack to eat between sections.

Along with sleep and diet, a third important part of physical health is exercise. Maintaining a steady workout schedule is helpful, but even taking 5-minute study breaks to walk can help get your blood pumping faster and clear your head. Exercise also releases endorphins, which contribute to a positive feeling and can help combat test anxiety.

When you nurture your physical health, you are also contributing to your mental health. If your body is healthy, your mind is much more likely to be healthy as well. So take time to rest, nourish your body with healthy food and water, and get moving as much as possible. Taking these physical steps will make you stronger and more able to take the mental steps necessary to overcome test anxiety.

Mental Steps for Beating Test Anxiety

Working on the mental side of test anxiety can be more challenging, but as with the physical side, there are clear steps you can take to overcome it. As mentioned earlier, test anxiety often stems from lack of preparation, so the obvious solution is to prepare for the test. Effective studying may be the most important weapon you have for beating test anxiety, but you can and should employ several other mental tools to combat fear.

First, boost your confidence by reminding yourself of past success—tests or projects that you aced. If you're putting as much effort into preparing for this test as you did for those, there's no reason you should expect to fail here. Work hard to prepare; then trust your preparation.

Second, surround yourself with encouraging people. It can be helpful to find a study group, but be sure that the people you're around will encourage a positive attitude. If you spend time with others who are anxious or cynical, this will only contribute to your own anxiety. Look for others who are motivated to study hard from a desire to succeed, not from a fear of failure.

Third, reward yourself. A test is physically and mentally tiring, even without anxiety, and it can be helpful to have something to look forward to. Plan an activity following the test, regardless of the outcome, such as going to a movie or getting ice cream.

When you are taking the test, if you find yourself beginning to feel anxious, remind yourself that you know the material. Visualize successfully completing the test. Then take a few deep, relaxing breaths and return to it. Work through the questions carefully but with confidence, knowing that you are capable of succeeding.

Developing a healthy mental approach to test taking will also aid in other areas of life. Test anxiety affects more than just the actual test—it can be damaging to your mental health and even contribute to depression. It's important to beat test anxiety before it becomes a problem for more than testing.

Study Strategy

Being prepared for the test is necessary to combat anxiety, but what does being prepared look like? You may study for hours on end and still not feel prepared. What you need is a strategy for test prep. The next few pages outline our recommended steps to help you plan out and conquer the challenge of preparation.

Step 1: Scope Out the Test

Learn everything you can about the format (multiple choice, essay, etc.) and what will be on the test. Gather any study materials, course outlines, or sample exams that may be available. Not only will this help you to prepare, but knowing what to expect can help to alleviate test anxiety.

Step 2: Map Out the Material

Look through the textbook or study guide and make note of how many chapters or sections it has. Then divide these over the time you have. For example, if a book has 15 chapters and you have five days to study, you need to cover three chapters each day. Even better, if you have the time, leave an extra day at the end for overall review after you have gone through the material in depth.

If time is limited, you may need to prioritize the material. Look through it and make note of which sections you think you already have a good grasp on, and which need review. While you are studying, skim quickly through the familiar sections and take more time on the challenging parts.

Write out your plan so you don't get lost as you go. Having a written plan also helps you feel more in control of the study, so anxiety is less likely to arise from feeling overwhelmed at the amount to cover.

Step 3: Gather Your Tools

Decide what study method works best for you. Do you prefer to highlight in the book as you study and then go back over the highlighted portions? Or do you type out notes of the important information? Or is it helpful to make flashcards that you can carry with you? Assemble the pens, index cards, highlighters, post-it notes, and any other materials you may need so you won't be distracted by getting up to find things while you study.

If you're having a hard time retaining the information or organizing your notes, experiment with different methods. For example, try color-coding by subject with colored pens, highlighters, or post-it notes. If you learn better by hearing, try recording yourself reading your notes so you can listen while in the car, working out, or simply sitting at your desk. Ask a friend to quiz you from your flashcards, or try teaching someone the material to solidify it in your mind.

Step 4: Create Your Environment

It's important to avoid distractions while you study. This includes both the obvious distractions like visitors and the subtle distractions like an uncomfortable chair (or a too-comfortable couch that makes you want to fall asleep). Set up the best study environment possible: good lighting and a comfortable work area. If background music helps you focus, you may want to turn it on, but otherwise keep the room quiet. If you are using a computer to take notes, be sure you don't have any other windows open, especially applications like social media, games, or anything else that could distract you. Silence your phone and turn off notifications. Be sure to keep water close by so you stay hydrated while you study (but avoid unhealthy drinks and snacks).

Also, take into account the best time of day to study. Are you freshest first thing in the morning? Try to set aside some time then to work through the material. Is your mind clearer in the afternoon or evening? Schedule your study session then. Another method is to study at the same time of day that you will take the test, so that your brain gets used to working on the material at that time and will be ready to focus at test time.

Step 5: Study!

Once you have done all the study preparation, it's time to settle into the actual studying. Sit down, take a few moments to settle your mind so you can focus, and begin to follow your study plan. Don't give in to distractions or let yourself procrastinate. This is your time to prepare so you'll be ready to fearlessly approach the test. Make the most of the time and stay focused.

Of course, you don't want to burn out. If you study too long you may find that you're not retaining the information very well. Take regular study breaks. For example, taking five minutes out of every hour to walk briskly, breathing deeply and swinging your arms, can help your mind stay fresh.

As you get to the end of each chapter or section, it's a good idea to do a quick review. Remind yourself of what you learned and work on any difficult parts. When you feel that you've mastered the material, move on to the next part. At the end of your study session, briefly skim through your notes again.

But while review is helpful, cramming last minute is NOT. If at all possible, work ahead so that you won't need to fit all your study into the last day. Cramming overloads your brain with more information than it can process and retain, and your tired mind may struggle to recall even previously learned information when it is overwhelmed with last-minute study. Also, the urgent nature of cramming and the stress placed on your brain contribute to anxiety. You'll be more likely to go to the test feeling unprepared and having trouble thinking clearly.

So don't cram, and don't stay up late before the test, even just to review your notes at a leisurely pace. Your brain needs rest more than it needs to go over the information again. In fact, plan to finish your studies by noon or early afternoon the day before the test. Give your brain the rest of the day to relax or focus on other things, and get a good night's sleep. Then you will be fresh for the test and better able to recall what you've studied.

Step 6: Take a Practice Test

Many courses offer sample tests, either online or in the study materials. This is an excellent resource to check whether you have mastered the material, as well as to prepare for the test format and environment.

Check the test format ahead of time: the number of questions, the type (multiple choice, free response, etc.), and the time limit. Then create a plan for working through them. For example, if you have 30 minutes to take a 60-question test, your limit is 30 seconds per question. Spend less time on the questions you know well so that you can take more time on the difficult ones.

If you have time to take several practice tests, take the first one open book, with no time limit. Work through the questions at your own pace and make sure you fully understand them. Gradually work up to taking a test under test conditions: sit at a desk with all study materials put away and set a timer. Pace yourself to make sure you finish the test with time to spare and go back to check your answers if you have time.

After each test, check your answers. On the questions you missed, be sure you understand why you missed them. Did you misread the question (tests can use tricky wording)? Did you forget the information? Or was it something you hadn't learned? Go back and study any shaky areas that the practice tests reveal.

Taking these tests not only helps with your grade, but also aids in combating test anxiety. If you're already used to the test conditions, you're less likely to worry about it, and working through tests until you're scoring well gives you a confidence boost. Go through the practice tests until you feel comfortable, and then you can go into the test knowing that you're ready for it.

Test Tips

On test day, you should be confident, knowing that you've prepared well and are ready to answer the questions. But aside from preparation, there are several test day strategies you can employ to maximize your performance.

First, as stated before, get a good night's sleep the night before the test (and for several nights before that, if possible). Go into the test with a fresh, alert mind rather than staying up late to study.

Try not to change too much about your normal routine on the day of the test. It's important to eat a nutritious breakfast, but if you normally don't eat breakfast at all, consider eating just a protein bar. If you're a coffee drinker, go ahead and have your normal coffee. Just make sure you time it so that the caffeine doesn't wear off right in the middle of your test. Avoid sugary beverages, and drink enough water to stay hydrated but not so much that you need a restroom break 10 minutes into the test. If your test isn't first thing in the morning, consider going for a walk or doing a light workout before the test to get your blood flowing.

Allow yourself enough time to get ready, and leave for the test with plenty of time to spare so you won't have the anxiety of scrambling to arrive in time. Another reason to be early is to select a good seat. It's helpful to sit away from doors and windows, which can be distracting. Find a good seat, get out your supplies, and settle your mind before the test begins.

When the test begins, start by going over the instructions carefully, even if you already know what to expect. Make sure you avoid any careless mistakes by following the directions.

Then begin working through the questions, pacing yourself as you've practiced. If you're not sure on an answer, don't spend too much time on it, and don't let it shake your confidence. Either skip it and come back later, or eliminate as many wrong answers as possible and guess among the remaining ones. Don't dwell on these questions as you continue—put them out of your mind and focus on what lies ahead.

Be sure to read all of the answer choices, even if you're sure the first one is the right answer. Sometimes you'll find a better one if you keep reading. But don't second-guess yourself if you do immediately know the answer. Your gut instinct is usually right. Don't let test anxiety rob you of the information you know.

If you have time at the end of the test (and if the test format allows), go back and review your answers. Be cautious about changing any, since your first instinct tends to be correct, but make sure you didn't misread any of the questions or accidentally mark the wrong answer choice. Look over any you skipped and make an educated guess.

At the end, leave the test feeling confident. You've done your best, so don't waste time worrying about your performance or wishing you could change anything. Instead, celebrate the successful completion of this test. And finally, use this test to learn how to deal with anxiety even better next time.

Review Video: Test Anxiety
Visit mometrix.com/academy and enter code: 100340

Important Qualification

Not all anxiety is created equal. If your test anxiety is causing major issues in your life beyond the classroom or testing center, or if you are experiencing troubling physical symptoms related to your anxiety, it may be a sign of a serious physiological or psychological condition. If this sounds like your situation, we strongly encourage you to seek professional help.

Online Resources

Due to our efforts to try to keep this book to a manageable length, we've created a link that will give you access to all of your online resources:

mometrix.com/resources719/ccrnneonatal

It's Your Moment, Let's Celebrate It!

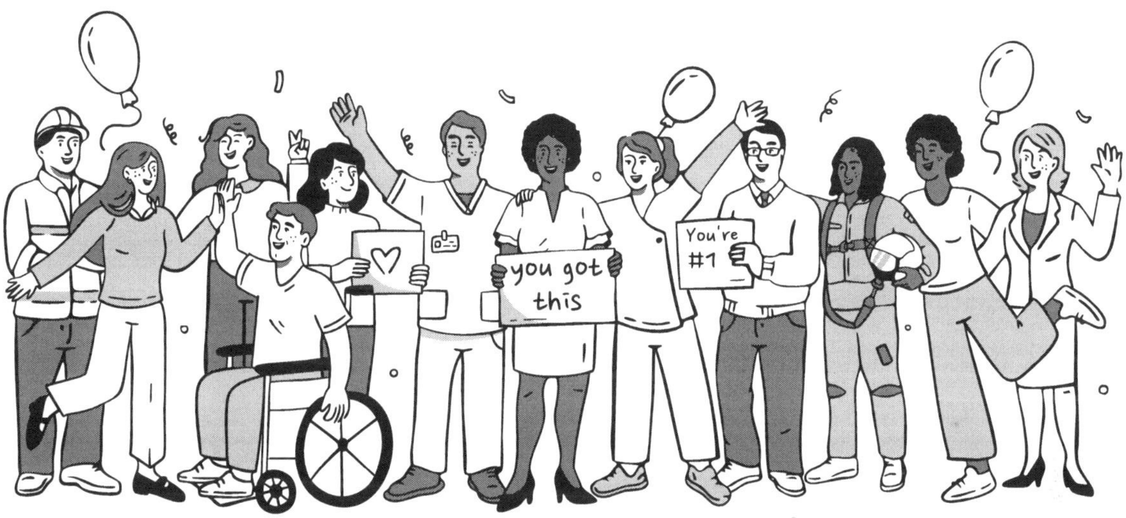

Share your story @mometrixtestpreparation

Mometrix
TEST PREPARATION

Neonatal CCRN® Exam Secrets Study Guide Part 1 of 2

Dear Future Exam Success Story

First of all, **THANK YOU** for purchasing Mometrix study materials!

Second, congratulations! You are one of the few determined test-takers who are committed to doing whatever it takes to excel on your exam. **You have come to the right place.** We developed these study materials with one goal in mind: to deliver you the information you need in a format that's concise and easy to use.

In addition to optimizing your guide for the content of the test, we've outlined our recommended steps for breaking down the preparation process into small, attainable goals so you can make sure you stay on track.

We've also analyzed the entire test-taking process, identifying the most common pitfalls and showing how you can overcome them and be ready for any curveball the test throws you.

Standardized testing is one of the biggest obstacles on your road to success, which only increases the importance of doing well in the high-pressure, high-stakes environment of test day. Your results on this test could have a significant impact on your future, and this guide provides the information and practical advice to help you achieve your full potential on test day.

Your success is our success

We would love to hear from you! If you would like to share the story of your exam success or if you have any questions or comments in regard to our products, please contact us at **800-673-8175** or **support@mometrix.com**.

Thanks again for your business and we wish you continued success!

Sincerely,
The Mometrix Test Preparation Team

Need more help? Check out our flashcards at:
http://MometrixFlashcards.com/CCRN

Written and edited by the Mometrix Exam Secrets Test Prep Team
Printed in the United States of America

TABLE OF CONTENTS

Introduction

Thank you for purchasing this resource! You have made the choice to prepare yourself for a test that could have a huge impact on your future, and this guide is designed to help you be fully ready for test day. Obviously, it's important to have a solid understanding of the test material, but you also need to be prepared for the unique environment and stressors of the test, so that you can perform to the best of your abilities.

For this purpose, the first section that appears in this guide is the **Secret Keys**. We've devoted countless hours to meticulously researching what works and what doesn't, and we've boiled down our findings to the five most impactful steps you can take to improve your performance on the test. We start at the beginning with study planning and move through the preparation process, all the way to the testing strategies that will help you get the most out of what you know when you're finally sitting in front of the test.

We recommend that you start preparing for your test as far in advance as possible. However, if you've bought this guide as a last-minute study resource and only have a few days before your test, we recommend that you skip over the first two Secret Keys since they address a long-term study plan.

If you struggle with **test anxiety**, we strongly encourage you to check out our recommendations for how you can overcome it. Test anxiety is a formidable foe, but it can be beaten, and we want to make sure you have the tools you need to defeat it.

Secret Key #1 – Plan Big, Study Small

There's a lot riding on your performance. If you want to ace this test, you're going to need to keep your skills sharp and the material fresh in your mind. You need a plan that lets you review everything you need to know while still fitting in your schedule. We'll break this strategy down into three categories.

Information Organization

Start with the information you already have: the official test outline. From this, you can make a complete list of all the concepts you need to cover before the test. Organize these concepts into groups that can be studied together, and create a list of any related vocabulary you need to learn so you can brush up on any difficult terms. You'll want to keep this vocabulary list handy once you actually start studying since you may need to add to it along the way.

Time Management

Once you have your set of study concepts, decide how to spread them out over the time you have left before the test. Break your study plan into small, clear goals so you have a manageable task for each day and know exactly what you're doing. Then just focus on one small step at a time. When you manage your time this way, you don't need to spend hours at a time studying. Studying a small block of content for a short period each day helps you retain information better and avoid stressing over how much you have left to do. You can relax knowing that you have a plan to cover everything in time. In order for this strategy to be effective though, you have to start studying early and stick to your schedule. Avoid the exhaustion and futility that comes from last-minute cramming!

Study Environment

The environment you study in has a big impact on your learning. Studying in a coffee shop, while probably more enjoyable, is not likely to be as fruitful as studying in a quiet room. It's important to keep distractions to a minimum. You're only planning to study for a short block of time, so make the most of it. Don't pause to check your phone or get up to find a snack. It's also important to **avoid multitasking**. Research has consistently shown that multitasking will make your studying dramatically less effective. Your study area should also be comfortable and well-lit so you don't have the distraction of straining your eyes or sitting on an uncomfortable chair.

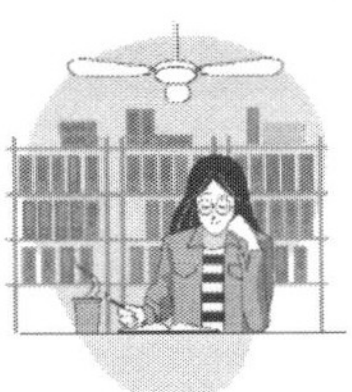

The time of day you study is also important. You want to be rested and alert. Don't wait until just before bedtime. Study when you'll be most likely to comprehend and remember. Even better, if you know what time of day your test will be, set that time aside for study. That way your brain will be used to working on that subject at that specific time and you'll have a better chance of recalling information.

Finally, it can be helpful to team up with others who are studying for the same test. Your actual studying should be done in as isolated an environment as possible, but the work of organizing the information and setting up the study plan can be divided up. In between study sessions, you can discuss with your teammates the concepts that you're all studying and quiz each other on the details. Just be sure that your teammates are as serious about the test as you are. If you find that your study time is being replaced with social time, you might need to find a new team.

Secret Key #2 – Make Your Studying Count

You're devoting a lot of time and effort to preparing for this test, so you want to be absolutely certain it will pay off. This means doing more than just reading the content and hoping you can remember it on test day. It's important to make every minute of study count. There are two main areas you can focus on to make your studying count.

Retention

It doesn't matter how much time you study if you can't remember the material. You need to make sure you are retaining the concepts. To check your retention of the information you're learning, try recalling it at later times with minimal prompting. Try carrying around flashcards and glance at one or two from time to time or ask a friend who's also studying for the test to quiz you.

To enhance your retention, look for ways to put the information into practice so that you can apply it rather than simply recalling it. If you're using the information in practical ways, it will be much easier to remember. Similarly, it helps to solidify a concept in your mind if you're not only reading it to yourself but also explaining it to someone else. Ask a friend to let you teach them about a concept you're a little shaky on (or speak aloud to an imaginary audience if necessary). As you try to summarize, define, give examples, and answer your friend's questions, you'll understand the concepts better and they will stay with you longer. Finally, step back for a big picture view and ask yourself how each piece of information fits with the whole subject. When you link the different concepts together and see them working together as a whole, it's easier to remember the individual components.

Finally, practice showing your work on any multi-step problems, even if you're just studying. Writing out each step you take to solve a problem will help solidify the process in your mind, and you'll be more likely to remember it during the test.

Modality

Modality simply refers to the means or method by which you study. Choosing a study modality that fits your own individual learning style is crucial. No two people learn best in exactly the same way, so it's important to know your strengths and use them to your advantage.

For example, if you learn best by visualization, focus on visualizing a concept in your mind and draw an image or a diagram. Try color-coding your notes, illustrating them, or creating symbols that will trigger your mind to recall a learned concept. If you learn best by hearing or discussing information, find a study partner who learns the same way or read aloud to yourself. Think about how to put the information in your own words. Imagine that you are giving a lecture on the topic and record yourself so you can listen to it later.

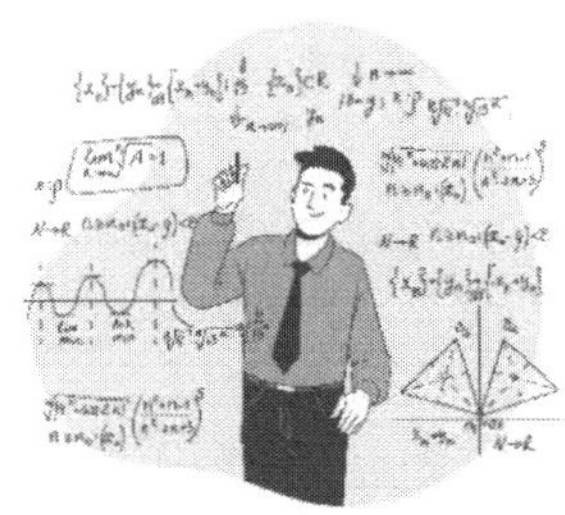

For any learning style, flashcards can be helpful. Organize the information so you can take advantage of spare moments to review. Underline key words or phrases. Use different colors for different categories. Mnemonic devices (such as creating a short list in which every item starts with the same letter) can also help with retention. Find what works best for you and use it to store the information in your mind most effectively and easily.

Secret Key #3 – Practice the Right Way

Your success on test day depends not only on how many hours you put into preparing, but also on whether you prepared the right way. It's good to check along the way to see if your studying is paying off. One of the most effective ways to do this is by taking practice tests to evaluate your progress. Practice tests are useful because they show exactly where you need to improve. Every time you take a practice test, pay special attention to these three groups of questions:

- The questions you got wrong
- The questions you had to guess on, even if you guessed right
- The questions you found difficult or slow to work through

This will show you exactly what your weak areas are, and where you need to devote more study time. Ask yourself why each of these questions gave you trouble. Was it because you didn't understand the material? Was it because you didn't remember the vocabulary? Do you need more repetitions on this type of question to build speed and confidence? Dig into those questions and figure out how you can strengthen your weak areas as you go back to review the material.

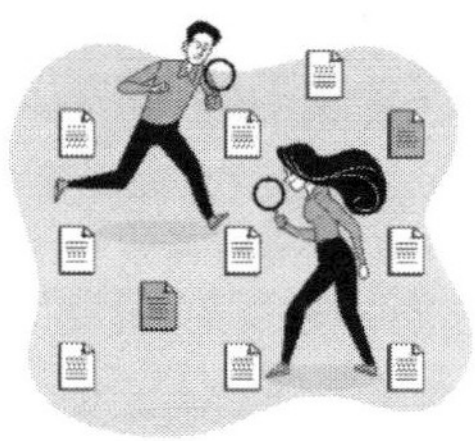

Additionally, many practice tests have a section explaining the answer choices. It can be tempting to read the explanation and think that you now have a good understanding of the concept. However, an explanation likely only covers part of the question's broader context. Even if the explanation makes perfect sense, **go back and investigate** every concept related to the question until you're positive you have a thorough understanding.

As you go along, keep in mind that the practice test is just that: practice. Memorizing these questions and answers will not be very helpful on the actual test because it is unlikely to have any of the same exact questions. If you only know the right answers to the sample questions, you won't be prepared for the real thing. **Study the concepts** until you understand them fully, and then you'll be able to answer any question that shows up on the test.

It's important to wait on the practice tests until you're ready. If you take a test on your first day of study, you may be overwhelmed by the amount of material covered and how much you need to learn. Work up to it gradually.

On test day, you'll need to be prepared for answering questions, managing your time, and using the test-taking strategies you've learned. It's a lot to balance, like a mental marathon that will have a big impact on your future. Like training for a marathon, you'll need to start slowly and work your way up. When test day arrives, you'll be ready.

Start with the strategies you've read in the first two Secret Keys—plan your course and study in the way that works best for you. If you have time, consider using multiple study resources to get different approaches to the same concepts. It can be helpful to see difficult concepts from more than one angle. Then find a good source for practice tests. Many times, the test website will suggest potential study resources or provide sample tests.

Practice Test Strategy

If you're able to find at least three practice tests, we recommend this strategy:

Untimed and Open-Book Practice

Take the first test with no time constraints and with your notes and study guide handy. Take your time and focus on applying the strategies you've learned.

Timed and Open-Book Practice

Take the second practice test open-book as well, but set a timer and practice pacing yourself to finish in time.

Timed and Closed-Book Practice

Take any other practice tests as if it were test day. Set a timer and put away your study materials. Sit at a table or desk in a quiet room, imagine yourself at the testing center, and answer questions as quickly and accurately as possible.

Keep repeating timed and closed-book tests on a regular basis until you run out of practice tests or it's time for the actual test. Your mind will be ready for the schedule and stress of test day, and you'll be able to focus on recalling the material you've learned.

Secret Key #4 – Pace Yourself

Once you're fully prepared for the material on the test, your biggest challenge on test day will be managing your time. Just knowing that the clock is ticking can make you panic even if you have plenty of time left. Work on pacing yourself so you can build confidence against the time constraints of the exam. Pacing is a difficult skill to master, especially in a high-pressure environment, so **practice is vital**.

Set time expectations for your pace based on how much time is available. For example, if a section has 60 questions and the time limit is 30 minutes, you know you have to average 30 seconds or less per question in order to answer them all. Although 30 seconds is the hard limit, set 25 seconds per question as your goal, so you reserve extra time to spend on harder questions. When you budget extra time for the harder questions, you no longer have any reason to stress when those questions take longer to answer.

Don't let this time expectation distract you from working through the test at a calm, steady pace, but keep it in mind so you don't spend too much time on any one question. Recognize that taking extra time on one question you don't understand may keep you from answering two that you do understand later in the test. If your time limit for a question is up and you're still not sure of the answer, mark it and move on, and come back to it later if the time and the test format allow. If the testing format doesn't allow you to return to earlier questions, just make an educated guess; then put it out of your mind and move on.

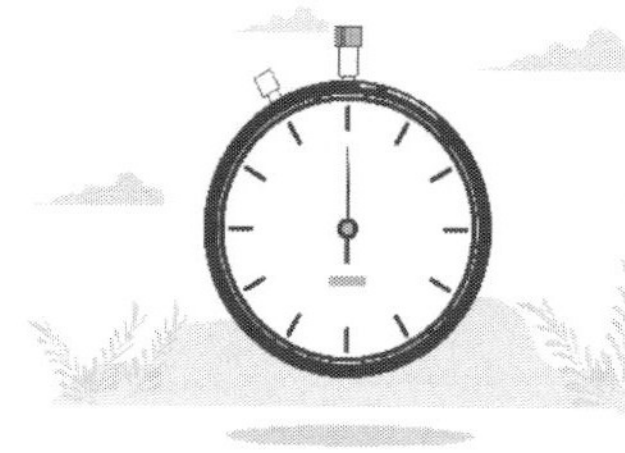

On the easier questions, be careful not to rush. It may seem wise to hurry through them so you have more time for the challenging ones, but it's not worth missing one if you know the concept and just didn't take the time to read the question fully. Work efficiently but make sure you understand the question and have looked at all of the answer choices, since more than one may seem right at first.

Even if you're paying attention to the time, you may find yourself a little behind at some point. You should speed up to get back on track, but do so wisely. Don't panic; just take a few seconds less on each question until you're caught up. Don't guess without thinking, but do look through the answer choices and eliminate any you know are wrong. If you can get down to two choices, it is often worthwhile to guess from those. Once you've chosen an answer, move on and don't dwell on any that you skipped or had to hurry through. If a question was taking too long, chances are it was one of the harder ones, so you weren't as likely to get it right anyway.

On the other hand, if you find yourself getting ahead of schedule, it may be beneficial to slow down a little. The more quickly you work, the more likely you are to make a careless mistake that will affect your score. You've budgeted time for each question, so don't be afraid to spend that time. Practice an efficient but careful pace to get the most out of the time you have.

Secret Key #5 – Have a Plan for Guessing

When you're taking the test, you may find yourself stuck on a question. Some of the answer choices seem better than others, but you don't see the one answer choice that is obviously correct. What do you do?

The scenario described above is very common, yet most test takers have not effectively prepared for it. Developing and practicing a plan for guessing may be one of the single most effective uses of your time as you get ready for the exam.

In developing your plan for guessing, there are three questions to address:

- When should you start the guessing process?
- How should you narrow down the choices?
- Which answer should you choose?

When to Start the Guessing Process

Unless your plan for guessing is to select C every time (which, despite its merits, is not what we recommend), you need to leave yourself enough time to apply your answer elimination strategies. Since you have a limited amount of time for each question, that means that if you're going to give yourself the best shot at guessing correctly, you have to decide quickly whether or not you will guess.

Of course, the best-case scenario is that you don't have to guess at all, so first, see if you can answer the question based on your knowledge of the subject and basic reasoning skills. Focus on the key words in the question and try to jog your memory of related topics. Give yourself a chance to bring the knowledge to mind, but once you realize that you don't have (or you can't access) the knowledge you need to answer the question, it's time to start the guessing process.

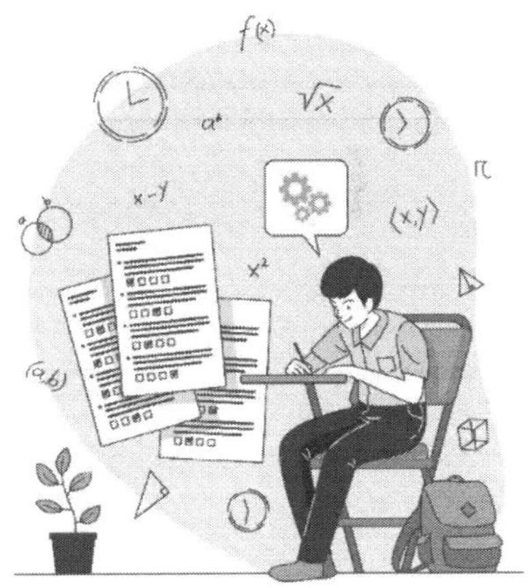

It's almost always better to start the guessing process too early than too late. It only takes a few seconds to remember something and answer the question from knowledge. Carefully eliminating wrong answer choices takes longer. Plus, going through the process of eliminating answer choices can actually help jog your memory.

Summary: Start the guessing process as soon as you decide that you can't answer the question based on your knowledge.

How to Narrow Down the Choices

The next chapter in this book (**Test-Taking Strategies**) includes a wide range of strategies for how to approach questions and how to look for answer choices to eliminate. You will definitely want to read those carefully, practice them, and figure out which ones work best for you. Here though, we're going to address a mindset rather than a particular strategy.

Your odds of guessing an answer correctly depend on how many options you are choosing from.

Number of options left	5	4	3	2	1
Odds of guessing correctly	20%	25%	33%	50%	100%

You can see from this chart just how valuable it is to be able to eliminate incorrect answers and make an educated guess, but there are two things that many test takers do that cause them to miss out on the benefits of guessing:

- Accidentally eliminating the correct answer
- Selecting an answer based on an impression

We'll look at the first one here, and the second one in the next section.

To avoid accidentally eliminating the correct answer, we recommend a thought exercise called **the $5 challenge**. In this challenge, you only eliminate an answer choice from contention if you are willing to bet $5 on it being wrong. Why $5? Five dollars is a small but not insignificant amount of money. It's an amount you could afford to lose but wouldn't want to throw away. And while losing $5 once might not hurt too much, doing it twenty times will set you back $100. In the same way, each small decision you make—eliminating a choice here, guessing on a question there—won't by itself impact your score very much, but when you put them all together, they can make a big difference. By holding each answer choice elimination decision to a higher standard, you can reduce the risk of accidentally eliminating the correct answer.

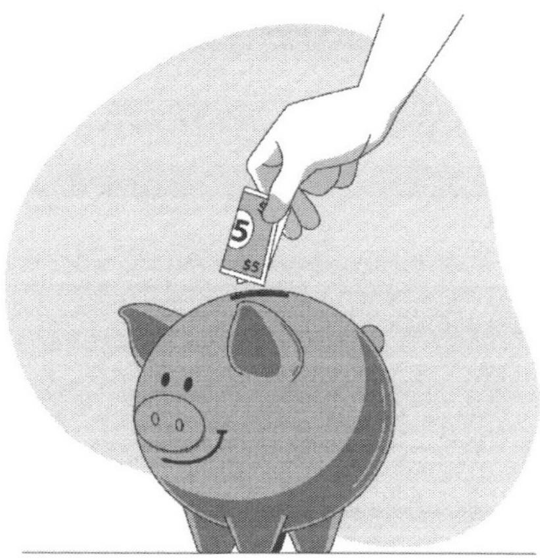

The $5 challenge can also be applied in a positive sense: If you are willing to bet $5 that an answer choice *is* correct, go ahead and mark it as correct.

Summary: Only eliminate an answer choice if you are willing to bet $5 that it is wrong.

Which Answer to Choose

You're taking the test. You've run into a hard question and decided you'll have to guess. You've eliminated all the answer choices you're willing to bet $5 on. Now you have to pick an answer. Why do we even need to talk about this? Why can't you just pick whichever one you feel like when the time comes?

The answer to these questions is that if you don't come into the test with a plan, you'll rely on your impression to select an answer choice, and if you do that, you risk falling into a trap. The test writers know that everyone who takes their test will be guessing on some of the questions, so they intentionally write wrong answer choices to seem plausible. You still have to pick an answer though, and if the wrong answer choices are designed to look right, how can you ever be sure that you're not falling for their trap? The best solution we've found to this dilemma is to take the decision out of your hands entirely. Here is the process we recommend:

Once you've eliminated any choices that you are confident (willing to bet $5) are wrong, select the first remaining choice as your answer.

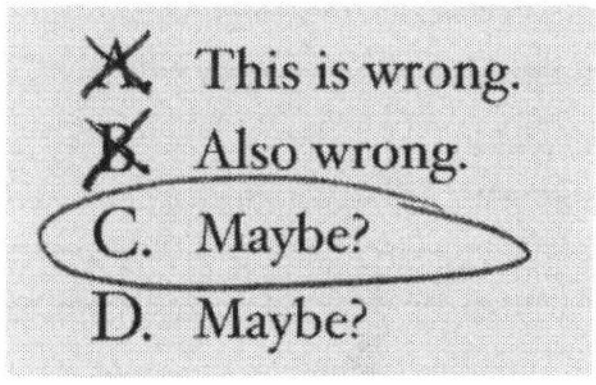

Whether you choose to select the first remaining choice, the second, or the last, the important thing is that you use some preselected standard. Using this approach guarantees that you will not be enticed into selecting an answer choice that looks right, because you are not basing your decision on how the answer choices look.

This is not meant to make you question your knowledge. Instead, it is to help you recognize the difference between your knowledge and your impressions. There's a huge difference between thinking an answer is right because of what you know, and thinking an answer is right because it looks or sounds like it should be right.

Summary: To ensure that your selection is appropriately random, make a predetermined selection from among all answer choices you have not eliminated.

Test-Taking Strategies

This section contains a list of test-taking strategies that you may find helpful as you work through the test. By taking what you know and applying logical thought, you can maximize your chances of answering any question correctly!

It is very important to realize that every question is different and every person is different: no single strategy will work on every question, and no single strategy will work for every person. That's why we've included all of them here, so you can try them out and determine which ones work best for different types of questions and which ones work best for you.

Question Strategies

✓ Read Carefully

Read the question and the answer choices carefully. Don't miss the question because you misread the terms. You have plenty of time to read each question thoroughly and make sure you understand what is being asked. Yet a happy medium must be attained, so don't waste too much time. You must read carefully and efficiently.

✓ Contextual Clues

Look for contextual clues. If the question includes a word you are not familiar with, look at the immediate context for some indication of what the word might mean. Contextual clues can often give you all the information you need to decipher the meaning of an unfamiliar word. Even if you can't determine the meaning, you may be able to narrow down the possibilities enough to make a solid guess at the answer to the question.

✓ Prefixes

If you're having trouble with a word in the question or answer choices, try dissecting it. Take advantage of every clue that the word might include. Prefixes can be a huge help. Usually, they allow you to determine a basic meaning. *Pre-* means before, *post-* means after, *pro-* is positive, *de-* is negative. From prefixes, you can get an idea of the general meaning of the word and try to put it into context.

✓ Hedge Words

Watch out for critical hedge words, such as *likely, may, can, often, almost, mostly, usually, generally, rarely*, and *sometimes*. Question writers insert these hedge phrases to cover every possibility. Often an answer choice will be wrong simply because it leaves no room for exception. Be on guard for answer choices that have definitive words such as *exactly* and *always*.

✓ Switchback Words

Stay alert for *switchbacks*. These are the words and phrases frequently used to alert you to shifts in thought. The most common switchback words are *but, although*, and *however*. Others include *nevertheless, on the other hand, even though, while, in spite of, despite*, and *regardless of*. Switchback words are important to catch because they can change the direction of the question or an answer choice.

✓ FACE VALUE

When in doubt, use common sense. Accept the situation in the problem at face value. Don't read too much into it. These problems will not require you to make wild assumptions. If you have to go beyond creativity and warp time or space in order to have an answer choice fit the question, then you should move on and consider the other answer choices. These are normal problems rooted in reality. The applicable relationship or explanation may not be readily apparent, but it is there for you to figure out. Use your common sense to interpret anything that isn't clear.

Answer Choice Strategies

✓ ANSWER SELECTION

The most thorough way to pick an answer choice is to identify and eliminate wrong answers until only one is left, then confirm it is the correct answer. Sometimes an answer choice may immediately seem right, but be careful. The test writers will usually put more than one reasonable answer choice on each question, so take a second to read all of them and make sure that the other choices are not equally obvious. As long as you have time left, it is better to read every answer choice than to pick the first one that looks right without checking the others.

✓ ANSWER CHOICE FAMILIES

An answer choice family consists of two (in rare cases, three) answer choices that are very similar in construction and cannot all be true at the same time. If you see two answer choices that are direct opposites or parallels, one of them is usually the correct answer. For instance, if one answer choice says that quantity *x* increases and another either says that quantity *x* decreases (opposite) or says that quantity *y* increases (parallel), then those answer choices would fall into the same family. An answer choice that doesn't match the construction of the answer choice family is more likely to be incorrect. Most questions will not have answer choice families, but when they do appear, you should be prepared to recognize them.

✓ ELIMINATE ANSWERS

Eliminate answer choices as soon as you realize they are wrong, but make sure you consider all possibilities. If you are eliminating answer choices and realize that the last one you are left with is also wrong, don't panic. Start over and consider each choice again. There may be something you missed the first time that you will realize on the second pass.

✓ AVOID FACT TRAPS

Don't be distracted by an answer choice that is factually true but doesn't answer the question. You are looking for the choice that answers the question. Stay focused on what the question is asking for so you don't accidentally pick an answer that is true but incorrect. Always go back to the question and make sure the answer choice you've selected actually answers the question and is not merely a true statement.

✓ EXTREME STATEMENTS

In general, you should avoid answers that put forth extreme actions as standard practice or proclaim controversial ideas as established fact. An answer choice that states the "process should be used in certain situations, if..." is much more likely to be correct than one that states the "process should be discontinued completely." The first is a calm rational statement and doesn't even make a definitive, uncompromising stance, using a hedge word *if* to provide wiggle room, whereas the second choice is far more extreme.

⊘ BENCHMARK

As you read through the answer choices and you come across one that seems to answer the question well, mentally select that answer choice. This is not your final answer, but it's the one that will help you evaluate the other answer choices. The one that you selected is your benchmark or standard for judging each of the other answer choices. Every other answer choice must be compared to your benchmark. That choice is correct until proven otherwise by another answer choice beating it. If you find a better answer, then that one becomes your new benchmark. Once you've decided that no other choice answers the question as well as your benchmark, you have your final answer.

⊘ PREDICT THE ANSWER

Before you even start looking at the answer choices, it is often best to try to predict the answer. When you come up with the answer on your own, it is easier to avoid distractions and traps because you will know exactly what to look for. The right answer choice is unlikely to be word-for-word what you came up with, but it should be a close match. Even if you are confident that you have the right answer, you should still take the time to read each option before moving on.

General Strategies

⊘ TOUGH QUESTIONS

If you are stumped on a problem or it appears too hard or too difficult, don't waste time. Move on! Remember though, if you can quickly check for obviously incorrect answer choices, your chances of guessing correctly are greatly improved. Before you completely give up, at least try to knock out a couple of possible answers. Eliminate what you can and then guess at the remaining answer choices before moving on.

⊘ CHECK YOUR WORK

Since you will probably not know every term listed and the answer to every question, it is important that you get credit for the ones that you do know. Don't miss any questions through careless mistakes. If at all possible, try to take a second to look back over your answer selection and make sure you've selected the correct answer choice and haven't made a costly careless mistake (such as marking an answer choice that you didn't mean to mark). This quick double check should more than pay for itself in caught mistakes for the time it costs.

⊘ PACE YOURSELF

It's easy to be overwhelmed when you're looking at a page full of questions; your mind is confused and full of random thoughts, and the clock is ticking down faster than you would like. Calm down and maintain the pace that you have set for yourself. Especially as you get down to the last few minutes of the test, don't let the small numbers on the clock make you panic. As long as you are on track by monitoring your pace, you are guaranteed to have time for each question.

⊘ DON'T RUSH

It is very easy to make errors when you are in a hurry. Maintaining a fast pace in answering questions is pointless if it makes you miss questions that you would have gotten right otherwise. Test writers like to include distracting information and wrong answers that seem right. Taking a little extra time to avoid careless mistakes can make all the difference in your test score. Find a pace that allows you to be confident in the answers that you select.

✓ Keep Moving

Panicking will not help you pass the test, so do your best to stay calm and keep moving. Taking deep breaths and going through the answer elimination steps you practiced can help to break through a stress barrier and keep your pace.

Final Notes

The combination of a solid foundation of content knowledge and the confidence that comes from practicing your plan for applying that knowledge is the key to maximizing your performance on test day. As your foundation of content knowledge is built up and strengthened, you'll find that the strategies included in this chapter become more and more effective in helping you quickly sift through the distractions and traps of the test to isolate the correct answer.

Now that you're preparing to move forward into the test content chapters of this book, be sure to keep your goal in mind. As you read, think about how you will be able to apply this information on the test. If you've already seen sample questions for the test and you have an idea of the question format and style, try to come up with questions of your own that you can answer based on what you're reading. This will give you valuable practice applying your knowledge in the same ways you can expect to on test day.

Good luck and good studying!

Clinical Judgment: General

Gestational Age Assessment

Estimating Gestational Age

Accurate determination of gestational age (GA) predicts neonatal morbidity and mortality. Compare GA with the birth weight to determine if the patient is large or small for GA. Respiratory distress syndrome affects 1% of neonates. The prognosis for a premature infant with respiratory distress who is an appropriate weight for GA (e.g., 33 weeks and 2,000 grams), is better than the prognosis for a full term, small for gestational age (SGA) baby (e.g. 40 weeks and 2,000 grams). These infants have identical birth weights, but the SGA baby is more likely to require mechanical ventilation and has a greater chance of mortality.

The obstetrician **calculates prenatal GA** throughout a pregnancy by the:

- Reported date of last menstrual period (LMP)
- Periodic physical examinations of the mother
- Ultrasound examinations of the fetus
- Date the fetal heartbeat is first heard
- Date fetal movements are first felt (quickening)

The **Modified Ballard examination** is the first comprehensive postnatal test of the neonate, and when scored correctly, it gives a very accurate estimate of the GA.

Initial Methods for Gestational Age Estimation

The initial marker for measuring gestational age is the date of the last menstrual period (LMP). Various calculators are available for this, but they are limited by both the reliability of the mother's report of the dates of her LMP and the typical variability in menstrual periods and ovulatory times. Ultrasound that utilizes various measurements of fetal dimensions is a more accurate method of estimating gestational age. Ultrasound is most accurate during the first trimester, when it has been shown to have a 95% accuracy of ±6 days. As the fetus grows, its size becomes more dependent on the environment, rather than the date of conception, making ultrasound dating during the second and third trimesters less accurate. Clinical examination by the obstetrician is less accurate in determining gestational age than ultrasound.

Modified Ballard Score Overview

The Modified Ballard Score is used to estimate **maturity and gestational age** in newborn infants. It is most reliable when performed within the first 12 hours of life. The Ballard Score was modified to include evaluation of extremely premature infants with gestational ages as low as 20 weeks (score 10) and as high as 50 weeks (score 44). It scores 6 measurements of **neuromuscular maturity** and 6 signs of **physical maturity** on a scale of -1 to +4 or +5, depending upon the category. The total score indicates the estimated gestational age for the infant.

Neuromuscular Measurements

- Observation of the **infant's posture** while lying supine indicates the total amount of muscle tone the infant possesses. Increased amounts of flexion of the elbows and knees correlates with increased gestational age.

- **Square window test** measures the resistance to stretching of extensor muscles in the infant's forearm. Increased ability for the tester to flex the infant's wrist correlates with greater gestational age.
- **Arm recoil test** measures the tone of the biceps muscle. Increased amount of arm recoil (flexion by the infant after the infant's arms are extended) correlates with greater gestational age.
- **Popliteal angle measurement** assesses the flexor tone of the knee joint. Increased resistance to flexion at the knee is associated with greater gestational age.
- **Scarf sign test** measures the tone of shoulder flexor muscles. Increased resistance to movement of the infant's arm across the chest is associated with greater gestational age.
- **Heel-to-ear test** measures the tone of pelvic girdle muscles. Increased resistance to movement of the infant's foot to its ear is associated with greater gestational age.

Physical Signs of Maturity

- **Skin**: Immature infants have thin, transparent skin. The vernix caseosa begins development at the beginning of the third trimester. Dried, cracked skin occurs as this protective coating disappears after the fortieth week.
- **Lanugo**: Fine, usually unpigmented hairs begin to appear at 24-25 weeks of gestation and thin as the neonate matures.
- **Plantar surface of feet:** Very immature infants have no creases on the soles of their feet. Creases develop first on the anterior portion, and more mature infants will have creases over the entire sole.
- **Breast buds**: These are fatty tissue underneath the areola which increase in size as the fetus matures.
- **Ears**: Increased cartilage content produces a more rigid pinna; ear recoil increases as the infant matures.
- **Genitalia**
    - **Male**: The testes descend from the abdomen into the scrotum at 30 weeks of gestation, and the scrotum develops rugae as the fetus matures.
    - **Female**: Initially, the female fetus has a large clitoris and small labia majora. As the fetus matures, the labia majora enlarge, while the clitoris shrinks.

Preterm Infant

A preterm infant is one born prior to 37 weeks gestational age. In the United States, preterm birth is the most important factor influencing infant mortality; preterm infants account for 75-80% of all neonatal morbidity and mortality. **Health problems associated with premature birth** include:

- Respiratory distress syndrome because of inadequate surfactant production (hyaline membrane disease)
- Hypothermia because of inadequate subcutaneous fat, small amounts of brown fat, and large skin surface area to mass ratio
- Hypoglycemia secondary to poor nutritional intake, poor nutritional stores, and increased glucose consumption associated with sepsis
- Skin trauma or infection secondary to fragile, immature skin
- Periods of apnea because of an immature respiratory center in the brain
- Intraventricular hemorrhage

The original cause of the preterm birth (such as maternal infection) may also play an integral role in the likely health problem associated with prematurity.

Characteristics of Late Preterm Infants

Late preterm infants are those born between 34 weeks 0 days and 36 weeks 6 days of gestation. These infants are often similar in size and appearance to full-term infants but have needs similar to those of other preterm infants because of the immaturity of their organ systems. Common characteristics include:

- **Respiratory disorders**: Increased risk of respiratory distress syndrome and transient tachypnea of the newborn; may need oxygen via nasal cannula or continuous positive airway pressure to support respiratory function.
- **Feeding difficulties**: Poor suck-swallow coordination, weak latch, increased risk of hypoglycemia because of inadequate intake; may need fortified formula or expressed milk. Feedings should be every 2–3 hours, and intake is closely monitored. Need frequent blood glucose monitoring.
- **Thermoregulatory disorders**: Prone to hypothermia because of immature skin and fat stores. Usually need kangaroo care, a radiant warmer, or an incubator.
- **Infection risk**: Immature immune system. Need temperature checks every 3 to 4 hours and observation for signs of infection, sepsis.
- **Neurological impairment**: System immature, brain is 65% the size of a full-term infant, prone to apnea, poor muscle tone, irritability, increased risk for long-term developmental delays. Need careful observation and assessment.
- **Hyperbilirubinemia**: Immature liver and increased turnover of red blood cells. Need frequent bilirubin counts and may need phototherapy. Exchange transfusions are rarely needed.

Characteristics of Preterm Infants Born at 24-25 Weeks

Characteristics of preterm infants born at 24-25 weeks include the following:

- **Skin**: very thin with visible veins; absent or minimal vernix caseosa as it is just beginning to be secreted at 2 weeks
- **Lanugo**: sparse
- **Feet**: smooth plantar surfaces or faint marks on the anterior surfaces
- **Areolae**: newly developing, breast bud not yet present
- **Eyes**: open
- **Ears**: no or very limited recoil
- **Posture**: immature, indicated by limited flexion of the limbs while the infant is in a supine position
- **Square window sign**: shows decreased flexion at the wrist of approximately 60-90°
- **Range of motion**: increased ROM (lone tone) when performing the popliteal angle, scarf sign, and heel to ear examinations
- **Arm recoil**: limited or no recoil

Neuromuscular Characteristics of Full-Term Infants

Neuromuscular characteristics of full-term infants include the following:

- **Supine resting posture**: hips, knees, and arms all flexed past 90°, indicating mature muscular tone
- **Square window**: wrist flexes to 0°, reflecting very little resistance to the extensor muscles of the wrist

- **Arm recoil**: arms recoil past 90°; contact between the infant's fist and face demonstrates mature tone in the biceps muscles
- **Popliteal angle**: <90° knee flexion
- **Scarf sign**: the arms cannot be drawn past the ipsilateral axillary line because of the mature tone of the posterior shoulder girdle flexor muscles
- **Heel to ear**: resistance is felt in the knee and hip when the heel is at the femoral crease because of the tone of the posterior pelvic girdle flexor muscles

Characteristics of Postterm Infants

Postterm infants are those born >42 weeks of gestation. Many are normal in size and appearance, but some continue to grow *in utero* and weigh >4000 g. Some may exhibit post-maturity syndrome (about 5%), which puts the infant at increased risk. **Characteristics** include:

- **Appearance**: alert (this may indicate intrauterine hypoxia)
- **Skin**: loose, dry, cracking, parchment-like, and lacking lanugo or vernix; may have meconium staining, yellow to green (indicating recent meconium release)
- **Fingernails**: long (sometimes with meconium staining)
- **Scalp hair**: long and thick
- **Body**: long and thin (fat layers absent)
- **Hypoglycemia** from nutritional deprivation
- **Hypothermia** due to decreased brown fat and liver glycogen
- **Meconium aspiration** (risk increases with oligohydramnios), increasing risk of impaired gas exchange
- **Polycythemia** as response to hypoxia, increasing risk of impaired tissue perfusion
- **Seizures** resulting from hypoxia
- **Cold stress** (lack of fat stores)
- **Congenital anomalies**

Birth Weight and Gestational Age Acronyms

These terms do not take into account the estimated gestational age of the infant:

- **ELBW (Extremely Low Birth Weight)**: birth weight of less than 1,000 g (2.2 lb)
- **VLBW (Very Low Birth Weight)**: birth weight of less than 1,500 grams (3.3 lb)

The following terms take into account the estimated gestational age of the infant in comparison to the birth weight:

- **SGA (small for gestational age)**: below the tenth percentile for gestational age
- **AGA (appropriate for gestational age)**: between the tenth and ninetieth percentiles for gestational age
- **LGA (large for gestational age)**: above the ninetieth percentile for gestational age

SGA

Small for gestational age (SGA) infants are those whose weight places them below the 10th percentile for their gestational age. SGA is also called dysmaturity and intrauterine growth restriction. SGA babies commonly aspirate meconium and have a low APGAR score, asphyxia, hypoglycemia, and polycythemia. Common **causes of SGA** include:

- Multiple gestation (twins, triplets, quadruplets)
- Constitutional SGA because both parents are small
- Many genetic defects, such as trisomy 18 (Edwards syndrome), Down syndrome, and Turner syndrome
- Placental malfunction or misplacement (inadequate fetal nutrition from reduced blood flow, sepsis, placenta previa, or abruptio placentae)
- Maternal disease (pre-eclampsia; high blood pressure; malnutrition; advanced diabetes mellitus; chronic kidney, heart, or respiratory disease; and anemia)
- Infections such as cytomegalovirus, toxoplasmosis, and rubella
- Maternal tobacco, illegal drug, or alcohol use during pregnancy
- Birth defects

LGA

Large for gestational age (LGA) infants are those whose weight places them above the 90th percentile for their gestational age. The main pathologic cause for LGA is maternal diabetes (either gestational diabetes or diabetes mellitus). Infants exposed to elevated levels of glucose produce elevated amounts of insulin, which has an anabolic effect on the developing fetus, causing macrosomia (large body). Poor control of diabetes during pregnancy generally results in a larger infant with these **common health problems**:

- Delivery complications (shoulder dystocia, clavicle fracture, prolonged vaginal exit requiring use of forceps or Cesarian section, and perinatal asphyxia)
- Abnormal blood test results (hypoglycemia developing within 1-2 hours of birth, hyperbilirubinemia, hypocalcemia, hypomagnesemia, hyperviscosity [thickened blood] secondary to polycythemia [elevated hemoglobin])
- Jaundice
- Feeding intolerance
- Lethargy
- Respiratory distress
- Birth defects

Intrauterine Growth Restriction

When a fetus does not fulfill his or her growth potential for any reason, the diagnosis is **intrauterine growth restriction (IUGR)**. Prenatal ultrasound is used to diagnose IUGR, which is associated with oligohydramnios (decreased amniotic fluid) and preeclampsia (pregnancy-induced hypertension and proteinuria). IUGR is classified as symmetric or asymmetric, based on the size of the newborn's head:

- **Symmetric IUGR**
    - Both head and body are small (growth-restricted).
    - The restriction occurs early in pregnancy.
    - Common causes are chromosomal abnormalities and infections.
- **Asymmetric IUGR**
    - The head is large in proportion to the body; the head is spared.
    - The head is normal in size for gestational age, while the body is growth-restricted.
    - Restriction occurs late in pregnancy.
    - Common causes include placental insufficiency and preeclampsia.

Physical Assessment

Physical Assessment

The neonate should undergo three different types of physical assessment:

- **Immediate**: The first examination is done in the delivery room to determine the need for resuscitation or other intervention. This includes the APGAR assessment.
- **1-4 hours after birth**: The second examination includes gestational age assessment, which must be completed within 24 hours for accuracy, and brief physical assessment to determine if there are any problems that might place the infant at risk. This includes assessment of respiratory and cardiac status, cord color, skin color, and movement. The Modified Ballard scoring system is often used.
- **≥24 hours after birth (or prior to discharge)**: The final examination should include a complete physical and behavioral assessment that includes all systems and evaluation of reflexes. All weights and measurements are taken and reviewed. This exam requires observation, palpation, and auscultation. In some cases, instead of a separate examination at 1-4 hours, only this complete physical examination is completed.

Rapid Assessment

The infant should be given a rapid assessment within seconds of birth to determine if the infant is at term, if the amniotic fluid is clear, if there is muscle tone, and if there are respirations or crying. If any of these conditions are not met, then the child should be placed under radiant heat and further resuscitation done. The basic **steps to resuscitation** include:

- Warming the infant after drying
- Positioning the infant and clearing the airway if necessary
- Stimulating and repositioning the infant

The child should be evaluated throughout the initial procedures:

- **Respirations**: Rate and character of respirations should be noted as well as observation of chest wall movement.
- **Heart rate**: Should be >100 bpm, assessed with stethoscope or at the base of the umbilical cord.

APGAR Delivery Room Assessment

Dr. Virginia Apgar developed the **APGAR** test in 1952. APGAR stands for **A**ppearance, **P**ulse, **G**rimace, **A**ctivity, and **R**espiration. The APGAR is the first test given to a newborn. It is used as a quick evaluation of a newborn's physical condition to determine if any emergency medical care is needed and is administered 1 minute and 5 minutes after birth. The test is administered more than once, as the baby's condition may change rapidly. It may be administered for a third time 10 minutes after birth if needed. The baby is rated on the five subscales and the scores are added together. A total score of ≥7 is a sign of good health.

Scoring Chart

Sign	0	1	2
Appearance (Skin Color)	Cyanotic or pallor over entire body	Normal, except for the extremities	Entire body normal
Pulse (Heart Rate)	Absent	<100 bpm	>100 bpm
Grimace (Reflex Irritability)	Unresponsive	Grimace	Infant sneezes, coughs, and recoils
Activity (Muscle Tone)	Absent	Flexed limbs	Infant moves freely
Respiration (Breathing Rate and Effort)	Absent	Bradypnea, dyspnea	Good breathing and crying

Review Video: Newborn APGAR Score
Visit mometrix.com/academy and enter code: 253451

Appearance, Weight, Measurements, and Vital Signs

The neonate's general appearance, measurements, and VS should be evaluated:

- **Head**: disproportionately large for body
- **Body**: long
- **Extremities**: short and in flexed position (Feet are usually dorsiflexed after breech birth.)
- **Hands**: clenched
- **Neck**: short and chin resting on chest
- **Abdomen**: prominent
- **Hips**: narrow
- **Chest**: rounded
- **Weight**: 2500-4000 g (average about 3400); physiologic weight loss is 5-10% for full term and up to 15% for preterm
- **Length**: 45-55 cm (average 50 cm)
- **Head circumference**: 32-38 cm (usually 2 cm greater than chest circumference)

- **Chest circumference**: 30-36 cm
- **Temperature**: Temperature drops rapidly (skin temperature falls 0.3 °C/minute) after birth with exposure to ambient room temperature but stabilizes within 8-12 hours. Temperature is usually measured by axillary method (for 3 minutes) and ranges from 36.3-37.0 °C.
- **Blood pressure**: 56-77/33-50 mmHg
- **Pulse**: 120-160 bpm awake; 100 bpm asleep; 180 bpm crying
- **Respiration**: 30-60 per minute

Cardiac Rates

Normal cardiac rates can vary widely from one neonate to another, so it's important to understand the normal range in order to determine if the infant has an abnormal pulse. Rates will also vary depending upon whether the infant is awake, sleeping, or active. Pulse rate should be taken with a stethoscope, because the pulse may be difficult to palpate or count accurately manually. The neonatal **point of maximal intensity (PMI)** is located at the intersection between the 4th intercostal space and the midclavicular line (versus the adult PMI located at the 5th intercostal). Additionally, this allows for assessment of heart murmurs.

Newborn infant:

- At rest: 100-180
- Asleep: 80-160
- Active/sick: ≤220

1-12 weeks:

- At rest: 100-220
- Asleep: 80-200
- Active/sick: ≤220

Monitoring of heart rate is particularly important as alterations of heart rate occur with periods of apnea. A period of apnea is usually followed by decreased heart rate, as well as decreased oxygen saturation. Respiratory rates should be monitored as well as heart rate. **Color** should be noted. Pink coloring indicates good perfusion. Generalized mottling or central cyanosis should be investigated further.

Blood Pressure

Normal blood pressure values for **term infant**:

- Systolic: 56-77 mmHg
- Diastolic: 33-50 mmHg
- MAP: 42-60 mmHg
- Hypertension: Systolic >90 and diastolic >60.

In a **preterm infant**, normal systolic and diastolic values will vary depending on the gestational age and size of the infant. A preterm infant should have a mean arterial pressure that is a number matching the gestational age in weeks of that infant. For example, an infant born at 28 weeks gestation should have an MAP of 28 mmHg. Hypertension in this instance would be systolic >80 and diastolic >50.

Proper **fit of the blood pressure cuff** is imperative to obtain an accurate reading. One must measure the width of the infant's arm in the area that the cuff will be applied. The cuff should be approximately 25% wider than this measurement. A cuff too small results in a BP reading too high and a cuff too large results in a BP reading too low.

HEART SOUNDS

S1

S1 is the heart sound heard as the mitral and tricuspid valves close at the beginning of the contraction of the ventricle (systole). S1 is easiest to hear if the stethoscope is placed at the fourth intercostal space while the infant is supine and calm. If the S1 heard is louder than normal, that means **cardiac output** and **blood flow** are higher than normal. The conditions that can cause this are:

- Patent ductus arteriosus
- Ventricular septal defect
- Tetralogy of Fallot

If the S1 heard is softer or quieter than normal, this is an indication of **lowered cardiac output**, which could be caused by these problems:

- Congestive heart failure
- Myocarditis

S2

S2 is the sound heard when the pulmonic valve and the aortic valve close at the end of the contraction of the ventricles (systole). S2 is easiest to hear at the upper left border of the sternum. S2 is normally split, as the aortic valve closes slightly ahead of the pulmonic valve. In the presence of a cardiac defect, the S2 split becomes wider (the difference in time between the closing of the aortic and pulmonic valve becomes greater). Conditions that cause a **widened S2 split** include:

- Atrial septal defect
- Tetralogy of Fallot
- Pulmonary stenosis
- Ebstein anomaly

Conditions that cause **no split** in the S2 (the two valves close at the same time or one is not closing) include:

- Pulmonary or aortic atresia
- Aortic or pulmonary stenosis
- Persistent pulmonary hypertension

PERIPHERAL PULSES

Peripheral pulses, usually palpated at the brachial or femoral arteries, are graded according to strength. Peripheral pulses may be difficult to palpate in a neonate and should not be relied upon for cardiac assessment. Pulses should always be verified by auscultation:

- 0 = absent
- 1+ = weak
- 2+ = weak to average

- 3+ = strong
- 4+ = bounding

Weak pulses are noted in conditions that cause a decrease in cardiac output. Some of these conditions include:

- Any defect resulting in obstructed blood flow leaving the left ventricle
- Failure of the heart muscle itself
- Shock

Bounding pulses (4+) are noted when there is too much blood coming from the aorta. Some of the conditions that would cause this are:

- Patent ductus arteriosus
- Aortic insufficiency
- Shunts

Respiratory Rate of Neonate and Breath Sounds Found on Auscultation

The average **respiratory rate** for newborns is about 35-40 (ranging from 30 to 60) times per minute. Tachypnea (>60/min) may occur within the first hour after birth and during the second period of reactivity, but it should not be prolonged. While mild substernal retractions may occur during the first hour, they should not persist, and movement of the chest should be symmetric (asymmetry may indicate pneumothorax). Nasal flaring may also occur during the first hour, but continued flaring may indicate inadequate oxygenation. After birth, the **lungs should be auscultated anteriorly and posteriorly** with almost all lung fields clear. However, during the first hour or two after birth, some fluid may remain in the lungs, so fine rales may be noted. If the newborn was delivered by Cesarean, more fluid may remain in the lungs, so the rales may sound coarse. If the breath sounds are absent (apneic periods of more than 20 seconds) or diminished, breathing is labored, seesaw respirations are evident, or expiratory grunting occurs, these are indications of respiratory distress.

Chest and Respiratory Assessment

The neonate's chest and respiratory status should be evaluated by observation and auscultation. The chest should be symmetric and the ribs flexible. The xiphoid process may protrude slightly. Breasts are sometimes engorged, and the nipples may secrete small amounts of white fluid. Accessory nipples may be noted. Pulmonary function assessment should include anterior and posterior auscultation. Abdominal movement should synchronize with respirations. Periodic breathing is common, but apneic periods should be <20 seconds or they can result in cyanosis or bradycardia. The **Silverman-Anderson Index** is used to evaluate respiratory status. A score of 0 indicates normal findings, and higher scores indicate respiratory distress.

Characteristic	0	1	2
Chest/Abdomen	Rise together with inspiration	Rising abdomen with sinking or lagging upper chest	See-saw movement
Intercostals	No retraction	Minimal retraction	Pronounced retraction
Xiphoid Process	No retraction	Minimal retraction	Pronounced retraction
Nasal Flaring	None	Minimal flaring	Pronounced flaring
Grunt (Expiratory)	None	Grunt heard with auscultation	Audible grunt

Gastrointestinal Assessment

As the neonate breathes, air enters the **GI system**—first the stomach and then the intestines—within 2-12 hours and enters the colon within 24 hours. Bowel sounds are usually present within 30-60 minutes of birth. The stomach has a capacity of about 50-60 mL and empties intermittently, usually beginning a few minutes after feeding begins and continuing for 2-4 hours after; however, because of immaturity of the cardiac sphincter, the neonate may regurgitate the first few feedings. If regurgitation becomes continuous, further evaluation is indicated. Infants produce little saliva until the salivary glands mature in about 3 months. Term neonates usually pass **meconium** within 8-24 hours, although they may not do so for 48 hours. First meconium is thick, dark, and tarry. **Transitional stools** for the next few days are usually brown to green, after which the child should pass normal stools. Stools of breastfed babies are usually yellow-gold and mushy, and those of formula-fed babies are pale yellow and pasty.

Abdominal and Rectal Assessment

The **abdomen** should be soft, symmetric, and rounded. A distended abdomen with engorged vessels may indicate GI abnormalities. Bowel sounds (present about an hour after birth) should be auscultated prior to palpation. The liver is usually palpable 1-2 cm below the right costal margin, and the tip of the spleen may be palpable in preterm infants only in the left lateral upper quadrant. It should not extend >1 cm below the costal margin. The umbilical cord should be white or blue-white, with two umbilical arteries and one umbilical vein observed and no discharge or bleeding. The presence of only one umbilical artery is associated with GI/GU congenital anomalies. Green/yellow discoloration may indicate meconium staining. The abdomen should be examined carefully for hernias while the infant is at rest and crying.

The **rectal area** should be examined to determine if the anus is present and patent. Meconium is usually passed within 24 hours of birth. Soft swelling in the femoral area may indicate hernia or undescended testicle.

Genitourinary Assessment

Genitourinary assessment requires evaluation of **urinary output**. Many neonates void immediately after birth, although the small amount of urine may be overlooked. About 92% void within 24 hours and 99% by 48 hours. Neonates with **edema** may have higher urinary output as edema recedes. In the first 2 days, most infants void 2-6 times daily, with an output averaging about 15 mL/kg/day. After this, the infant should urinate 5-25 times per day, with volume increasing to 25 mL/kg/day. Urine may appear cloudy because of mucus, and initial voidings have high **specific gravity**, but specific gravity returns to normal levels when the child feeds. Pink stains, referred to as "brick dust spots" often show on the diapers, but these **urate deposits** are of no concern. Female infants may exhibit **pseudomenstruation**—slight bleeding—as maternal hormones are withdrawn.

MALE GENITALIA ASSESSMENT

Male genitalia should be carefully examined to determine if they are clearly male or ambiguous:

- **Penis**: The normal penis is usually about 2.5-3.5 cm long and 1 cm wide with the urinary meatus at the distal end in the glans. Displacement of the urethra is found with epispadias/hypospadias. Micropenis may indicate congenital anomaly. The urethral opening should not be inflamed. The foreskin should adhere to the glans and is tight (if uncircumcised). Small white cysts are sometimes evident on the prepuce.
- **Scrotum**: Skin may be loose/hanging or tight/small with normal slightly darkened skin color and extensive rugae. A large scrotum should be examined by transillumination for hydrocele. If the skin is red and shiny, this may indicate orchitis. Discoloration (bruising) may be present with breech presentation.
- **Testes**: Should be descended and 1.5-2.0 cm in diameter, but may not be in scrotum and may be retractile (moving into the upper scrotum or inguinal canal on stimulation).

FEMALE GENITALIA ASSESSMENT

Female genitalia should be assessed to determine if there are indications of gender ambiguity, as enlarged clitoris and micropenis may be similar in appearance:

- **Mons**: The labia majora should be symmetric and should cover the clitoris and labia minora in full-term and post-term infants although the labia minora and clitoris are exposed with preterm infants. The urinary meatus should be positioned below the clitoris. Bruising of the labia majora may be evident after vaginal birth.
- **Clitoris**: The clitoris is enlarged in the neonate, and bruising and edema may occur with breech birth. Hypertrophy may indicate hermaphroditism.
- **Vagina**: The vaginal opening should be evident (0.5 cm). Hymenal tag may be observed in the vagina. White or pink-tinged vaginal discharge is common for 2-4 weeks after birth. An imperforate hymen may be indicated by suprapubic mass or mass between labia majora.

SKIN ASSESSMENT

Skin colors vary with race, but all should be pink-tinged to some degree, as skin pigmentation is slight after birth. Skin characteristics include:

- **Birthmarks**: Dark-skinned infants may have **Mongolian spots** on the buttocks and dorsal area. **Nevus flammeus** (port-wine stain) is a demarcated unraised red-purple lesion caused by capillaries below the epidermis. **Nevus vasculosus** (strawberry mark) is a capillary hemangioma and is a raised, demarcated dark red lesion.
- **Acrocyanosis**: Slight cyanosis of the hands and feet during the 2-6 hours after birth, especially if chilled. Color returns rapidly when skin blanched.
- **Mottling**: Common for hours to weeks after birth and may relate to long periods of apnea/chilling.
- **Harlequin sign**: Deep color on one side of body only for 1-20 minutes; usually transient.
- **Erythema toxicum**: Perifollicular lesions (1-3 mm) white or yellow with pustule appears suddenly over body (except palms and soles); usually transient, cause unknown.
- **Milia**: Small raised white spots on face from exposed sebaceous glands; transient.

Skin Appearance of Neonate

Newborns' skin appearance depends on the development and thickening of their dermis, epidermis, and vernix caseosa. When skin develops during week 15 of gestation, it is initially thin and translucent. By week 20, vernix caseosa production begins. Vernix is a thick, waxy substance secreted by the sebaceous glands and mixed with sloughed-off skin cells, often described as "cheesy." The stratum corneum (protective top layer of the epidermis) develops from weeks 20-24. The epidermis continues to develop and thicken, and is able to form a water barrier by week 32. Near term, the vernix washes away and the skin becomes more wrinkled without its protection:

Gestational Age	Skin Appearance
24-26 Weeks	Translucent, red, many visible blood vessels, and scant vernix
35-40 Weeks	Deep cracks, no visible blood vessels, and thick vernix
42-44 Weeks	Dry, peeling skin, no vernix, and loss of subcutaneous fat

Musculoskeletal Assessment

The **musculoskeletal system** should be assessed for muscle tone. Maintenance of fetal position or limp tone may indicate hypoxia, CNS abnormalities, or hypoglycemia. Joint movement should be spontaneous with good muscle tone. Spasticity or floppiness indicates cerebral palsy or other disorders. Jitteriness may indicate hypoglycemia or hypocalcemia.

Extremities should be short, flexed, and able to move symmetrically through range of motion, but without full extension. Arms/legs should be equal in length with feet and hands of normal size (5 digits each). Feet should be flat. Hips should abduct to >60°. Cyanosis or clubbing of nails indicates cardiac anomalies, and yellow-green discoloration indicates meconium staining.

The **back and spine** are examined with the infant in a prone position. The spine should be straight, without a sacral or lumbar curve, which develops only after the child begins to sit. Obvious anomalies, such as spina bifida, and indications of a pilonidal dimple, skin lesions, or tufts of hair that may indicate abnormalities should be noted. C-shaped spine may indicate spina bifida occulta, and lumbar lordosis may indicate myelomeningocele.

Assessment of Muscular Tone

Determining the quality of **muscle tone** in a neonate is an important part of neuromuscular assessment. The child is placed supine with the head in neutral position and the LRN nurse moves body parts (arms, legs, head) to determine if the muscle tone is flaccid, jittery, or hypertonic. Neonates are slightly hypertonic so that some resistance should be felt to movement, such as when moving a leg or straightening an arm. Tone should be symmetric. The extremities are usually flexed and legs abducted to the abdomen. This assessment allows the LRN nurse to differentiate common fine tremors or jitteriness found in neonates from seizure activity or nervous system disorders that cause muscular twitching. Normal fine tremors are usually halted by holding or flexing the extremity while seizure activity or twitching does not resolve in this way.

Assessment of Neonatal Reflexes

Reflex	Eliciting Reflex	Normal Response	Discussion
Palmar Grasping	Stroke the infant's palm.	The infant responds by grasping the finger.	Grasp reflex is stronger in premature infants and fades away at 2 to 3 months of age. Absence indicates CNS deficit or muscle injury.
Rooting	Stroke the side of the infant's cheek.	The infant turns the head in the direction of the touch, and opens mouth to feed.	Rooting reflex helps the infant find and latch onto the mother's breast.
Sucking	Touch the infant's mouth.	The infant sucks.	Premature infants may have an absent or weak suck reflex, as it usually develops around week 32 of gestation. Weak or absent reflex indicates CNS deficit or depression.
Moro (Startle)	Make a loud sound or give the infant a gentle jolt.	The infant extends arms, legs, and neck, then pulls back arms and legs. May also cry.	Moro reflex disappears at 5 to 6 months of age. Asymmetric response indicates peripheral nerve injury, or fracture of long bones, clavicle, or skull.
Blinking	Flash light at eyes.	Eyelids close.	Absence or delay may indicate cerebral palsy, hydrocephalus, and developmental delay.
Tonic Neck (Fencing)	With infant supine, turn head to one side.	Extremities flex on opposite side and extend on same side.	May be incomplete immediately after birth and should diminish by 4 months. Persistence >4 months may indicate neurological abnormalities.
Babinski (Plantar)	Stroke the lateral aspect of the sole from heel to ball of foot.	Hyper-extension of all toes.	Persists until ≤2 years, after which the toes flex.
Trunk Incurvation (Galant)	With infant prone, stroke down one side of the spine (1 inch from spine).	Pelvis turns to stimulated side.	Absence indicates CNS depression or lesion of spinal cord. Should disappear by 4 months.
Tongue Extrusion	Touch tip of tongue.	Neonate pushes tongue out of mouth.	Continuous or repetitive extrusion indicates CNS abnormalities or seizure activity.

Stepping Reflex

If a newborn is held upright with the feet touching a horizontal surface, the contact should make the infant lift one foot and then the other, giving the appearance of walking. This reflex promotes the development of muscles and usually disappears by 4 months. If this reflex is missing, then may be an indication that the infant has a motor nerve defect or other neurological abnormality.

Anal Wink

The anocutaneous reflex is the reflexive contraction of the anus in response to gentle stroking or stimulation of the skin around the rectum. It occurs in both females and males. Pulling the penis elicits the response in males as well; at one time, this response was believed indicative of sexual abuse, but that has been disproved. Failure of this response indicates that there in an interruption in the reflex arc in the sensory or motor nerves.

Assessing Motor Development

Pull-to-Sit

This test, also known as the head lag test, is conducted with the infant lying in supine position. The infant's arms are grasped with the elbows slightly flexed and the infant pulled into sitting position. The head should be observed carefully as it may lag behind the trunk but should not be completely flexed backward. When the infant reaches the sitting position, the infant should be able to at least briefly bring the head into upright position. If the head consistently lags, this may be an indication of cerebral injury and/or neurobehavioral abnormalities.

Truncal Tone

This test is used to assess hypotonia/floppy infant syndrome. The infant is suspended face down by the abdomen and draped over the examiner's hand. A normal response is for the infant to straighten the back, flex the limbs, and straighten the head while an abnormal response is for the infant to hang in place with the head down and the extremities extended. An abnormal response may indicate CNS disorders or neuromuscular disorders. The most common cause of hypotonia is hypoxic-ischemic encephalopathy.

Eyes, Nose, Neck, and Throat Assessments

The appearance and movement of the **face** should be symmetric in the neonate and a number of different characteristics examined:

- **Eyes**: Usually blue to blue/gray with white to bluish-white sclera. Small conjunctival hemorrhages and transient strabismus or squint may be evident. Pupils should be equal and reactive. Red retinal reflex should be present. Tears are usually absent during crying. Eye blink test causes lids to close.
- **Nose**: Infants usually breathe through their nose and should be able to breathe easily if mouth is closed. If not, the child should be examined for choanal atresia. Sense of smell is determined if the infant turns toward milk source or away from strong smells, such as alcohol.
- **Neck**: The infant should be able to hold head up slightly while prone, but the head lags when lifted from the supine position because of weak muscles. Neck rigidity may indicate injury to sternocleidomastoid injury.
- **Throat**: The palate should be highly arched, mucous membranes moist, and uvula midline (if bifid, this can indicate submucosal cleft). The infant should exhibit the sucking, rooting, gag, and extrusion reflexes.

Mouth Assessment

The mouth should be carefully examined with a gloved finger pressing against the tongue to open the mouth:

- **Lips**: Should be pink, normal-shaped, and symmetric. Thin upper lip with smooth philtrum and short palpebral fissures may indicate fetal alcohol syndrome.
- **Sucking**: Sucking (symmetrical) should occur if lips are touched. Asymmetric movement of the mouth may indicate injury to facial nerve.
- **Gums**: Examined for precocious teeth and Epstein's pearls (keratin-containing cysts).
- **Tongue**: Examined for ridge of frenulum tissue on underside (tongue-tied), although this is not clipped and evidence of protrusion or hypertrophy, which can indicate various disorders, such as Down syndrome and hypothyroidism. Bluish swelling of the frenulum may indicate mucus/salivary gland retention cyst.
- **Mucus membranes**: Examined for color and moisture as cyanosis may indicate respiratory distress and dryness or dehydration. Excessive salivation and drooling may indicate esophageal atresia. White patches on mucus membranes/tongue indicate infection with *Candida albicans.*

Structures of the Ear

The **tympanic membrane** is the eardrum, a thin, semitransparent membrane that separates the external auditory canal from the middle ear. Sound waves cause the membrane to vibrate, transmitting sounds to structures in the middle ear. Three **auditory ossicles** help to transmit the vibrations from the ear drum to structures in the inner ear. These three bones are named the malleus (hammer), incus (anvil), and stapes (stirrup) and are connected to each other by synovial joints. The **cochlea** (snail shell) is located in the inner ear and translates vibrations received from the auditory ossicles into signals that are transmitted to the brain via the vestibulocochlear nerve (cranial nerve VIII).

The following are **structures of the external ear**:

- **Pinna**: All the structures that make up the external ear
- **Helix**: The outermost, curved portion of the ear, which is posterior/superior and has a folded edge
- **Antihelix**: 'C' shaped cartilage that runs on the inside of the helix, separated from the helix by a scooped-out section, called the scapha
- **Tragus**: Small projection just anterior to the external auditory ear canal
- **Antitragus**: Lower cartilaginous portion of the concha, just superior to the fleshy lobe of the ear
- **Concha**: Bowl that surrounds the external auditory canal
- **Lobe**: Fleshy lower portion of the ear that is the traditional site of ear piercing

Ear Assessment

The ears should be carefully examined for a number of different characteristics:

- **Position**: The insertion point of the top of the ear should be parallel to the inner and outer canthus of the eye. Low-set ears may relate to a number of disorders, such as trisomy 13 and trisomy 18, intellectual disability, and various other disorders.
- **Shape/size**: Ears should be proportionate to head size and symmetric.
- **Pliability**: Ears should be soft and pliable. Cartilage is lacking in premature infants, and the pinna is soft. Cartilage should be firm by 38 to 40 weeks with 2/3 of pinna curving inward.

- **Hearing**: Hearing may be initially assessed by observing response to sudden loud sound. Evoked otoacoustic emissions (EOAE) and auditory brainstem response (ABR) are used for universal hearing screening.
- **Tympanic membrane**: Usually not examined with otoscope because of occlusion with vernix and blood after birth, but should appear gray-white and vascular.

Screening for Hearing Loss

Neonatal hearing tests include:

- **Otoacoustic emissions** (OAE) are sounds generated by the cochlea. They are a measure of the integrity of the middle and inner ear—or, more specifically, the outer hair cells of the cochlea. The audiologist measures the OAE by inserting a probe into the infant's external auditory canal and stimulating the cochlea with several clicking noises. The audiologist uses a microphone to measure the evoked OAE sent off by the cochlea.
- **Auditory brainstem response** examination measures the brain's reaction to sound (middle and inner ear and nerve pathway). The audiologist places electrodes on the infant's scalp, positions a device that makes sounds outside the ear, and measures the brain's response to the sound with measured waveforms that are compared to the normal, expected pattern.

Both hearing examinations are scored as pass or fail. If the infant fails an audiology screening examination, further testing must be arranged by an otorhinolaryngologist to confirm if a problem truly exists and to determine the nature of the hearing loss.

Head Assessment

Fontanels

The newborn has 8 skull bones and 14 facial bones. Their adjoining edges are bone sutures. Soft spots where the skull flexes along sutures to exit the vagina are **fontanels**. The newborn has 6 fontanels:

- Diamond-shaped anterior fontanel (AF)
- Triangular posterior fontanel (PF)
- Sphenoid fontanels (2)
- Mastoid fontanels (2)

The AF is the largest and most informative during clinical examination, with a normal size falling between 1 and 3 cm at birth. Fontanels **bulge** when the newborn cries, vomits, lies down, or has hydrocephalus, intracranial tumor, hemorrhage, or meningitis. Fontanels should return to normal when the NNP holds the baby head up and the infant is calm. **Depressed fontanels** indicate the newborn is dehydrated. Conditions associated with an abnormally large AF include hypothyroidism, Down syndrome, achondroplasia, rickets, and increased intracranial pressure. Infants with Down syndrome may have an extra fontanel between the AF and posterior fontanel.

Craniotabes

Craniotabes is an area of softened skull found in 30% of newborns. It is softer and more pliable than surrounding tissue and gives way when pressure is applied, as though one is pushing on a ping-pong ball. It is more commonly in premature infants, but can also be found in full-term infants. Usually, craniotabes occurs in the posterior occipital or posterior parietal bones or along the suture lines. Craniotabes is considered to be a normal finding that requires no treatment because it usually resolves by one month of age. Craniotabes may persist longer when it is positioned along a suture line. No work-up is required, but the infant should be carefully examined for indications of disease-related causes of craniotabes, including other conditions that affect bone growth or hardness, such as rickets, syphilis, marasmus, or osteogenesis imperfecta.

Caput Succedaneum and Cephalohematoma

Caput succedaneum and cephalohematoma are both examples of head molding resulting from head trauma during birthing. They can be observed during the newborn period and appear similar upon physical examination because the neonate's head is swollen:

- **Caput succedaneum** is more common. It is a collection of fluid beneath the skin, but superficial to the periosteum. It often occurs when the head presses against the dilating cervix during the birth process. Vacuum-assisted deliveries also contribute to caput succedaneum. The swelling crosses suture lines. Complications are rare. Swelling usually resolves over several days.
- **Cephalohematoma** occurs when blood vessels between the skull and the periosteum rupture, causing a subperiosteal collection of blood. The swelling appears several hours after birth. It does not cross suture lines. Complications such as anemia or hypovolemia may occur if the amount of bleeding is large. The blood will eventually be resorbed and may cause jaundice secondary to the breakdown of red blood cells.

Clinical Laboratory Tests

Capillary Blood Sampling

Neonatal capillary blood sampling is a common procedure used to acquire small samples of blood for testing of glucose and drug levels, blood gases, electrolytes, urea, blood counts, and other screening tests. If done incorrectly, it can cause pain, trauma, and nerve damage. The lancet for a full-term neonate should be 2.5 mm deep with an insertion depth of 1mm. The lancet for a preterm neonate should be 1.75 mm with an insertion depth of 0.85 mm. Automatic lancets are preferred over manual ones, as they have proven to cause less pain to the neonate. The baby should be supine. The nurse grasps the foot with one hand holding the ankle with the thumb and index finger and supporting the leg with the other fingers. The infant's heel (bottom, lateral aspect only to avoid nerves in the middle of the foot) should be cleansed thoroughly with water (not alcohol) and air-dried. The skin of the heel should be held tense until after the puncture, and then it is relaxed and the heel lightly compressed to express a drop of blood, which is collected in a capillary tube. Relaxing the pressure and then compressing again will "milk" additional drops. Pressure is applied to the puncture site until bleeding stops and then a dressing is applied.

Microbiological Testing

Neonates with exposure to microbiological agents before, during, or after birth may require microbiological testing:

- Blood cultures are done to isolate causative agents in order to begin appropriate antibiotic treatment.
- In some cases, microbiological testing of expressed human milk may be indicated.
- Microscopic examination of urine and urine culture may be done to identify urinary pathogens.
- Stool cultures may be done to identify GI pathogens.

- Tracheal secretions may be cultured to identify pathogens causing pneumonia, especially in infants who are ventilated. The findings should be reviewed along with chest radiographs to ensure that positive findings don't just represent tracheal colonization alone.
- Gram stain and scraping of conjunctiva may be done to identify gonococcal conjunctivitis.
- Skin culture may be indicated for the infant with a skin infection.

Urine Testing

Urine testing includes:

- **pH** should range from 4.5 to 9.0. An alkaline (high) pH can be caused by urinary tract infections, diarrhea, or kidney infection. An acidic (low) pH may reflect lung disease, hyperglycemia, or diarrhea with dehydration.
- **Specific gravity** ranges from 1.001 to 1.040 (usually about 1.015).

Asymptomatic bacteremia is rare in neonates, and urinalysis alone is not an effective test to determine if an infant has a urinary tract infection because the neonate's urine usually contains leukocytes ($\geq 25/mm^3$ in males and $\geq 50/mm^3$ in females), so urine cultures of infants younger than 3 days often show poor results, even in the presence of infection. Thus, blood cultures (and in some cases cultures of CSF) are preferred if infection is suspected, as neonates are more likely to develop kidney infections and sepsis from cystitis than older infants. The most common infective agent is *Escherichia coli* although *Candida* and *Staphylococcus* are common with prolonged hospitalization.

Serum Creatinine Levels and Renal Function

Serum creatinine is a marker of renal function. Creatinine is a byproduct of creatine phosphate metabolism in muscle. **Serum creatinine levels** reflect the balance between the production of creatinine and its clearance by the kidneys. Creatinine is filtered by the kidneys and generally not reabsorbed by the tubules, so it is a good indicator of the glomerular filtration rate (GFR). Elevated serum creatinine at birth may reflect elevated maternal levels, especially if the mother has toxemia. The serum creatinine level normally drops in the first few weeks of life. Premature infants often have a higher serum creatinine level and take longer to reach a normal level, because the GFR is lower in premature infants and immature kidneys allow creatinine to be reabsorbed across leaky tubules. Certain disease states (such as respiratory distress syndrome with mechanical ventilation) are associated with decreased GFR.

ABG Testing

Arterial blood gases (ABGs) are monitored to assess the effectiveness of oxygenation, ventilation, and acid-base status and to determine oxygen flow rates. Partial pressure of a gas is that exerted by each gas in a mixture of gases, proportional to its concentration, based on total atmospheric pressure of 760 mmHg at sea level. Normal values for children include:

- Acidity/alkalinity (pH): 7.26-7.44
- Partial pressure of carbon dioxide ($PaCO_2$): 35-45 mmHg
- Partial pressure of oxygen (PaO_2): >80 mmHg
- Bicarbonate concentration (HCO_3^-): 22-28 mEq/L
- Oxygen saturation (SaO_2): >92%

The relationship between these elements, particularly the $PaCO_2$ and the PaO_2, indicates respiratory status. For example, $PaCO_2$ >55 and the PaO_2 <60 in an infant previously in good health indicates respiratory failure. There are many issues to consider. Ventilator management may require a higher

$PaCO_2$ to prevent barotrauma and a lower PaO_2 to reduce oxygen toxicity. Premature infants may need lower PaO_2 to prevent retinopathy of prematurity.

Invasive Blood Gas Monitoring

Invasive blood gas monitoring options include the following:

- **Arterial blood gas (ABG)** is the most informative measurement of blood gas status. If an infant has an umbilical artery catheter, it is easily obtained by aspirating 1-2 mL of blood.
- **Venous blood gas (VBG)** is easier to obtain if an arterial catheter is not in place. In order to compare the values in the VBG with an ABG, make the following calculations:
  - Add 0.05 to the pH of the VBG.
  - Subtract 5-10 mmHg from the $PaCO_2$ of the VBG.
- **Capillary Blood Gas (CBG)** can be obtained with a heel stick, without a venous or arterial line, but the values obtained in a CBG are the least accurate and are rarely useful. The oxygen status of the neonate (reflected in the PaO_2) can be estimated by clinical evaluation of the neonate and a noninvasive pulse oximeter reading.

Review Video: Newborn Cord Blood Gases
Visit mometrix.com/academy and enter code: 188117

RBC Testing

Red blood cells (RBCs or erythrocytes) are biconcave disks that contain hemoglobin, which carries oxygen throughout the body. The heme portion of the cell contains iron, which binds to the oxygen. RBCs live about 120 days in adults but this is reduced 20-25% in neonates and 50% in preterm infants. The RBCs are destroyed and their hemoglobin is recycled or excreted. **Normal values of red blood cell** count vary by age:

- Neonate: 4.1-6.1 million per mm^3
- 2-6 months: 3.8-5.6 million per mm^3

The most common disorders of RBCs are those that interfere with production, leading to various types of **anemia**:

- Blood loss
- Hemolysis
- Bone marrow failure

The **morphology** of RBCs may vary depending upon the type of anemia:

- Size: normocytes, microcytes, macrocytes
- Shape: spherocytes (round), poikilocytes (irregular), drepanocytes (sickled)
- Color (reflecting the concentration of hemoglobin): normochromic, hypochromic

Hgb, Hct, MCV, Reticulocyte Count, and Platelets

Additional laboratory tests specific to red blood cells include the following:

- **Hemoglobin:** carries oxygen and is decreased in anemia and increased in polycythemia
  - Neonate: 14.5-22.5 g/dL
  - 2 months: 9.0-14.0 g/dL

- **Hematocrit:** indicates the proportion of RBCs in a liter of blood (usually about 3 times the hemoglobin number)
  - Neonate: 48-69%
  - 3 days: 44-75%
  - 2 months: 28-42%
- **Mean corpuscular volume (MCV):** indicates the size of RBCs and can differentiate types of anemia (For adults, <80 is microcytic and >100 is macrocytic, but this varies with age.)
  - Neonate: 95-121 μm^3
  - 0.5-2 years: 70-86 μm^3
- **Reticulocyte count:** measures marrow production and should rise with anemia
  - 0.5-1.5% of total RBCs
- **Platelets:** essential for clotting
  - 150,000-400,000
  - may increase to >1 million with iron deficiency anemia or decrease to <100,000 during acute infection

WBC Testing

Leukocytes are white blood cells (WBCs). Normal total values vary according to age. The differential is the percentage of each type of WBC out of the total. The differential will shift with infection or allergies, but should return to normal values:

Item	Neonate	1 Day	2 Weeks	1 Month
WBCs (1000s/mm^3)	9.0-30.0	9.4-34.0	5.0-20.0	5.0-19.5.
Myelocytes	0%	0%	0%	0%
Neutrophils (Bands)	9.1%	9.2%	5.5%	4.5%
Neutrophils (Segs)	52%	52%	34%	30%
Lymphocytes	31%	31%	48%	56%
Monocytes	5.8%	5.8%	8.8%	6.5%
Eosinophils	2.2%	2.0%	3.1%	2.8%
Basophils	0.6%	0.5%	0.4%	0.5%

Pituitary Hormone Testing

The **anterior pituitary gland (adenohypophysis)** produces hormones that are critical for growth and development:

- **Growth hormone** (GH) promotes growth of bones and muscles and promotes protein synthesis and metabolism of fat but decreases carbohydrate metabolism. Normal values:
  - Cord blood: 8-40 μg/L
  - 1 day:5-50 μg/L
  - 1 week: 5-25 μg/L
- **Thyroid stimulating hormone** (TSH) stimulates secretion of thyroid hormones. Normal values:
  - 0-3 days: <20 mIU/L
- **Adrenocorticotropic hormone** (ACTH) stimulates the adrenal glands to produce glucocorticoids, androgens, and mineralocorticoids. Abnormalities can result in Cushing's disease or Addison's disease. Normal values:

- Cord blood: 11-25 pmol/L
- Neonate: 2-41 pmol/L

The **posterior pituitary gland (neurohypophysis)** stores hormones produced by the hypothalamus, critical to renal function. **Antidiuretic hormone (ADH)** controls the reabsorption of fluids in the kidney tubules. Changes in serum osmolality stimulate or depress ADH secretion, so values vary:

- Serum osmolality 270-280 mOsm/kg: ADH 0-1.4 pmol/L
- Serum osmolality 280-285 mOsm/kg: ADH 0.5-2.3 pmol/L
- Serum osmolality 285-290 mOsm/kg: ADH 0.9-4.6 pmol/L

Thyroid Hormone Testing

The **thyroid gland** produces hormones critical for metabolism and growth. They are amino acids that contain iodine and are stored in the thyroid until needed by the body. The thyroid gland takes iodide from the blood and utilizes it to produce hormones. Thyroid hormone production is controlled by the thyroid-stimulating hormone (TSH) produced by the pituitary gland and the thyrotropin-releasing hormone (TRH) produced by the hypothalamus. Together, the thyroid hormones increase metabolic rate and protein and bone turnover. They are necessary for the growth and development of the fetus and infant. Thyroid hormones include:

- **Thyroxine** (T_4) is a weak hormone that maintains the body's metabolism in a steady state.
  - Neonate: 10-36 pmol/L
- **Triiodothyronine** (T_3) is about 5 times stronger than thyroxine and can respond quickly to metabolic needs.
  - All ages: 4.0-7.4 pmol/L
- **Thyrocalcitonin** is secreted in response to serum calcium levels and reduces the serum level of calcium and phosphate by increasing deposits in bones, aiding ossification and bone development.
  - Male: <19 ng/L
  - Female: <14 ng/L

Testing for Infants with HIV-Positive Mothers

The immunological status of infants with **HIV-positive mothers** is assessed in a series of tests performed over the first two years in order to institute treatment and decrease likelihood of transmission to 2% or less.

Virologic assays (most commonly ELISA) and rapid tests are used to identify those neonates who are HIV-positive at birth. Confirmatory testing is done with the neonate's blood (not cord blood due to possibility of maternal contamination), usually using DNA PCR, which is about 99% sensitive by 1 month, but does NOT detect very recent infection (for instance, infection acquired during the birth). RNA PCR may be used for some subtypes of HIV infection.

In the United States, testing is based on identifying mothers with HIV. If the mother's status is not known, then some states require mandatory testing of the infant, but laws vary. Based on positive findings, treatment is begun within 24 hours without waiting for confirmatory test results. Subsequent testing is done at 2, 4, 12, and 18 months.

Neonatal Pharmacology

Principles of Drug Administration to Neonates

Dosage and Interval

The half-life of a drug ($t_{1/2}$) is the time required to reduce serum concentrations by half, and half-life must be considered when determining **dosage and interval** of drugs for neonates. Steady state is usually achieved within 4-5 half-lives. Half-life is a factor of clearance, and small or preterm infants often have reduced clearance because of slow metabolism, resulting in longer half-life. In determining dosage, the infant's weight, gestational age, and post-natal age must be considered.

One major problem with dosing and interval for neonates is that most drugs are not tested on infants, so about 98% are prescribed off-label. There are a number of reference tools available, including software programs, to assist with determining proper dosage and interval for neonatal medications.

Neonatal Tolerance and Weaning

Tolerance and weaning from drugs are often concerns with the administration of opiates. **Tolerance** occurs after repeated administration results in a lessening of effects, requiring an increase in dosage to achieve the same results. When a neonate is weaned from a medication or a dosage is decreased, only one class of medications should be involved. Thus, if the infant is receiving both an opiate and a benzodiazepine, they should not be weaned from both at the same time. The infant should be evaluated for level of pain prior to weaning and reassessed at least every 4 hours during the weaning process. Usually medications are reduced at a rate of 10% per day or 20% every other day. Infants often tolerate an initial reduction in dose better than subsequent reductions, so careful observation for signs of increased pain or withdrawal must be made. Careful control of the environment—temperature, light, and noise—should be done to reduce infant stress during the **weaning process**.

Principles of Neonatal Absorption

Principles of neonatal absorption can be discussed specific to various elements of the process of absorption:

- **GI tract**: Medications may have increased or decreased rates of absorption depending on the rate of gastric emptying, the acidity of the GI tract, the availability of pancreatic or other enzymes, the presence of intestinal bacteria, and GI perfusion as well as disease processes, such as vomiting or diarrhea, and medical procedures, such as GI suctioning.
- **Skin/muscle**: Skin maturation occurs between 23 and 33 weeks of gestation and continues to mature in the weeks after birth. The neonate's skin is thinner and more readily absorbs topical preparations because of increased permeability. Muscle is thinner and generally has less perfusion, so absorption may be slow in the premature or seriously ill neonate, but if perfusion increases, the faster absorption of retained medication may result in overdose.
- **Blood drug levels**: Medications are absorbed immediately but distribution to some organs may vary, and therapeutic levels must be monitored carefully as toxic concentrations may occur if medication administered by IV push or over a short period. Dosage and concentration may be inconsistent because clearance is prolonged.
- **Drug incompatibilities**: Occur when two drugs undergo a reaction when combined that results in the deterioration of one or both of the drugs and can result in inadequate therapeutic effect. Parenteral drugs/solutions may appear cloudy or develop precipitates. The greater the number of drugs administered, the greater the risk of incompatibilities.

- **Drug withdrawal** (therapeutic drugs): Withdrawal protocols vary according to the medication. Some medications, such as some heart medications, must be withdrawn slowly in decreasing doses to avoid a negative response while others can be stopped abruptly. Because clearance may be slowed, the effects of the drug may continue after the medication has been discontinued, so this must be considered when changing medications.
- **Drug resistance**: Ineffectiveness of a drug to treat an infection or condition. For example, some forms of *Staphylococcus* are resistant to vancomycin because of antimicrobial resistance.

Protein Binding in Neonatal Drug Therapy

Protein binding is an important consideration for neonatal drug therapy because when drugs are bound by proteins in the blood, they are not available to be biologically active. The portion of the drug that is **not** bound to a plasma protein is the active portion. **Protein binding** is significant in premature neonates because they typically have:

- Lower levels of plasma proteins, such as albumin.
- Lower binding capacity.
- Susceptibility to competition from endogenous substances like bilirubin, which also attaches to plasma proteins.

Drugs that are normally highly protein bound in the adult have a higher free percentage (activity) in the neonate. Lower than expected dosages may give clinical results. Examples of drugs that are highly protein bound include phenobarbital and indomethacin. If a drug with a high affinity for plasma proteins is administered, it may displace bilirubin from binding sites, increasing the neonate's risk for kernicterus.

Placental Transfer of Drugs

The **placenta** acts as a barrier to protect the fetus, but its main function is to provide oxygen and nutrients for the fetus by linking the maternal and fetal circulation. Virtually all **drugs** cross the barrier to some degree, some by active transport. Some drugs are readily diffused across the placental barrier and can affect the fetus. Drugs that are non-ionized, fat-soluble and have low molecular weight diffuse easily as glucose does. Once a substance crosses the barrier, the lower pH of the fetal blood allows weakly basic drugs, such as local anesthetics and opioids, to cross into fetal circulation where they become ionized and accumulate because they can't pass back into maternal circulation (ion trapping). Giving an intravenous injection during a contraction, when uterine blood flow decreases, reduces the amount of the drug that crosses the placental barrier. A few drugs with large molecules (heparin, insulin) have minimal transfer, and lipid soluble drugs transfer more readily than water-soluble.

Anticoagulants

Neonates may require **anticoagulant therapy** for thrombosis, sometimes associated with catheters used for critical care or thrombocytosis associated with iron-deficiency anemia. Anticoagulant therapy poses fewer risks than fibrinolytic therapy although excessive bleeding may occur. Anticoagulants include:

- **Unfractionated heparin**:
  - Preterm infants: initial bolus of 50 units/kg and maintenance of 15–35 units/kg/hr to maintain level of 0.3–0.7 units/mL
  - Full-term infants: initial bolus of 100 units/kg and maintenance of 25–50 units/kg/hr to maintain level of 0.3–0.7 unit/mL

- **Low-molecular-weight heparin**: 1.7 mg/kg subcutaneously every 12 hours or as needed to maintain level of 0.5–1.0 units/mL 4 hours after administration
- **Warfarin**: may be used in rare cases, such as genetic deficiencies of protein C or S (purpura fulminans), for long-term therapy

Infants that are heparin resistant may be administered fresh frozen plasma (1 mL/kg every 24–48 hours) or AT concentrate (50–150 units/kg every 24–48 hours) to enhance effect of heparin.

Anticonvulsants

Anticonvulsants are used to treat seizures, which often indicate central nervous system dysfunction. Seizures are more common during the neonatal period than later in infancy/childhood and are associated with low birth weight. Treatment is critical to prevent brain damage, but drugs may cause sedation, rash, and blood dyscrasias:

- **Phenobarbital** is the neonatal drug of choice. Loading dose is 20 mg/kg IV in 10–15 minutes and then 5 mg/kg to maximum 40 mg/kg to control seizures. Maintenance dose is 3–4 mg/kg/24 hours in 2 doses beginning ≥12 hours after loading dose. Infant should be provided oxygen and ventilation as needed.
- **Fosphenytoin** is used if phenobarbital is ineffective. It has high water solubility and neutral pH and does not cause tissue injury. It can be administered IV or IM. Loading dose is 15–20 mg PE/kg and maintenance is 4–8 mg PE/kg/day. Blood pressure should be monitored and caution exercised with hyperbilirubinemia.
- **Phenytoin** is sometimes used instead of fosphenytoin if phenobarbital is ineffective. It is incompatible with other drugs and glucose and can cause hypotension, bradycardia, and dysrhythmias if administered too quickly and cannot be given IM or in central lines. Loading dose is 15–20 mg/kg IV over 30 minutes, and maintenance is 4–8 mg/kg/day. Line must be flushed with NS.

In some cases, seizures are triggered by hypoglycemia, and treatment includes glucose 10% solution. Pyridoxine (B_6) deficiency may also cause seizures and is treated with IV or IM Vitamin B_6.

Antibiotics

Antibiotics are frequently prescribed to neonates with suspected infection or sepsis, but dosing must be carefully calculated to account for the larger volume of extracellular fluid and the clearance rate of their renal system. Neonatal exposure to antibiotics also increases the risk of future health problems (due to their influence on the development of the neonate's gastrointestinal system/gut) or antibiotic resistance. Antibiotics may be classified according to their chemical nature, origin, action, or range of effectiveness. **Broad-spectrum antibiotics** are useful against both gram-positive and gram-negative bacteria. **Medium-spectrum antibiotics** are usually effective against gram-positive bacteria, although some may also be effective against gram-negative bacteria. **Narrow-spectrum antibiotics** are effective against a small range of bacteria. Antibiotics kill the bacteria by interfering with their biological functions (bactericidal) or by preventing reproduction (bacteriostatic).

Antibiotic Therapy for Neonatal Sepsis

For the treatment of **early-onset sepsis**, the American Academy of Pediatrics recommends a broad-spectrum antibiotic (such as ampicillin) every 12 hours combined with an aminoglycoside (gentamicin) or cephalosporin every 24 hours until the causative bacteria is/are identified and treatment can be more specified. In the case of **late-onset sepsis,** ampicillin (or vancomycin if the neonate has remained hospitalized since birth) is usually combined with gentamicin. In either case, once blood cultures return negatively for infection, antibiotics should be discontinued no more than 48 hours from incubation.

Review Video: Antibiotics: An Overview
Visit mometrix.com/academy and enter code: 165628

Gentamicin

Gentamicin is an inexpensive aminoglycoside antibiotic commonly used to treat neonates with gram-negative bacterial infections, like *Staphylococci*. It works by interfering with bacterial protein synthesis, resulting in a defective bacterial cell membrane. **Gentamicin** is excreted unmetabolized by the kidneys and renal function is directly related to clearance. Clearance is slower in premature neonates secondary to immature kidneys. The peak level (highest concentration in the blood) of gentamicin is measured 30 minutes after infusion is completed, and trough level (lowest concentration of the drug in the blood) is measured 30 minutes prior to the next dose. Potential toxicities from elevated gentamicin levels are ototoxicity (ear damage potentiated by concurrent use of furosemide) and nephrotoxicity (kidney damage), so patients with renal failure may only require dosing once every several days. If the pre-dose level falls below 0.5 mg/L and the post-dose level falls below 4 mg/L, the gentamicin is sub-therapeutic and will not kill the bacterial infection.

Neonatal Anti-Viral Drugs

Drug	Dosage	Use
Acyclovir	IV: 60 mg/kg/day for 14–21 days	Indicated for herpes simplex and varicella zoster infections. Complications include rash, TTP, hemolytic uremic syndrome, increased liver enzymes, urea, and creatinine.
Ganciclovir	IV: 6 mg/kg every 12 hr for 6 weeks	Indicated for cytomegalovirus (disseminated, pneumonia). Complications include neutropenia, thrombocytopenia, phlebitis, rash, increased liver function tests, and seizures.
Palivizumab (Synagis)	IV or IM: 15 mg/kg monthly during season or while at risk	Humanized monoclonal antibody indicated to treat or protect against respiratory syncytial virus for neonates with severe respiratory disease, such as bronchopulmonary dysplasia. Complications include fever, poor feeding, bleeding, irritability, wheezing, and allergic reaction.
Respiratory Syncytial Virus Immune Globulin (RSVIG/RespiGam)	IV: 750 mg/kg (15 mL/kg) with slow infusion	Indicated for prophylaxis against respiratory syncytial virus but less potent than palivizumab and requires IV administration and larger volume. Complications include fever, wheezing, GI upset, allergic reaction, muscle rigidity.

Anti-Hypertensives and Other Cardiac Drugs

Antihypertensives are used to control congestive heart failure and reduce the cardiac workload:

- **Propranolol** is a beta-blocker used to control hypertension.
- **Labetalol** is an alpha-1 and beta-adrenergic blocker that slows the heart rate and decreases peripheral vascular resistance and cardiac output.

- **Esmolol** is a beta-blocker given intravenously after surgery to control systemic hypertension, arrhythmias, and outflow obstruction.
- **Nicardipine** is a calcium channel blocker used to control hypertension, particularly severe neonatal hypertension, through peripheral vasodilation.
- **Hydralazine** is a vasodilator used to treat moderate hypertension.

Miscellaneous cardiac drugs are used for specific purposes:

- **Calcium chloride/calcium gluconate** is given intravenously to treat electrolyte imbalances such as hyperkalemia and hypocalcemia.
- **Indomethacin** (Indocin) is a NSAID that is given intravenously to inhibit the production of prostaglandin, thereby speeding the closure of the ductus arteriosus.
- **Prostaglandin** is given intravenously before surgery to maintain the patency of the ductus arteriosus for structural cardiac abnormalities in conditions such as coarctation of the aorta or transposition of the great arteries.

Diuretics

Loop, Thiazide, and Potassium-Sparing Diuretics

Diuretics decrease the fluid load in infants with heart failure or lung disorders, such as bronchopulmonary dysplasia. Different **classes of diuretics** have different mechanisms of action and different side effect profiles:

- **Thiazide diuretics** (e.g., chlorothiazide) work by inhibiting Na+/Cl- transport in the distal convoluted tubule. They are less potent than loop diuretics, but are first-line treatment options for neonates requiring diuresis. Hyponatremia, hypokalemia, and hypomagnesemia are the adverse reactions from chronic use.
- **Loop diuretics** (e.g., furosemide) are the most potent of the diuretics and work on the ascending limb of the loop of Henle. They disrupt the Na+/K+/2Cl- transporter and also limit K+ reabsorption. Hypokalemia, hyponatremia, and increased calcium excretion are the adverse reactions seen with chronic use. Due to adverse effects that are more common in neonates, loop diuretics are not a first-line therapy.
- **Potassium-sparing diuretics** (e.g., spironolactone) work by inhibiting the action of aldosterone. Aldosterone promotes K+ secretion and Na+ reabsorption at the distal nephron. These diuretics are the least potent, but do not cause hypokalemia, and have proven effective for some neonates.

Review Video: What are Diuretics and How do they Work?
Visit mometrix.com/academy and enter code: 373276

Diuretic Use in Neonates

Diuretics are used in the cardiac patient to increase renal perfusion and filtration, thereby reducing preload. Dosages are weight and age related. Diuretics commonly used include:

- **Thiazide diuretics,** such as chlorothiazide and hydrochlorothiazide, are the diuretics of choice for neonates in the management of mild hypertension or bronchopulmonary dysplasia.
- **Furosemide** (Lasix) is a loop diuretic and is used for the control of congestive heart failure as well as renal insufficiency. Loop diuretics are not recommended as a first-line diuretic due to the risk for adverse effects.

- **Spironolactone** (Aldactone) is a potassium-sparing synthetic steroid diuretic that increases the secretion of both water and sodium and is used to treat congestive heart failure. It may be given orally or intravenously.

Vasodilators and Anti-Arrhythmics

Vasodilators may be used for arterial dilation or venous dilation. These drugs are used to treat pulmonary hypertension or generalized systemic hypertension. Dosages are weight and age related. Vasodilators include:

- **Hydralazine** can be administered orally or via IV and acts on the smooth muscles to decrease blood pressure.
- **Nitroprusside** is given intravenously for peripheral vascular dilation to decrease afterload and SVR in order to increase cardiac output.

Vasopressors/Inotropes

Drugs used to increase cardiac output and improve contractibility of the myocardium are the vasopressors/inotropes. Dosage and administration of pediatric medications is weight and age related. Inotropes include:

- **Dobutamine** is given intravenously to improve cardiac output and treat cardiac decompensation.
- **Dopamine** is given intravenously to increase cardiac output, blood pressure, and the excretion of urine.
- **Epinephrine** is given intravenously to increase blood pressure and cardiac output, but it must be used judiciously because it also increases consumption of oxygen.
- **Milrinone** is given to increase cardiac output and stroke volume, decrease systemic vascular resistance (SVR), and control congestive heart failure.

Digitalis

Digitalis is a cardiac glycoside that is used to treat stage C heart failure and several different cardiac arrhythmias. Digitalis slows and strengthens the heartbeat. It has both a direct action on the myocardium and an indirect action mediated through the autonomic nervous system. The direct effect on the myocardium works by inhibiting the action of the sodium/potassium pump across cardiac cell membranes. The net result is an increase in intracellular sodium and calcium and an increase in extracellular potassium. The intracellular calcium is responsible for the increased strength of contractions of the heart (positive ionotrope). The indirect action of digitalis causes the heart rate to slow (negative chronotrope) by decreasing electrical conduction through the AV node. Digoxin has a narrow therapeutic index, meaning the lethal dose is close to the therapeutic dose. Signs of **digitalis toxicity** in infants include:

- GI signs: anorexia, nausea, vomiting, and diarrhea
- Cardiac arrhythmias: most commonly conduction disturbances, such as first-degree heart block, a supraventricular tachyarrhythmia such as atrial tachycardia, or bradycardia

Assume any alteration in cardiac conduction in an infant taking digoxin is a consequence of digitalis toxicity.

Volatile Anesthetics

Small infants have a high water content (70–75%) compared to adults (50–60%), and a lower muscle mass. These factors, coupled with slow renal and hepatic clearance, increased rate of metabolism, decreased protein binding, and increased organ perfusion affect the pharmacological action of drugs. Pediatric doses are calculated according to the child's weight in kilograms, but other factors may affect dosage. **Anesthetic agents** must be chosen with care because of the potential for adverse effects:

Inhalational

Infants are more likely to develop hypotension and bradycardia with inhalational anesthetic agents. Inhalation induction is rapid because infants and young children have high alveolar ventilation and decreased FRC compared to older patients with depression of ventilation more common in infants. There is increased risk of overdose. Sevoflurane is usually preferred for induction and isoflurane or halothane for maintenance as desflurane and sevoflurane are associated with delirium on emergence.

Nonvolatile Anesthetics

Infants may need higher proportionate (based on weight) doses of propofol because it is eliminated more quickly than with adults. It should not be used for infants who are critically ill, as it has been correlated to increased mortality rate and severe adverse effects leading to multi-organ failure. Thiopental is also used in higher proportionate doses for infants and children although this is not true for neonates. Neonates are especially sensitive to opioids, and morphine should be avoided or used with caution. Clearance rates for some drugs (sufentanil, alfentanil) may be higher in infants. Ketamine combined with fentanyl may cause more hypotension in neonates and small infants than ketamine combined with midazolam. Midazolam combined with fentanyl can cause severe hypotension. Etomidate is not used for infants but is reserved for children >10.

Muscle Relaxants

Onset with muscle relaxants is about 50% shorter in infants than adults, and pediatric patients may have variable responses to muscle to non-depolarizing muscle relaxants. Drugs that are metabolized through the liver (vecuronium) have prolonged action, so atracurium and cisatracurium, which do not depend on the liver, are more reliable. Succinylcholine can cause severe adverse effects (rhabdomyolysis, malignant hyperthermia, hyperkalemia, arrhythmias), so its use requires premedication with atropine, but succinylcholine is usually avoided in pediatric patients except for rapid sequence induction for children with full stomach and laryngospasm. Rocuronium is frequently used for intubation because of fast onset, but it has up to 90 minutes duration, so mivacurium, atracurium, and cisatracurium may be preferred for shorter procedures. Nerve stimulators should be used to monitor incremental doses, which are usually 25–30% of the original bolus. Blockade by non-depolarizing muscle relaxants can be reversed with neostigmine or edrophonium and glycopyrrolate or atropine.

Review Video: Muscle Relaxants
Visit mometrix.com/academy and enter code: 862193

Bronchodilators and Respiratory Stimulants

Bronchodilators and respiratory stimulants are used to treat respiratory distress in the neonate:

- **Aminophylline and theophylline** both stimulate the sympathetic nervous system and dilate the bronchi. These medications are used for apnea of prematurity in the neonate and bronchospasm in infants with respiratory distress. Apnea of prematurity is treated with loading dose of 6 mg/kg aminophylline with maintenance doses of 2.5–3.5 mg/kg intravenously every 12 hours. Further treatment may be done orally with theophylline. Side effects include tachycardia, seizures, and irritability.

- **Albuterol** is a selective β2-adrenergic agonist bronchodilator that can be administered orally (100–300 μg/kg 3–4 times daily) or inhaled (100–500 μg/kg 4–8 times daily).
- **Caffeine citrate,** a stimulant, is the first line treatment for apnea of prematurity as it is safer than theophylline and can be administered orally. Loading dose is usually 20 mg/mg with one-time daily maintenance dose of 5mg/kg.
- **Epinephrine** is used to treat stridor with effect on β-adrenoreceptors. It is delivered with nebulizer at 50–100 μg/kg as needed.

Caffeine for Neonatal Apnea

Apnea of prematurity occurs when the neonate stops breathing for 20 seconds or longer because the respiratory centers are immature. Apnea of prematurity is an exclusionary diagnosis, arrived at only when all other causes have been ruled out. Treatment consists of respiratory support with supplemental oxygen, continuous positive airway pressure (CPAP), or a ventilator in severe cases. **Caffeine** has largely replaced theophylline as the pharmacological treatment of choice for apnea of prematurity. Both are methylxanthines, but caffeine has a wider therapeutic index and a slower excretion rate than theophylline. Caffeine is a **central nervous system stimulant** that naturally occurs in tea, coffee, and chocolate. Give 10 mg CAFCIT to the infant orally. Side effects include irritability, tremors, tachycardia, tachypnea, vomiting, fever, and hyperglycemia. Peak blood levels will be reached in 30–120 minutes and should not exceed 6–10 mg/L. Toxicity is 50 mg/L. If seizures occur with caffeine overdose, give diazepam or pentobarbital sodium. Mean half-life is 3–4 days. Monitor trough levels periodically.

Surfactants

Surfactants reduce surface tension to prevent collapse of alveoli. Beractant (Survanta) is derived from bovine lung tissue and calfactant (Infasurf) from calf lung tissue. Surfactant replacement therapy is used to prevent RDS for infants born at 27-30 weeks gestation. It is also used for infants showing signs of worsening lung disease. Surfactant has traditionally been given via the endotracheal tube (ETT) as an inhalant, but with advancing efforts to reduce mechanical ventilation in the context of RDS, other routes of administration are being considered, including minimally invasive surfactant therapy (MIST) through a thin catheter in the trachea while being oxygenated throug noninvasive means, or via nebulizer through a laryngeal mask. Both endoctracheal and MIST approaches have different protocol for determining the need of secondary doses, and facility policy for surfactant therapy should be followed closely.

Steroids

Steroids are commonly administered to mothers to promote fetal lung development for preterm births. These drugs include betamethasone and dexamethasone. Steroids may also be administered to the neonate, but they are associated with significant side effects:

- **Betamethasone** may be used for chronic lung disease (CLD) in the neonate and post-intubation airway edema, but high dose treatment has been associated with cerebral palsy, growth depression, hypertension, hyperglycemia, hypokalemia, and increased risk of infection. Airway edema is treated with 200 mcg/kg orally or IV every 8 hours beginning 4 hours before extubation. Dosages for other treatment vary widely with tapering of doses.
- **Hydrocortisone** may be used for physiologic replacement or acute hypotension. Replacement is begun with 1-2 mg orally every 8 hours and increased to 6-9 mg/m2/day. Hypotension is treated with 2 mg/kg IV loading dose and maintenance of 1 mg/kg IV every 8-12 hours.

Vitamin K

Vitamin K deficiency in newborns may cause vitamin K deficiency bleeding (VKDB), also called **hemorrhagic disease of the newborn**. Vitamin K is a fat-soluble vitamin produced in the gut. Vitamin K is required by the liver to produce four of the clotting factors—II, VII, IX, and X. At birth, all infants are Vitamin K deficient because of limited transfer of vitamin K across the placenta. Newborns are injected with one intramuscular (IM) dose of vitamin K1, 0.5-1.0 mg within six hours of birth. The injection quickly raises the infant's vitamin K level to normal and maintains the normal level for several months. Vitamin K should be given prior to circumcision. Infants who do not receive vitamin K prophylaxis at birth will take several weeks (formula-fed) to several months (breastfed) to attain normal vitamin K levels. Formula contains higher levels of vitamin K than human breast milk. VKDB occurs in two forms:

- **Early-onset form** occurs within the first 24 hours after birth and is related to maternal medications that interfere with Vitamin K.
- **Late-onset form** occurs after two weeks of age, because of exclusive breastfeeding, diarrhea, hepatitis, cystic fibrosis, alpha 1-antitrypsin disease, or celiac disease.

Neonatal Analgesics

Sucrose Analgesia

Sucrose analgesia (Sweet-Ease) is used to relieve stress and discomfort in infants before and during medical procedures, such as heel sticks, IV insertion, injections, suctioning, and insertion of NG tubes. Sweet-Ease, a commercially prepared product, is 24% sucrose in an oral solution into which a standard pacifier is dipped and given to the infant, usually 2 minutes before a procedure. The pacifier may be re-dipped every 2 minutes for a total of 4 times. If the infant cannot suck, 0.1 mL of solution is placed on the anterior tongue with a medical syringe with the same frequency. For more painful procedures, such as lumbar puncture and circumcision, sucrose analgesia may be used in conjunction with other forms of analgesia to provide comfort. Contraindications include <32 weeks gestation, hyperglycemia, history of asphyxia or intolerance to feedings, critical illness, paralysis, opioid sedation, and infants NPO for surgery unless cleared by an anesthesiologist.

Acetaminophen

Acetaminophen (Tylenol) is used both for control of mild to moderate pain and fever. Acetaminophen can be administered orally and rectally, but absorption is less reliable with the rectal route. Acetaminophen has a half-life of 4 hours, is conjugated in the liver, and is excreted through the kidneys. **Oral dosage** is typically 24 mg/kg as a loading dose and 12 mg/kg every four hours (or 8 hours in infants <32 weeks); **rectal dosage** is 36 mg/kg (loading), followed by 24 mg/kg every 8 hours. Serum levels should be checked if treatment is to continue for >24 hours. Serum levels of 12-24 mg/L are required for adequate pain control. Acetaminophen is commonly used for control of pain after **circumcision**, although it is not sufficient for pain control during the procedure.

Fentanyl and Morphine

Fentanyl and morphine are opioid analgesics/narcotics that treat moderate-to-severe pain:

- **Fentanyl** is for painful dressing changes or procedures. Duration of action is 1-2 hours and half-life is 2-4 hours. Dosage is 0.5-1 mcg/kg every 1-2 hours or by continuous infusion. Rapid tolerance develops, requiring higher doses to create the same relief, and increasing the chance of overdose. Fentanyl is metabolized by the liver and excreted by the kidneys. *Side* effects of fentanyl include respiratory depression, peripheral vasodilatation, inhibition of intestinal peristalsis, and chest wall rigidity at higher doses, which compromises ventilation. Fentanyl is less likely to cause hypotension than morphine.
- **Morphine** is for postoperative pain. Duration of action is 3-4 hours, and half-life is 2-4 hours. Morphine is metabolized by the liver to an inactive metabolite and excreted by the kidneys; 2-12% is excreted unchanged in the urine. Dosage is 0.02-0.10 mg/kg every 1-4 hours or by continuous infusion. Side effects of morphine include respiratory depression, histamine release, and seizures.

Neuroprotective and Neurodevelopmental Care

Developmental Care

Developmental care is neonatal nursing that acknowledges environmental conditions and behavioral cues. Minimize noises and bright lights to decrease excessive stimuli. Observe the patient for cues regarding his or her feeding requirements and emotional state. The goal is to provide the optimum environment and treatment modalities that are the least stressful to the neonate, allowing for positive growth and development. Encourage parental involvement to foster attachment and competence in caring for the neonate. **Key components of developmental care** include:

- Observe, interpret, and respond to infant cues during care.
- Alter care based on neonatal developmental changes (e.g., the needs of a neonate at 26 weeks gestational age are different from those of one at 38 weeks gestational age).
- Time, pace, and handle the infant based on observed cues during care.
- Position infants based on their needs.
- Modify the environment based on the infant's needs.
- Foster parental participation in the care of their infant.

Neurobehavioral Development

Terms related to neurobehavioral development:

- **Habituation**: A decreasing response to repeated stimuli. For example, if a child is exposed to repeated sounds, the child will over time become used to the sound and show less reaction.
- **Motor organization**: Motor organization involves 3 different levels:
  - The spinal cord (which mediates automatic movement and reflexes)
  - The brain stem (which includes the medial descending systems that control body movement and antigravity reflexes and the lateral descending systems that control voluntary limb movements)
  - The cerebral cortex (which regulates movement)
- **State organization**: The brain has the ability to respond differently in different states or conditions, suggesting that the neonate's brain is active and not just passive.

- **Sensory/interaction capabilities**: The ability to respond to stimuli and to interact with the environment and others. The interactions the neonate has after birth with others (dyadic interactions) help the child to learn patterns of interactions and responses.

Sleep States

Infants spend a high percentage of their time in **sleep states**. Sleep periods are divided into active sleep or quiet sleep by observing the infant's behavior:

- **Quiet sleep** is restorative and fosters anabolic growth. Quiet sleep is associated with increased cell mitosis and replication, lowered oxygen consumption, and the release of growth hormone. During quiet sleep, the infant appears relaxed, moves minimally, and breathes smoothly and regularly. The eyelids are still. The infant only responds to intense stimuli during quiet sleep.
- **Active sleep** is associated with processing and storing of information. Rapid eye movement (REM sleep) occurs during active sleep, but it is unknown if newborn infants are able to dream. During active sleep, the infant moves occasionally and breathes irregularly. Eye movements can be seen beneath the eyelids. Infants spend most of their sleep time in active sleep, and it usually precedes wakening.

Awake States

Infants have different levels of consciousness in the 4 **awake states**. Infants respond differently to outside stimuli and interaction from caregivers, depending on which state they are in:

- **Drowsy:** This is characterized by variable activity, mild startles, and smooth movement. There is some facial movement. Eyes open and close, breathing is irregular, and response to stimuli may be delayed.
- **Quiet alert:** The infant rarely moves, breathing is regular, and the infant focuses intently on individuals or objects that are within focal range, widening eyes. The face appears bright and alert, breathing is regular, and the infant focuses on stimuli.
- **Active alert:** The infant moves frequently and has much facial movement although the face not as bright and alert, eyes may have a dull glaze, breathing is irregular, and there are variable responses to outside stimuli.
- **Crying:** Characterized by grimacing, eyes shut, irregular breathing, increased movement with color changes and marked response to both internal and external stimuli.

Neonatal Behavioral Assessment Scale

The Neonatal Behavioral Assessment Scale, developed by Dr. Berry Brazelton, is a multi-dimensional scale that is used to assess a neonate's state, temperament, and behavioral patterns. It includes the assessment of 20 reflexes and 28 behaviors, and is divided into four categories: autonomic regulation, motor development, state regulation, and social engagement. It is usually completed on day 3 with an attempt to elicit the most positive response, usually when the infant is comforted and in a quiet dim room. Scoring correlates to the child's awake or sleep state. Infants are scored according to response in many areas, including:

- **Habituation**: Ability to diminish response to repeat stimuli
- **Visual and auditory orientation**: Ability to respond to stimuli, fixate, and follow a visual object
- **Motor activity**: Assessment of body tone in various activities
- **Variations**: Changes in color, state, activity, alertness, and excitement during the exam

- **Self-quieting activities**: Frequency and speed of self-calming activities, such as sucking on their hand, putting their hand to mouth, and focusing on objects or sounds
- **Social behaviors**: Ability to cuddle, engage, and enjoy physical contact

A condensed version of this tool, the Newborn Behavioral Observations (NBO) system, was created in 2000. The NBO is made to be given in a variety of settings, both at home and in the healthcare environment, and consists of 18 observable neurobehavioral items.

Stress Responses

The neonate may exhibit a number of different stress responses:

- **Motoric responses:** Instead of normal and consistent muscle tone, the neonate may exhibit hypotonia with flaccid extremities and jaw. Some may exhibit hypertonicity with extremities hyperextended and/or hyperflexion of extremities. Some neonates may exhibit flailing, twitching, and tremors.
- **Attentional responses:** The neonate may react poorly to auditory, social, and visual stimuli and may exhibit poor sleeping, inability to be consoled, and staring or eye-roving behavior. The neonate may appear stressed and panicked or close eyes and withdraw.
- **Self-regulating/comforting responses:** The neonate may exhibit a number of behaviors to attempt to reduce stress. Motor activities may include grasping hands, moving hands toward the mouth, sucking, grasping blankets and tubing, moving about, and bracing feet against blankets or other barriers. The neonate may cry loudly and rhythmically to reduce stress and induce sleep. These tactics help the neonate to modulate responses to stimuli so that the newborn is not overwhelmed by the stress response.

Autonomic Stress Response

The autonomic nervous system is part of the peripheral nervous system and includes sympathetic nerves. The sympathetic nervous system (T1 to L2) activates in times of stress and is implicated in pain. The nerves innervate deep structures, viscera, and skin. The autonomic nervous system mediates the body's organs and maintains homeostasis. When a neonate is stressed, the neonate typically responds by crying. Other signs of the **autonomic stress response** in the newborn include:

- **Change in skin color**: flushing, pallor, mottling rather than stable pink color
- **Respiratory changes**: when stable, respirations are regular and smooth; with stress, the neonate may exhibit gasping, sighing, apneic periods, and tachypnea
- **Cardiovascular changes**: heart rate and blood pressure increase
- **Visceral/GI response**: hiccups, gagging, coughing, vomiting, sneezing, passing flatus, choking, grunting

The caregiver must recognize the signs of stress, respond to the neonate's needs, and reduce stimuli. For example, a combination of stimuli, such as sound, lights, and touch, may overwhelm a newborn. Additionally, newborns may react to the stress of caregivers.

Stress Related to Light

Light is a necessary component of caring for both sick and healthy neonates in the delivery room and nursery. Adequate lighting is required to evaluate the at-risk neonate, to assess color, to complete procedures such as intubation, or to give medications. Light also discourages the growth of pathogens. However, constant bright light interferes with the development of natural diurnal rhythms because it arouses the central nervous system and stresses the infant. Controlling light helps to stabilize the infant. Some simple methods to protect the neonate from light over-stimulation and to establish a normal sleep cycle include:

- Reducing overhead light levels when direct visualization is not necessary
- Covering incubator hoods to reduce light entering the incubator
- Dimming the lights at night to help establish a natural day/night pattern (circadian rhythm)

STRESS RELATED TO NOISE

Excessive **noise** causes agitation in all neonates, but especially in preterm neonates. The preterm neonate has less ability to self-calm, and over-stimulation results in decompensation, as demonstrated by increased oxygen requirements and increased apnea and bradycardia episodes. The American Academy of Pediatrics (AAP) recommends noise levels in the nursery and NICU be kept at **≤45 decibels**. A normal speaking voice is 50–60 decibels. Noise levels above 80 decibels can damage the cochlea and cause hearing loss in adults. To keep noise acceptably low:

- Turn radios/TVs off or down.
- Designate a daily quiet time.
- Close incubator portholes gently, because closing a plastic porthole can spike the decibel level more than 80 dB.
- Whisper and, as much as possible, avoid speaking loudly.
- Remove bubbling water from ventilator tubing.
- Educate parents about the deleterious effects of over-stimulating their infant with loud noises.

ENVIRONMENTAL STRESSORS AND "TIME OUT"

Premature neonates have a very limited ability to deal with **environmental stressors,** but these stressors can affect all neonates. Signs of stress in neonates include:

- Color changes, such as mottling or cyanosis
- Episodes of apnea and bradycardia
- Activity changes, such as tremors, twitches, frantic activity, arching, and gaze-averting
- Flaccid posture (sagging trunk, extremities, and face)
- Easy fatigability

When the infant shows signs of stress, a **time-out** recovery period is indicated:

- Stop the activity causing the stress.
- Reduce unnecessary stimuli (e.g., lower the lights and postpone non-essential manipulation of the neonate).
- Give the neonate a chance to calm down or self-soothe.
- Bundle the neonate and place him/her in a comforting, side-lying position with the shoulders drawn forward and the hands brought to the midline.

NON-NUTRITIVE SUCKING

Non-nutritive sucking occurs when an infant sucks on an item such as a pacifier or his/her own fist. Non-nutritive sucking is not associated with nutritional intake, but it is an important method of self-quieting and begins in the uterus at about 29 weeks of gestation. Extremely premature infants often lack basic neurodevelopmental capabilities, and cannot coordinate sucking, swallowing, and breathing simultaneously. Typically, the ability to suck and swallow in a coordinated fashion is not present until 32–34 weeks of gestation. Premature infants should be encouraged to perform non-nutritive sucking during the gavage feeding process if they can accomplish it. Benefits of non-nutritive sucking include:

- Improved digestion of enteral feeds because digestive enzyme release is stimulated
- Facilitated development of coordinated nutritive sucking behavior
- Calming of the distressed infant

Positioning of the Premature Neonate

Correct positioning of the premature neonate minimizes outside stimuli and mimics the enclosed and calming environment of the womb, helping with the transition to extrauterine life:

- Place the neonate in a flexed position, with his hands close to midline and near his face.
- Create a nest of blankets or pillows to:
    - Help block out light and noise.
    - Give him the impression of a closed environment.
    - Minimize abnormal molding of the head from prolonged pressure on one side.
- Cover the incubator to further keep out sound and light.
- Place the neonate in the prone position (on his stomach) to help to stabilize the chest wall, improve ventilation, and increase the amount of time the infant is in quiet sleep. However, infants should be placed supine (on the back) most of the time, to decrease the chance of SIDS.

Clustering Care

The concept of clustering care for the premature neonate centers on allowing the neonate to have prolonged periods of rest or sleep in between required care procedures and manipulations. Long periods of rest and quiet simulate the uninterrupted and fairly constant environment of the womb. Clustering care means performing multiple tasks at the same time, such as feeding, bathing, wound care, drawing laboratory samples, or examining the infant. However, the premature infant may not be able to tolerate multiple manipulations and may show signs of decompensation before all the planned procedures are completed. The premature infant may need a time-out period to recover before performing more stressful procedures. Balance clustering care with observing the infant for cues of stress.

Provision of Sensory Experiences

While sensory interventions are important for neurobehavioral development, preterm neonates or those who are seriously ill may be able to tolerate only one or two types of sensory interventions, so each neonate must be assessed individually and carefully observed for signs of stress. **Sensory experiences** that benefit the neonate can include:

- **Auditory**: Talking to the neonates in a calm and soothing high-pitched tone of voice or providing toys that produce soft or low sounds (such as music) may be used, but loud or sudden noises should be avoided.
- **Tactile**: Gently massaging the neonate, starting from the head down to the extremities, abdomen, and back as the neonate can tolerate is highly beneficial for the neonate; however, light touch should be avoided. Neonatal hand-to-mouth activity should be encouraged.
- **Visual**: Keeping eye contact with the child during all interactions, providing other visual items (mirrors, bright red item, mobiles), and keeping lights low benefits the infant's visual development.

- **Vestibular** (middle ear/brain) **and proprioceptive** (position): Swaddling (legs flexed and hands near mouth), holding, and slowly rocking the neonate back and forth for at least 5 minutes benefits the neonate.

Genetic Complications

Metabolic Screening of the Newborn

Metabolic screening of the newborn to detect genetic diseases varies somewhat from one state to another, but some states test for as many as 80 conditions. Because approximately 1 in 200 newborns has chromosomal abnormalities, screening is an important tool, although many birth defects are not genetic in origin, such as defects caused by maternal alcohol abuse or vitamin deficiency. A few drops of blood are placed on special filter paper from a heel stick with the sample collected between 24 and 48 hours of birth. Each of five circles on the filter paper must be saturated with a drop of blood, and the paper is then placed in a horizontal position to air dry for 3 hours before it is forwarded to a laboratory for testing. Screening tests generally include the following:

- Biotinidase deficiency (autosomal recessive)
- Congenital adrenal hyperplasia (autosomal recessive)
- Congenital hearing loss (autosomal recessive, autosomal dominant, or mitochondrial)
- Congenital hypothyroidism (autosomal recessive or autosomal dominant)
- Cystic fibrosis (autosomal recessive)
- Galactosemia (autosomal recessive)
- Homocystinuria (autosomal recessive)
- Maple syrup urine disease (autosomal recessive)
- Medium-chain Acyl-CoA dehydrogenase (autosomal recessive)
- Phenylketonuria (autosomal recessive)
- Sickle cell disease (autosomal recessive)
- Tyrosinemia (Two types are autosomal recessive; a third type is unclear)

Autosomal Inheritance Patterns

Autosomal inheritance patterns involve genetic **abnormalities in chromosome pairs 1-22**:

- **Autosomal recessive***:* This occurs when two parents (without active disease) each have a copy of the same abnormal recessive gene, and both pass the abnormal copy to offspring. The **recurrence risk** (the chance to have affected offspring) for two carrier parents with the same abnormal gene mutation is 25% for each pregnancy and 50% chance the child will become a carrier. Autosomal recessive disorders, such as cystic fibrosis, Tay Sachs, and sickle cell anemia, are seen more frequently among certain ethnic groups and in offspring of related parents.
- **Autosomal dominant***:* This means that only one abnormal dominant gene needs to be inherited to cause the condition. Autosomal dominant diseases include Huntington's disease and Marfan syndrome. The recurrence risk for an affected parent to pass the disease to a child is 50% with each pregnancy, but there is no carrier state.

Sex-Linked Inheritance

Sex-linked inheritance involves the sex chromosomes (**chromosome 23**). Y-linked disorders such as Klinefelter syndrome are rare, but they will be passed from the father to all male children. X-linked diseases, such as hemophilia and Duchenne muscular dystrophy, usually occur in males because males have only one X chromosome, so a single recessive gene on that X chromosome causes the disease. Females have two X chromosomes, so the normal gene on an unaffected X chromosome can usually compensate. Although the Y chromosome is the other half of the XY chromosome pair in the male, the Y chromosome is much smaller than the X chromosome and doesn't contain most of the genes of the X chromosome—it's not a complete match—so there is no compensating gene to protect the male. Thus, females carry the disease and males inherit the disease. A man with an X-linked recessive disorder will not pass the disease to his sons (because they don't inherit his X chromosome), but his daughters will inherit the mutated gene, so they have one abnormal X (from the father) and one normal (from the mother). These daughters then have a 50% chance of having sons who are affected and a 50% chance of having daughters who carry one copy of the mutated gene. X-linked dominant inheritance also differs depending upon whether the mother or father carries the defective gene. There is no carrier state with X-linked dominant disorders. If the father has the disease, such as Rett's syndrome, all daughters will inherit. If the mother has the disease, each child, regardless of gender, has a 50% chance of inheriting.

Multifactorial Inheritance

Complex or multifactorial inheritance relates to an interaction of many different genes, as well as the environment and lifestyle choices. Thus, a genetic disorder may depend upon genes inherited from both parents as well as unidentified environmental factors (smoking, drug use, diet) interacting in such a way as to produce an abnormality. This type of inheritance pattern is much less predictable than the others. Neural tube defects, for example, are caused by multifactorial inheritance. In some cases, an infant may inherit only a tendency toward a disease, such as diabetes type 2, but development of the disease may depend up weight, diet, smoking, and other factors as the child matures. Complex diseases include such things as asthma, heart disease, and osteoarthritis. Multifactorial traits often run in families, with risk 50% in first-degree relatives (parents), 25% in second-degree (grandparents, aunts, uncles), and 12.5% in third-degree (cousins).

Cystic Fibrosis

Cystic fibrosis (mucoviscidosis or CF) is a progressive congenital disease that particularly affects the pancreas and lungs, causing digestive and respiratory problems. It is caused by a genetic defect that affects sodium chloride movement in cells, including mucosal cells that line the lungs, causing the production of thick mucus that clogs the lungs and provides a rich medium for bacteria. While most patients with cystic fibrosis at one time died in childhood, the life expectancy is now about 30 years. About 15-20% of neonates with CF have meconium ileus (obstruction of small intestine with meconium) at birth. Other infants have no symptoms at first but show failure to thrive in the first 4-6 weeks and may develop a cough and wheezing. Cystic fibrosis patients usually suffer from recurrent respiratory infections of the lower respiratory tract. The most common infective agents are *Pseudomonas aeruginosa* and *Burkholderia cepacia* complex. The screening test for CF is IRT/DNA. If the IRT/DNA is positive, the infant is scheduled for a sweat test and buccal swab.

G6PD Deficiency

Glucose-6-phosphate dehydrogenase (G6PD) deficiency is an X-linked recessive disease and can often present as, or similar to, hyperbilirubinemia. Because female infants inherit two X chromosomes, it's rare that both are defective, and the normal chromosome compensates, so X-linked recessive disorders affect primarily male children (who get the X chromosome from the mother, not the father) but are passed on by the mother. G6PD is an enzyme utilized to process carbohydrates and to protect red blood cells. G6PD results in premature destruction of red blood cells and hemolytic anemia, which can be triggered by infection, some medications (antimalarial drugs, sulfa, ASAS, NSAIDS, quinidine, quinine, and nitrofurantoin), and eating or inhaling the pollen of fava beans (favism). Infants may be asymptomatic, although some may exhibit increased jaundice. In the United States, G6PD is most common in African American males (1 out of 10) and those with Middle Eastern heritage. Treatment includes avoiding triggers, treating infections, and transfusions if necessary.

Chromosome Abnormalities

Chromosomal abnormalities (alterations in the structure or number of chromosomes) can result in various types of congenital anomalies. Common chromosomal abnormalities include:

- Trisomy 21 (Down syndrome): Cognitive impairment, hypotonia, palmar crease, flat facial profile, CHD
- Trisomy 18 (Edwards syndrome): Severe cognitive impairment, microcephaly, clenched fist/overlapping fingers, rocker-bottom feet, CHD
- Turner syndrome (45,X): Short stature, webbed neck, broad chest, coarctation of the aorta

Physical Assessment

Physical assessment of the neonate with chromosomal abnormalities includes:

- General: Measure the head circumference, length, weight, and note deviations from standard percentiles.
- Craniofacial: Note the head shape and size, abnormalities of the skull, space between the eyes, and ear abnormalities (low set, malformed), nonflat nasal bridge, micrognathia, cleft lip/palate.
- Neck: Note webbing or increased nuchal translucency.
- Thoracic: Note broad/shield shape, wide-spaced nipples, listen for heart murmurs.
- Abdomen: Palpate and note hepatosplenomegaly and abdominal wall defects (e.g., omphalocele, gastroschisis).
- Genitourinary: Note ambiguous genitalia.
- Extremities: Note limb abnormalities (e.g., polydactyly, syndactyly, differences in limb lengths), note sign of palmar crease.
- Neurological: Assess muscle tone for hypertonia or hypotonia and primitive reflexes.
- Dermatological: Note pigmentation anomalies (e.g., café au lait, hypopigmentation) and vascular anomalies (e.g., hemangiomas).
- Eye/Ear: Fundoscopy should be done to assess for ocular anomalies and auditory screening for hearing loss.

Trisomy 13

Trisomy 13 (Patau syndrome) may occur with complete trisomy, mosaicism, or partial trisomy, so symptoms may vary depending upon the amount of extra genetic material in **chromosome 13**. Diagnosis can be made prenatally with amniocentesis. This disorder occurs in 1 of every 20,000 live births in both males and females. **Indications** include:

- Cleft lip/palate
- Polydactyly and clenched fists
- Microcephaly, abnormal brain structure, profound intellectual disability, seizures
- Small or absent close-set eyes (may be fused into one eye), vision impairment
- Coloboma (split or hole in iris)
- Low-set ears and deafness
- Umbilical/inguinal hernias
- Cardiac abnormalities with heart on right side of chest and congestive heart disease (80%)
- Rocker-bottom feet
- Micrognathia
- Multiple system disorders

Treatment is supportive and symptomatic, but despite interventions, about 80% die ≤1 month. Infants may have profound dyspnea, seizures, and difficulty feeding.

Trisomy 18

Trisomy 18 occurs when the infant has **three number 18 chromosomes**, instead of the normal two. Trisomy 18 is an aneuploidy second only to Down syndrome (trisomy 21) for frequency. Trisomy 18 occurs in 1 of every 6,000-8,000 live births, and is associated with severe malformations and high infant mortality. Only 5-10% of affected children survive beyond the first year of life. **Malformations** include:

- **Neurological**: Microcephaly, anencephaly, hydrocephaly, Arnold-Chiari malformation, hypoplasia of the corpus callosum, wide occipitoparietal skull diameter with narrow frontal diameter, called "strawberry sign" because of its appearance on ultrasound.
- **Facial**: Epicanthal folds, short palpebral fissures, cataracts, short nose with upturned nares, micrognathia, narrow palate, cleft palate, and low-set ears.
- **Skeletal**: Clenched fists, radial hypoplasia, rocker-bottom feet, hypoplastic nails, and short neck with excessive skin folds.
- **Cardiac**: Ventricular septal defect is most common, but some heart problem is present over 90% of the time.
- **Other**: Pulmonary hypoplasia, omphalocele, esophageal atresia, multicystic kidneys, cryptorchidism, and intrauterine growth restriction.

Trisomy 21

Trisomy 21 (**Down syndrome**) occurs in 1 out of every 800 live births. Trisomy 21 is the most common chromosomal disorder in humans. Advanced maternal age is a risk factor. The definitive diagnosis is made by cytogenetic examination of the infant's DNA from amniocentesis or chorionic villi sampling. Common **physical characteristics** of infants born with Down syndrome are listed below in decreasing order of incidence:

- Low birth weight
- Brachycephaly (head is short in diameter from front to back and disproportionately broad)
- Upslanting palpebral fissures (openings between the eyelids)
- Wide gap between first and second toes
- Small, low set ears
- Hypotonia
- Epicanthic skin folds (redundant skin folds in the upper eyelid from the nose to the inner side of the eyebrow)
- Brushfield's spots (small white or gray spots on the periphery of the iris)
- Short, wide hands
- Single transverse palmar crease
- Heart disease (40-50%); murmur may be heard on physical exam

DiGeorge Syndrome

DiGeorge syndrome is a series of congenital defects that results from a deletion of part of the long arm of **chromosome 22**. This same area of the chromosome is also missing in infants with velo-cardio-facial syndrome and conotruncal anomalies face syndrome, so use the preferred name

22q11 deletion syndrome to describe all three syndromes. The basic **defects** in 22q11 deletion syndrome are:

- Conotruncal heart defects: Tetralogy of Fallot, ventricular septal defect, or interrupted aortic arch (80%)
- Cleft lip or palate (70%)
- Hypocalcemia secondary to hypoparathyroidism (20-60%), which causes seizures
  - Note: Hypocalcemia is often temporary; many children do not require calcium supplementation after their first year of life
- Microcephaly, small ears, hooded eyelids, small mouth, and small chin
- Mild to borderline intellectual disability, with IQs in the 70-90 range (40%)
- Hypoplastic or absent thymus, resulting in T-cell dysfunction, recurrent infections secondary to immune deficiencies, and rarely, severe immune deficiency

Turner Syndrome

Turner syndrome is one of the most common chromosomal abnormalities, occurring in approximately 1 in 2,000 live female births (male fetuses die). **Turner syndrome** is caused by the absence of a set of genes that form the short arm of one of the X chromosomes. Most infants are missing the entire second chromosome (45X). Most pregnancies in which the infant has Turner syndrome end in spontaneous abortions. **Clinical signs** present at birth include:

- Webbed neck from fetal lymphedema; after the swelling resolves, loose folds of skin are still present on the neck
- Broad chest with wide spaced nipples (shield chest)
- Swollen hands and feet
- Short 4th or 5th metacarpals or metatarsals
- Increased incidence of congenital hip dislocation
- Increased incidence of coarctation of the aorta and bicuspid aortic valve

The **diagnosis** of Turner syndrome is confirmed by a karyotype. All infants with Turner syndrome must have their hearts evaluated.

Beckwith-Wiedemann Syndrome

Beckwith-Wiedemann syndrome is a congenital imprinting disorder (80% caused by defect of chromosome 11) of infants that exhibit overgrowth, affecting multiple body systems. Most cases are sporadic, although 10–15% are autosomal dominant transmission. Characteristics may include the following:

- Preterm delivery of LGA infants
- Macrosomia
- Height and weight >95% for age
- Hemihyperplasia
- Macroglossia
- Forehead ridge
- Increased risk of Wilms tumors, adrenal carcinoma, and liver tumors
- Nevus flammeus (erythema of the eyelids and forehead)
- Seizures
- Cryptorchidism
- Abdominal wall defects with enlarged organs (kidneys, adrenal glands, spleen, liver, and pancreas)
- Omphalocele or umbilical hernia, often needing surgical intervention
- Hypoglycemia
- Hemihypertrophy (overgrowth of only one side of body)
- Cardiac abnormalities.
- Hypoglycemia after birth, which can cause seizures
- Ear anomalies, sometimes result in hearing loss

Treatment includes surgical repair of abnormalities (such as abdominal wall defects) and removal of tumors (such as Wilms tumors), with chemotherapy as needed and control of hypoglycemia. Tongue reduction surgery and orthopedic repair may be done. Children who survive infancy have a good prognosis. Intelligence is usually normal although some may have slight cognitive impairment. Children must be monitored for tumor development.

Potter Sequence

Potter sequence or syndrome is a congenital disorder related to oligohydramnios or anhydramnios resulting from renal disease, such as bilateral renal agenesis (BRA), other urinary obstruction, or premature amniotic sac rupture. There are five different classifications of Potter syndrome:

- Classic: BRA present
- Type I: autosomal recessive polycystic kidney disease
- Type II: one kidney missing and the other abnormal
- Type III: autosomal dominant polycystic kidney disease
- Type IV: hydronephrosis from obstruction (rarely causes death)

The lack of amniotic fluid causes the fetus to be compressed by the uterus, resulting in a number of physical manifestations, including the following:

- Potter's facies: parrot-beak nose, micrognathia, low-set ears, flattened nose, wide-set eyes, and skin fold from edge of eye across cheek
- Clubfeet, tibial bowing, or fused legs (sirenomelia)
- Genitourinary and gynecological abnormalities (small bladder, absence or abnormality of reproductive organs)
- Pulmonary abnormalities (underdeveloped alveoli), resulting in severe respiratory distress at birth
- Diaphragmatic hernia
- Genitourinary anomalies, including absent or malformed kidneys

Treatment is supportive and symptomatic, but survival is extremely rare for most types. At birth, immediate respiratory support is needed, including intubation and ventilation or ECMO.

VATER Syndrome (VACTERL Association)

VATER syndrome is a subset of VACTERL association with fewer abnormalities. VATER/VACTERL is an acronym for several different birth defects that often occur together. The letters in the acronym stand for:

- **V**—Vertebral defects (70%): usually consist of smaller than normal vertebrae that may predispose the infant to develop scoliosis
- **A**—Anal atresia or imperforate anus (55%): often requires surgical correction at birth
- **C**—Cardiovascular defects (75%): common heart defects include ventral septal defect, atrial septal defect, and tetralogy of Fallot
- **T**—Tracheoesophageal fistula (70%)
- **E**—Esophageal atresia (70%)
- **R**—Renal anomalies (50%): anomalies can be severe, including incomplete formation of the kidneys or obstruction of urine outflow
- **L**—Limb anomalies (70%): defects include absent or displaced thumbs, extra digits, fusion of digits, and forearm defects

For VACTERL diagnosis, the infant must have 3 of the 7 malformations. An infant with any one of these birth defects must also be evaluated for other defects in the association. For VATER diagnosis, the infant must have 3 of 5 malformations.

CHARGE Syndrome

CHARGE syndrome is a multi-organ autosomal dominant (or new mutation) disorder. The CHARGE acronym represents common features of the syndrome, although abnormalities may vary in different neonates:

- **C**olomba: a hole or gap in eye structures that can affect the iris, retina, optic disc or choroid and can result in impairment of vision or blindness; eyes may be small and underdeveloped
- **H**eart defects: may include tetralogy of Fallot, VSD, ASD, or PDA
- **A**tresia, choanal: one or both nasal passages may be blocked; since neonates are obligate nasal breathers, this can lead to difficulty breathing in the neonate
- **R**etardation of growth/development: delay in meeting milestones
- **G**enitourinary anomalies: hypogonadism and reduced hormone production may result in males with micropenis and cryptorchidism although female external genitalia usually appear normal; puberty may be delayed in both genders
- **E**ar abnormalities/hearing loss: abnormalities in the middle and inner ear, abnormalities of the external ear, and varying decrease of hearing loss

A square-shaped face is common. Other less common disorders associated with the syndrome include cranial nerve abnormalities, impaired sense of smell, difficulty swallowing, tracheoesophageal fistula, renal abnormalities, scoliosis, kyphosis, polydactyly, oligodactyly, club foot, and long-bone abnormalities.

Skeletal Dysplasia

Skeletal dysplasias are a large group (450+) of genetic disorders affecting the bones and cartilage, one bone, or a group of bones, and the mode of inheritance can vary. Some disorders may result from spontaneous mutations or exposure to toxins. For example, X-linked disorders may affect males and not females. Often parents have mild symptoms but the child has a more severe disorder. Some of these disorders, such as osteogenesis imperfecta, may be diagnosed in the fetus by screening or ultrasound during the first trimester, but others may not be diagnosed until the third trimester or birth of the infant. Common dysplasias include thanatophoric, campomelic, achondroplasia, and achondrogenesis. About half of infants with skeletal dysplasias are stillborn or die within a few weeks of birth. If the dysplasia is lethal, then the neonate is provided comfort care, but if the dysplasia is consistent with life, then the infant must be stabilized, consultation with genetic specialists conducted, and non-skeletal complications assessed.

Osteogenesis Imperfecta

Osteogenesis imperfecta (OI) is a genetic disorder of collagen synthesis that results in brittle, easily fractured bones. OI occurs in 1 in 20,000 live births. Collagen is a major component of bone that gives it both strength and flexibility. Infants with OI either produce defective collagen or deficient amounts of collagen. Four different types of OI have been identified, with symptoms ranging from very mild to lethality in the neonatal period. **Common features** of OI include:

- Brittle bones that fracture easily (fractures may be present at birth)
- Bowing of long bones
- Shortened limbs
- Discolored, brittle teeth
- Blue sclera
- Skeletal deformities, including scoliosis
- Respiratory difficulties
- Weak muscles

Generally, OI is inherited in a dominant fashion, but a new mutation may cause the disorder in approximately 25% of cases. Parents of children diagnosed with OI must be instructed on correct methods of handling and bathing their child and placing the child in the crib to minimize trauma and the development of fractures.

Osteopenia of Prematurity

Osteopenia of prematurity (OOP) is a disorder of decreased bone mineralization seen in premature infants. Infants born extremely premature are at greatest risk for developing OOP. During the last trimester of pregnancy, large amounts of calcium and phosphorus are provided to the developing fetus to aid in bone mineralization. Clinical findings that may not be apparent until 2 to 4 months of age are craniotabes and impaired linear growth. Pediatricians diagnose rickets (vitamin D deficiency) when the preterm infant shows thickening of wrists and ankles, rachitic rosaries, and cupping of bone metaphysics in x-rays, and elevated alkaline phosphatase in blood serum. **Risk factors** for the development of OOP include:

- Preterm (less than 34 weeks of gestation)
- Weight less than 1,500 grams
- Delayed onset of enteral feeds
- Chronic use of steroids or diuretics by the mother or infant, which increase excretion of minerals
- Feeding unfortified human milk or full term formulas to preterm infants

Treatment includes supplementing calcium, phosphorus, and vitamin D.

Chapter Quiz

Ready to see how well you retained what you just read? Scan the QR code to go directly to the chapter quiz interface for this study guide. If you're using a computer, simply visit the online resources page at **mometrix.com/resources719/ccrnneonatal** and click the Chapter Quizzes link.

Clinical Judgment: Cardiovascular

Cardiovascular Complications

Cyanotic and Acyanotic Congenital Cardiac Defects

Congenital heart disease is one of the leading causes of death in children within the first year of life. There are two main types of congenital heart disease: acyanotic and cyanotic. They may also be classified according to hemodynamics related to the blood flow pattern.

Cyanotic defects includes those with decreased pulmonary blood flow or mixed blood flow.

- **Decreased pulmonary blood flow**
  - Tetralogy of Fallot
  - Tricuspid atresia
  - Pulmonary atresia with intact ventricular septum
- **Mixed blood flow**
  - Ebstein anomaly
  - Hypoplastic left heart syndrome
  - Total anomalous pulmonary venous return
  - Transposition of great arteries
  - Truncus arteriosus

Acyanotic defects include those with increased pulmonary blood flow or obstructed ventricular blood flow.

- **Increased pulmonary blood flow**
  - Atrial septal defect
  - Atrioventricular canal defect
  - Patent ductus arteriosus
  - Ventricular septal defect
- **Obstructed ventricular blood flow**
  - Aortic stenosis
  - Coarctation of aorta
  - Pulmonic stenosis (may become cyanotic in critical states)

Screening the Newborn for Congenital Heart Defects (CHDs)

According to the CDC, the American Academy of Pediatrics, and the American Heart Association, screening for **congenital heart defects** (CHDs) should be done on all newborns at 24–48 hours after birth using pulse oximetry. This screening can detect seven critical CHDs, including cyanotic heart defects and ductal-dependent heart defects: hypoplastic left heart syndrome, pulmonary atresia, tetralogy of Fallot, total anomalous pulmonary venous return, transposition of the great arteries, tricuspid atresia, and truncus arteriosus. Procedures include:

- Pulse oximetry: Carry out testing when the infant is warm, calm, and awake but not moving excessively.
- Place neonatal oximeter on the right hand (preductal) and the right or left foot (postductal).
- Allow oximeters to stabilize for 30–60 seconds before recording the values.

Results:

- Pass: ≥95% in both readings and difference of ≤3%. (No further testing is needed.)
- Fail (Needs further testing): 90–94% in either the right hand or a foot with a difference >3% between them on three repeated tests, 1 hour apart. If the oxygen saturation remains low, there needs to be further evaluation.
- Critical fail (needs immediate intervention): <90% in either the right hand or a foot on any test.

Central and Peripheral Cyanosis

Cyanosis results from lack of oxygen and desaturated hemoglobin level of at least 4 g/dL. The two primary types of cyanosis are central and peripheral:

- **Central cyanosis**: Results from desaturated blood (decrease in oxygen transport from the lungs to the bloodstream), often because of a heart lesion, heart failure, or respiratory disorder. Because the arteries carry insufficient oxygen, cyanosis is apparent in the tongue, conjunctiva, and mucous membranes.
- **Peripheral cyanosis**: Results from peripheral vascular constriction from various causes, including hypothermia, stress, hypovolemia, or from conditions that interfere with blood flow to the extremities, such as cardiogenic shock or sepsis. Because blood supply to the extremities is inadequate, cyanosis becomes evident in the distal hands (fingers, nailbeds) and feet as well as the lips, tip of the nose, perioral areas, periorbital areas, and earlobes. However, PaO_2 levels generally remain normal.

Note that cyanosis may be more difficult to assess in dark-skinned neonates and may appear as a gray "ashy" discoloration rather than blue. **Acrocyanosis** (about mouth and extremities) is often a normal finding in neonates for up to 48 hours.

Cardiac and Pulmonary Cyanosis

Cyanosis can reflect underlying cardiac and pulmonary disease:

- **Cardiac cyanosis:** This generally presents as cyanosis without respiratory distress. Cyanotic heart disease is likely a factor if the neonate's PaO_2 remains <70 mmHg while the neonate breathes 100% oxygen. Typically, with cyanotic heart disease, central cyanosis is a diagnostic factor although the degree of cyanosis at onset may vary. With structural heart defects that result in right-to-left shunting, cyanosis is generally evident, often from birth, and heart murmurs or extra heart sounds are evident. In some cases, such as tetralogy of Fallot, the cyanosis is more noticeable during crying.
- **Pulmonary cyanosis**: The neonate often has obvious signs of respiratory distress, including grunting respirations and sternal retraction, as well as central cyanosis. PaO_2 usually remains >100 mmHg while on 100% oxygen. Pulmonary conditions that may cause cyanosis include pulmonary hypoplasia, pulmonary edema, pneumothorax, pleural effusion, pneumonia, phrenic nerve palsy, hypoventilation, and diaphragmatic hernia.

Tetralogy of Fallot

Tetralogy of Fallot (TOF) is a combination of 4 different defects:

- **Ventricular septal defect** usually with a large opening
- **Pulmonic stenosis** with decreased blood flow to lungs

- **Overriding aorta** (displacement to the right so that it appears to come from both ventricles, usually overriding the ventricular septal defect), resulting in the mixing of oxygenated and deoxygenated blood
- **Right ventricular hypertrophy**

Infants with TOF are often acutely cyanotic immediately after birth, while others with less severe defects may have increasing cyanosis over the first year.

Symptoms include:

- Intolerance to feeding or crying, resulting in increased cyanotic "blue spells" or "tet spells"
- Failure to thrive with poor growth
- Clubbing of fingers may occur over time
- Intolerance to activity as child grows
- Increased risk for emboli, brain attacks, brain abscess, seizures, fainting, or sudden death

Treatment: Total surgical repair at ≤1 year (ideally before 6 months of age, if tolerable) is now the preferred treatment rather than the palliative procedures formerly used.

Transposition of the Great Arteries

Transposition of the great arteries is a congenital heart defect in which the aorta is connected to the right ventricle instead of the left ventricle, and the pulmonary artery is connected to the left ventricle instead of the right ventricle. This transposition means that deoxygenated blood is being pumped back to the body and the oxygenated blood returns to the lungs instead of going to the body. Septal defects may also occur, allowing some mixing of blood, and the ductus arteriosus allows mixing until it closes.

Symptoms vary depending upon whether there is mixing of blood but may include:

- Mild-to-severe cyanosis
- Symptoms of congestive heart failure
- Cardiomegaly developing in the weeks after birth
- Heart sounds vary depending upon the severity of the defects

Treatment may include:

- Prostaglandin to keep the ductus arteriosus and foramen ovale open; balloon atrial septostomy to increase size of foramen ovale
- Surgical repair to transpose arteries to the normal position ("arterial switch") as well as to repair septal defects and other abnormalities

Acyanotic Heart Disease

PDA

Patent ductus arteriosus (PDA) is failure of the ductus arteriosus that connects the **pulmonary artery and aorta** to close after birth, resulting in left-to-right shunting of blood from the aorta back to the pulmonary artery. This increases the blood flow to the lungs and causes an increase in pulmonary hypertension that can result in damage to the lung tissue. While some infants may be essentially asymptomatic, **typical symptoms** include:

- Cyanosis
- Congestive heart failure

- Machinery-like murmur
- Frequent respiratory infections and dyspnea, especially on exertion
- Widened pulse pressure
- Bounding pulse
- Atrial fibrillation/palpitations
- Increased risk for bacterial endocarditis, congestive heart failure, and development of pulmonary vascular obstructive disease

Treatment includes:

- Pharmacologic therapy: Nonselective COX inhibitors such as ibuprofen and indomethacin have proven effective in closing PDA. Ibuprofen has shown to equally effective as the traditional pharmacologic approach of indomethacin, and less-likely to induce necrotizing enterocolitis or renal dysfunction. Both of these options carry a risk for bleeding. For patients with contraindications to nonselective COX inhibitors, acetaminophen is a supported option, but requires high dosages for maximal effect which places the neonate at risk for liver damage.
- Surgical repair can be done with ligation of the patent vessel.

Ventricular Septal Defect

Ventricular septal defect is an abnormal opening in the **septum** between the right and left ventricles. If the opening is small, the child may be asymptomatic, but larger openings can result in a left-to-right shunt because of higher pressure in the left ventricle. This shunting increases in the 6 weeks after birth, with symptoms becoming more evident, but the defect may close within a few years.

Symptoms include:

- Congestive heart failure with peripheral edema
- Tachycardia
- Dyspnea
- Difficulty feeding
- Heart murmur
- Recurrent pulmonary infections
- Increased risk for bacterial endocarditis and pulmonary vascular obstructive disease

Treatment includes:

- Mild cases: Diuretics, such as furosemide (Lasix), may be used for mild heart failure.
- Nutritional support may be required for infants struggling to gain weight.
- Surgery, including pulmonary banding or cardiopulmonary bypass, can be performed to repair the opening with sutures or a patch, depending upon the size.

Atrial Septal Defect

An atrial septal defect (ASD) is an abnormal opening in the **septum** between the right and left atria. Because the left atrium has higher pressure than the right atrium, some of the oxygenated blood returning from the lungs to the left atrium is shunted back to the right atrium, where it is again returned to the lungs, displacing deoxygenated blood.

Symptoms may be few or even absent depending upon the degree of the defect but can include:

- Congestive heart failure
- Heart murmur
- Increased risk for dysrhythmias and pulmonary vascular obstructive disease over time

Treatment may not be necessary for small defects, but larger defects require closure. Closure is usually deferred until 2 years of age, if possible, and can be accomplished two different ways:

- Preferred: Heart catheterization and placing of closure device (Amplatz device) across the atrial septal defect
- Open-heart surgical repair

Coarctation of the Aorta

Coarctation of the aorta is a stricture of the aorta, proximal to the ductus arteriosus intersection. The increased blood pressure caused by the heart attempting to pump the blood past the stricture causes the heart to enlarge and also increases blood pressure to the head and upper extremities while decreasing blood pressure to the lower body and extremities. With severe stricture, symptoms may not occur until the ductus arteriosus closes, causing sudden loss of blood supply to the lower body.

Symptoms include:

- Difference in blood pressure between upper and lower extremities
- Congestive heart failure symptoms in infants
- Headaches, dizziness, and nosebleeds in older children
- Increased risk of hypertension, ruptured aorta, aortic aneurysm, bacterial endocarditis, and brain attack

Treatment includes:

- Prostaglandin (alprostadil), such as Prostin VR Pediatric, to reopen the ductus arteriosus for infants
- Balloon angioplasty
- Surgical resection and anastomosis or graft replacement (usually at 3-5 years of age unless condition is severe); infants who have surgery may need later repair

Congestive Heart Failure

Types

Congestive heart failure results from the inability of the heart to adequately pump the blood the body needs. In infants, it is usually secondary to cardiac abnormalities with resultant increased blood volume and blood pressure:

- **Right-sided failure** occurs if the right ventricle cannot effectively contract to pump blood into the pulmonary artery, causing pressure to build in the right atrium and the venous circulation. This venous hypertension causes generalized edema of lower extremities, distended abdomen from ascites, hepatomegaly, and jugular venous distension.

- **Left-sided failure** occurs if the left ventricle cannot effectively pump blood into the aorta and systemic circulation, increasing pressure in the left atrium and the pulmonary veins, with resultant pulmonary edema and increased pulmonary pressure. Symptoms include respiratory distress with tachypnea, grunting respirations, sternal retraction, rales, failure to thrive, and difficulty eating, often leaving the child exhausted and sweaty.

Children often have some combination of right and left-sided failure. Increased pressure in the lungs after birth may delay symptoms for 1-2 weeks.

MANAGEMENT

Management of congestive heart failure (CHF) in infants can be difficult. It is extremely important to establish the etiology and to treat the underlying cause. For infants with structural cardiac abnormalities, surgical repair may be needed to resolve the CHF. There are some medical treatments that can relieve symptoms:

- **Diuretics**, such as furosemide (Lasix), metolazone, or hydrochlorothiazide to reduce pulmonary and peripheral edema
- **Antihypertensives**, such as Captopril or Propranolol to decrease heart workload
- **Cardiac glycosides**, such as Lanoxin, may relieve symptoms if above medicines are not successful
- **High caloric feedings**, either by bottle or nasogastric feeding to provide sufficient nutrients
- **Oxygen** may be useful for some children with weak hearts
- **Restriction of activities** to reduce stress on the heart
- **Dopamine or dobutamine** may be given to increase the contractibility of the heart

HYPOTENSION

Hypotension is a systemic mean arterial blood pressure <2 standard deviations less that average values for gestational age. The lowest reading that is within normal limits for preterm infants is calculated as gestational age plus five. Thus, a 31-week preterm acceptable low BP would be 31-36 mmHg. Hypotension in the neonate most often relates to dysregulation of peripheral vascular tone and/or myocardial dysfunction. Hypotension may also occur as the result of hypocalcemia, hypovolemic, cardiogenic, or distributive shock, so determining the cause of hypotension is critical to planning appropriate intervention. Early signs of hypotension are those of compensated shock and later signs of decompensated shock. Tachycardia, respiratory distress, pallor, lethargy, and cyanosis may be evident. Dopamine (2-20 μg/kg/min) is the most commonly used drug to treat neonatal hypotension as it improves myocardial function and improves peripheral vascular tension without causing vasodilation. Oxygen is administered to combat hypoxia as well as saline bolus (10-20 mL/kg).

HYPERTENSION

Hypertension is a relatively rare finding in the neonate. Signs of elevated blood pressure include lethargy, increased apnea episodes, seizures, irritability, tachypnea, and intracranial hemorrhage. The nurse often discovers elevated blood pressure through a routine check of vital signs. Most **causes of hypertension** in the neonate are **renal** in origin and include:

- **Thrombus formation in the kidneys** from an umbilical artery catheter (the most common cause in the NICU)
- **Other vascular causes**, such as renal vein thrombosis, or renal artery stenosis, or coarctation of the aorta
- **Compression of renal artery** by a mass

Non-renal causes include:

- **Iatrogenesis**, due to administration of dopamine, Aminophylline, or glucocorticoids
- **Neurological**, secondary to seizures or intraventricular hemorrhage
- **Endocrine**, secondary to congenital adrenal hyperplasia or hyperthyroidism
- **Pulmonary**, secondary to pneumothorax or bronchopulmonary dysplasia

SHOCK

Shock is the result of circulatory failure in which there is inadequate perfusion to meet the metabolic needs of the body. There are a number of different causes, but the **physiologic responses** are essentially the same:

- Hypotension (which may not be present initially because of reactive vasoconstriction)
- Hypoxemia resulting in hypoxic tissue
- Metabolic acidosis

There are essentially **3 stages** in the progression of the shock response:

1. **Compensated shock**: The sympathetic nervous response causes vasoconstriction, which may mask essential underlying hypotension but serves to provide blood flow for vital organ functions, although there may be decreased circulation at the microvascular (small vessel) level.
2. **Decompensated shock**: The cardiovascular system is unable to adequately compensate and microvascular perfusion decreases.
3. **Irreversible/terminal shock**: Damage to internal organs, such as the heart and brain, is so extensive that therapeutic measures cannot reverse eventual death.

COMPENSATED SHOCK

During compensated shock, the blood pressure may remain normal initially as the compensatory sympathetic nervous response results in vasoconstriction and an increase in the heart rate and contractibility that combine to maintain cardiac output at a level adequate to supply the heart and brain while shifting circulation from other organs:

- **Skin:** Skin cold and clammy
- **Gastrointestinal tract**: Bowel sounds absent or decreased
- **Kidneys**: Urinary output decreased

Because of a decrease in tissue perfusion, lactic acid begins to build up, producing metabolic acidosis. The acidosis results in an increased respiratory rate, which serves to expel excess carbon dioxide. However, this also raises the pH of the blood and may result in respiratory alkalosis. Fluid replacement and medications to increase blood pressure and perfusion of the tissues are critical during this stage.

DECOMPENSATED SHOCK

Decompensated shock occurs as the body can no longer compensate, the blood pressure falls below normal, and all organ systems suffer from hypoperfusion. The heart is overworked and becomes dysfunctional, and chemical changes cause myocardial depression, so that the heart begins to fail.

The permeability of the capillaries increases with fluid buildup in the interstitial tissues and decreased venous return to the heart. Multi-system effects occur:

- **Respiratory**: Respirations become rapid and shallow as the hypoxemia causes an inflammatory response and pulmonary edema, with collapse of alveoli and fibrotic changes in the lung tissue.
- **Cardiovascular**: Dysrhythmias and ischemia of the myocardium result in tachycardia. The myocardium is depressed and ventricles may dilate.
- **Neurological**: Hypoperfusion of the brain leads to changes in mental status, including lethargy and loss of consciousness. Pupils may dilate or react sluggishly.
- **Renal**: Acute renal failure occurs with decrease in urinary output, increase in BUN and creatinine, and electrolyte shifts.
- **Hepatic**: The liver loses the ability to filter and metabolize medications and metabolic waste products. Liver enzymes rise, and the skin becomes jaundiced.
- **Gastrointestinal**: Mucosal ulcerations may occur, causing bleeding and bloody diarrhea. Bacterial toxins may invade the lymphatic system where they are carried to the bloodstream, causing infection and increasing adverse cardiovascular responses.
- **Hematologic**: Disseminated vascular coagulation (DIC) may occur with both clotting and bleeding. The skin may show ecchymoses and petechiae. Clotting times are prolonged.

Treatment during this stage is dependent upon the underlying cause but includes intravenous fluids, medications to control blood pressure, cardiac function, infection, and gastrointestinal ulcerations and bleeding. Ventilatory support with oxygen and administration of sodium bicarbonate may be needed to treat metabolic acidosis. The infant must be monitored constantly, including hemodynamic monitoring, blood gases, urinary function, EKG, fluid and electrolytes, blood chemistries, enzyme levels, and neurological status.

Irreversible/Terminal Shock

The irreversible/terminal stage of shock can be difficult to determine because the progression of shock is a continuum rather than clearly defined stages, so the usual strategy is to continue to treat the patient with fluids, vasoactive medications to improve cardiac function, and nutritional support. During this stage hypotension persists, and complete liver and renal failure occurs. As perfusion causes necrosis of tissue, the toxins created result in severe metabolic acidosis. There is also increased lactic acidosis. Adenosine triphosphate (ATP) levels are depleted and there are no mechanisms left to store energy. **Multiple organ dysfunction syndrome (MODS)** occurs. There is no specific treatment that can reverse MODS, so treatment at this point becomes supportive. The mortality rate for MODS ranges from 30-100%, depending upon the number of organ systems that are involved.

Cardiogenic Shock

Cardiogenic shock in infants usually relates to congenital heart disease (usually with systemic to pulmonary shunting), myocarditis, and dysrhythmias, such as AV block and paroxysmal atrial tachycardia. These disorders interfere with the pumping mechanism of the heart, decreasing oxygen perfusion. Cardiogenic shock has 3 **characteristics**:

- Increased preload
- Increased afterload
- Decreased contractibility

Together these result in a decreased cardiac output and an increase in systemic vascular resistance (SVR) to compensate and protect vital organs. This results in an increase of afterload in the left ventricle with increased need for oxygen. As the cardiac output continues to decrease, tissue perfusion decreases, coronary artery perfusion decreases, fluid backs up, and the left ventricle fails to adequately pump the blood, resulting in pulmonary edema and right ventricular failure.

Cardiac Dysrhythmias

Cardiac dysrhythmias (abnormal heart beats), although more common in adults, can occur in infants and are frequently the result of damage to the conduction system during major cardiac surgery.

Bradydysrhythmias are pulse rates that are abnormally slow:

- Complete atrioventricular block (A-V block) may be congenital or a response to surgical trauma.
- Sinus bradycardia may be caused by the autonomic nervous system or a response to hypotension and decrease in oxygenation.
- Junctional/nodal rhythms often occur in post-surgical patients when absence of P wave is noted but heart rate and output usually remain stable, and unless there is compromise, usually no treatment is necessary.

Tachydysrhythmias are pulse rates that are abnormally fast:

- Sinus tachycardia is often caused by illness, such as fever or infection.
- Supraventricular tachycardia (200-300 bpm) may have a sudden onset and result in congestive heart failure.

Conduction irregularities are irregular pulses that often occur post-operatively and are usually not significant. Premature contractions may arise from the atria or ventricles.

Cardioversion Procedures for Arrythmia Types

Cardioversion procedures for arrythmia types are as follows:

- **Stable tachyarrhythmia:** Vagal maneuver to increase parasympathetic input to the heart and slow it. Apply ice to the neonate's face, which triggers the diving response to slow the heart rate. If unsuccessful, try adenosine, digoxin, or propranolol.
- **Unstable arrhythmia with narrow QRS complex:** Synchronized electrical cardioversion is appropriate for atrial flutter or fibrillation, WPW, or PJRT. Set the defibrillator for 0.5-2.0 J/kg. Place two electrode pads on the infant's chest. Wait for the optimum moment in the cardiac cycle. Pass electrical current through the infant's heart.
- **Unstable arrhythmia with wide QRS complex:** Asynchronous cardioversion is appropriate for ventricular tachycardia or fibrillation, SVT with BBB, or antidromic SVT in WPW. Defibrillate because there is no R wave present to time the shock.
- **Stable arrhythmia with wide QRS complex:** Administer amiodarone or procainamide for rate control. If unsuccessful, consider adenosine (0.1 mg/kg, with a maximum of 6 mg, rapid IV push and up to 0.2 mg/kg or 12 mg for a second dose). If pharmacologic interventions are unsuccessful, consider cardioversion at 0.5-1.0 J/kg for the first attempt, and then 2 J/kg if the first attempt is unsuccessful.
- **Bradydysrhythmias:** For 1:1 sinus bradycardia, complete AV block, Wenckebach's phenomenon, and sinus exit block: Check airway, breathing, and circulation. Treat underlying cause. Give oxygen, atropine, and isoproterenol. Start transvenous pacing.

Chapter Quiz

Ready to see how well you retained what you just read? Scan the QR code to go directly to the chapter quiz interface for this study guide. If you're using a computer, simply visit the online resources page at **mometrix.com/resources719/ccrnneonatal** and click the Chapter Quizzes link.

Clinical Judgment: Respiratory

Respiratory Complications

Respiratory Distress Syndrome

Respiratory distress syndrome (RDS), formerly called hyaline membrane disease, has an incidence rate of approximately 90% for extremely preterm infants (gestational age 28 weeks or less). Incidence remains significant even for late preterm infants, being close to 10% in infants born at 34 weeks. RDS is caused by the absence or deficiency of surfactant. Surfactant is a lipoprotein that reduces surface tension in the alveoli. Surfactant causes the lungs to be more compliant (alveoli expand with less effort) and the alveoli do not collapse on end expiration. Surfactant production begins at 22 weeks of gestation, but levels are inadequate until 36 weeks of gestation. Lack of surfactant produces alveolar collapse (atelectasis) and less compliant lungs that cause laborious breathing. Collapsed areas of lung may still receive blood flow, but no exchange of gases occurs (ventilation perfusion mismatch). If RDS is left untreated, hypoxemia and hypercarbia develop, leading to respiratory acidosis. Acidosis and hypoxemia lead to a cycle of increased pulmonary vascular resistance and vasoconstriction, causing increased hypoxemia.

Air Leak Syndromes

Premature infants have more fragile lung tissue and often require respiratory resuscitative measures, such as positive pressure ventilation (PPV), ventilator support, and administration of pulmonary drugs (e.g., surfactant) that make them more susceptible to air leak syndrome. **Air leak syndrome** occurs when an alveolus ruptures and air leaks into a space that it normally does not occupy. Different syndromes occur, depending on the area that air leaks into.

- **Pneumothorax**: Air leakage into the pleural cavity that surrounds the lungs
- **Tension pneumothorax**: One-way air flow into the pleural cavity, with pressure build-up and significant collapse of lung tissue, causing respiratory compromise
- **Pneumomediastinum**: Air traveling along the pulmonary blood vessels that enters the mediastinum
- **Pneumopericardium**: Air in the sac that surrounds the heart
- **Pulmonary interstitial emphysema**: Air trapped in the lung's interstitial spaces

Pneumothorax

Pneumothorax is the most common type of air leak syndrome. In infants, increased air pressure caused by the use of mechanical ventilation is the most common cause, but infants may develop spontaneous pneumothorax. Infants with fragile lung tissue are at especially high risk:

- Infants with respiratory distress syndrome
- Premature infants
- Infants with meconium aspiration

Symptoms vary according to the type of pneumothorax (spontaneous, traumatic, or tension) but can include:

- Increased respiratory distress with tachypnea and chest wall retractions
- Absence of breath sounds on auscultation

- Paradoxical chest movement in which the chest contracts during inhalation and expands during exhalation
- Shift in maximum intensity sounds of heart
- Bradycardia and cyanosis

Treatment includes:

- Evacuating air with needle aspiration or chest tubes to water seal drainage
- Correction of underlying cause

Review Video: Pneumothorax
Visit mometrix.com/academy and enter code: 186841

Pneumomediastinum

A pneumomediastinum is an air leak in the mediastinum, the area of the chest between the sternum and the spine, and between the lungs. Causes of neonatal **pneumomediastinum** vary. Often, this complication arises after or in conjunction with neonatal respiratory distress, pneumonia, mechanical ventilation use, meconium aspiration, or as a result of birth-related trauma. While pneumomediastinum is often asymptomatic, it can also present with cyanosis, diminished heart sounds or shallow respirations. The condition often resolves spontaneously, but the patient must be monitored closely for complications and may require mechanical ventilation despite this being a common cause of the condition. Diagnosis of pneumomediastinum is through chest x-ray, with ABG's to evaluate the impact of the condition on the newborn's gas exchange and oxygenation.

Apnea of Prematurity

Premature infants (especially those <34 weeks) often exhibit **apnea of prematurity (AOP).** AOP begins at birth and is believed to be caused by immaturity of the nervous system, and improves as the brain matures. It may persist for 4–8 weeks. There are three **types of apnea**:

- **Central**: no airflow or effort to breathe
- **Obstructive**: no airflow, but effort to breathe
- **Mixed**: both central and obstructive elements (75% of AOP)

Symptoms include:

- Swallowing during apneic periods
- Apnea >20 seconds
- Apnea <20 seconds with bradycardia 30 beats <normal
- Oxygen saturation <85% persisting ≥5 seconds
- Cyanosis

Treatment includes:

- Tactile stimulation (rubbing limbs or thorax or gently slapping bottoms of feet) or gently lifting the jaw to relieve obstruction
- Oxygen or bag/mask ventilation for bradycardia and decreased oxygen saturation
- Continuous positive airway pressure (CPAP) for mixed or obstructive apnea
- Caffeine (for central apnea) to increase contractions of the diaphragm (Caffeine is preferred over theophylline due to having fewer adverse effects and requiring less monitoring.)

TTN

Transient tachypnea of the newborn (TTN) occurs when fluid in the lungs is not adequately absorbed after birth. The neonate usually exhibits symptoms within 36 hours of birth, and the condition typically resolves within 3 days. TTN is most common in infants delivered by Cesarean section, but premature birth and having a mother who smokes or has diabetes increases risk to the infant.

Symptoms include:

- Dyspnea (>60/min)
- Sternal retraction (mild)
- Expiratory grunt
- Nasal flaring
- Poor feeding (because of increased respiratory rate)

Laboratory findings include:

- ABGs: hypoxemia
- Chest radiograph: fluid in lungs

Treatment includes:

- Monitor oxygen saturation levels
- Provide supplemental oxygen as indicated
- Provide intravenous fluids or nasogastric feedings if infant is unable to take oral feedings

Meconium Aspiration Syndrome

Meconium aspiration syndrome (MAS) occurs when meconium, expelled in the amniotic fluid (occurring in about 20% of pregnancies), is aspirated by the fetus *in utero* or the neonate at first breath. Blood and amniotic fluids may be aspirated as well. Some infants may present with **symptoms** at birth, but sometimes symptoms are delayed for a number of hours:

- Tachypnea
- Lethargy, depressed state
- Hypoxemia and hypercapnia
- Metabolic acidosis may occur
- Hyperventilation may occur in early stages with hypoventilation in later stages

Symptoms are similar to transient tachypnea of the newborn (TTN) but they are more severe and the infant appears more compromised. Chest x-rays may show infiltrates, atelectasis, and hypoinflated areas as well as hyperinflated areas. Pulmonary hypertension may result. **Treatment** includes:

- Supplemental oxygen and/or mechanical ventilation as indicated
- Positive pressure ventilation or endotracheal intubation for infants with respiratory distress (weak respirations, bradycardia, hypotonia)

Note: Preventive suctioning of the nasopharynx as soon as the head is delivered is **no longer recommended**.

PPHN

Persistent pulmonary hypertension of the newborn (PPHN) occurs when the high pulmonary vascular pressure that keeps fetal blood from circulating through the lungs fails to reduce after birth, so that blood continues to bypass the lungs, and the foramen ovale and ductus arteriosus are forced by pressure to remain open with venous blood shunting into systemic circulation instead of being oxygenated in the lungs. Infants are usually near or full-term, but present at birth with respiratory distress and cyanosis. PPHN is the cause of about 50% of neonatal deaths. There are 3 **classifications**:

- **Primary** is idiopathic with normal lung tissue but arterial hyperplasia and/or premature constricting of ductus arteriosus *in utero.*
- **Secondary** is precipitated by another disorder, such as meconium aspiration pneumonia (MAP), transient tachypnea of the newborn (TTN) or hyaline membrane disease. This is the most common form.
- **Hypoplastic** is related to pulmonary hypoplasia with anatomic changes in alveoli and vasculature in the lung.

PPHN has been linked to maternal use of SSRIs and NSAIDs.

Symptoms are usually evident within the first 12 hours of birth and progress over the next 24–48 hours:

- Cyanosis with poor cardiac perfusion, tachycardia
- Hypoxemia, persisting even with supplemental oxygen
- Systolic murmur with regurgitation of the tricuspid valve
- Tachypnea and general respiratory distress

Treatment

Treatment for persistent pulmonary hypertension (PPHN) will be specific for the underlying cause, and can include:

- Intubation and mechanical ventilation with HFV especially with parenchymal lung disease
- Central venous lines for administration of solutions, such as calcium gluconate
- Arterial line to monitor arterial blood gas
- Surfactant to reduce surface tension in patients without primary PPHN
- High frequency ventilation (HFV) is used with underlying lung disease resulting in low volume
- Extracorporeal membrane oxygenation (ECMO) is used if other forms of support are not successful, and most often if the infant also has congenital diaphragmatic hernia
- Sodium bicarbonate is often used to correct metabolic acidosis in practice, however there is no evidence of short or long-term benefits
- Sedation (fentanyl) to reduce restlessness. Induced paralysis (pancuronium, vecuronium) has been used but is implicated in increased mortality rates, atelectasis, sensory hearing loss, and ventilation-perfusion mismatch
- Inhaled nitrous oxide

Pulmonary Hemorrhage

Pulmonary hemorrhage is bleeding within the alveoli. This usually is the result of some other event, such as intracranial hemorrhage, asphyxia, aspiration, heart disease, or sepsis. This can also be the result of a trauma from over-aggressive suctioning. **Pulmonary hemorrhage** presents as bright red blood from the trachea found with suctioning and as rapid, sudden respiratory deterioration. Pulmonary hemorrhage can cause rapid death if the bleeding is severe and is often only found during an autopsy. A more minor hemorrhage can be managed with blood transfusions and assisted ventilation. Pulmonary hemorrhage may result in hemothorax. In some cases, pneumothorax may also be present, resulting in mediastinal shift that increases the difficulty of identifying and repairing the bleeding vessel. If the infant is stabilized, computed tomography may provide accurate diagnosis to isolate the area of hemorrhage. The underlying cause of the hemorrhage must be discovered and treated.

CDH

Congenital diaphragmatic hernias (CDH) may cause severe respiratory distress. The primary CDHs that affect infants are **posterolateral** (Bochdalek hernia).

- **Left-sided** in 85% of cases; includes herniation of the large and small intestine and intra-abdominal organs into the thoracic cavity
- **Right-sided** in 13% of cases; may be asymptomatic or involve only the liver and part of the large intestine herniate

Neonates with left CDH may exhibit **severe respiratory distress** and **cyanosis**. The lungs may be underdeveloped because of pressure exerted from displaced organs during fetal development. There may be a left hemithorax with a mediastinal shift, with the heart pressing on the right lung, which may be hypoplastic. Bowel sounds are heard over the chest area. Pulmonary hypertension and cardiopulmonary failure may occur. **Treatments** include:

- Immediate surgical repair
- HFOV and nitric oxide for pulmonary hypoplasia
- Extracorporeal membrane oxygenation (ECMO) for cardiopulmonary dysfunction

Despite treatment, mortality rates are 50%, and children who survive may have emphysema, with a larger volume but inadequate number of alveoli.

Oxygen and Ventilation

Oxyhemoglobin Dissociation Curve

The oxyhemoglobin dissociation curve is a graph that plots the percentage of hemoglobin saturated with oxygen (*y*-axis) and different partial pressures of oxygen (PaO_2 levels, *x*-axis). A curve shift to the right represents conditions where hemoglobin has less affinity for oxygen (greater amounts of oxygen are released). A shift to the left has the opposite implications.

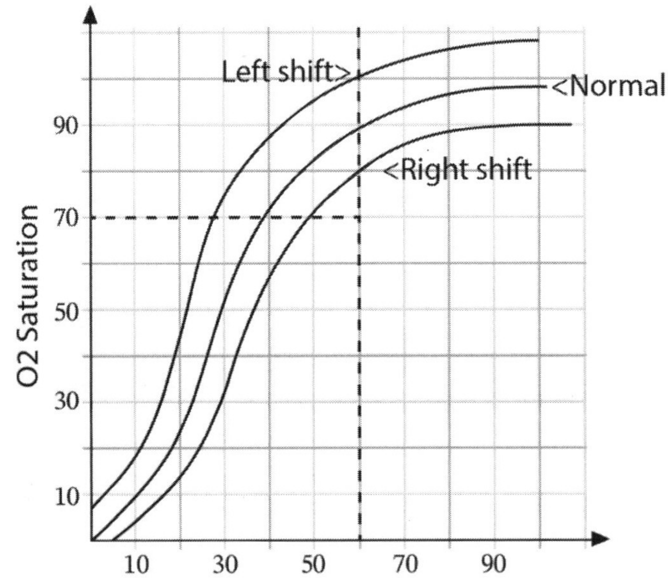

Low pH shifts the curve to the right, enabling increased unloading of hemoglobin to tissues. Elevated oxygen shifts the curve to the left, causing increased affinity of hemoglobin for oxygen in the lungs. Small changes in fetal PaO_2 result in greater loading or unloading of oxygen compared to adult hemoglobin. Because of the increased affinity for oxygen, lower tissue oxygen levels are needed to trigger the unload of oxygen. Thus, the infant will have a lower PaO_2 and oxygen saturation before cyanosis is evident. Normal PaO_2 is 80–100 mmHg, equal to 95–98% oxygen saturation. Levels less than 40 mmHg are dangerous.

Monitoring

Non-Invasive Monitoring of Infant on Oxygen

Non-invasive monitoring of the neonate receiving oxygen includes:

- **Heart rate monitor**: Should show beats per minute as well as a visual depiction of the heart rhythm.
- **Respiratory monitor**: Should show respiratory rate as well as a visual wave showing the pattern of breathing. Alarms should be turned on for apnea and tachypnea.
- **Blood pressure monitor**: Peripheral cuff type monitoring, this does not need to be continuous but needs to be done at regular intervals determined by the physician or practitioner.
- **Pulse oximetry**: Should be a continuous monitoring with alarms set for ordered lower limits.
- **Oxygen analyzer**: Shows the oxygen level being delivered to the neonate.

NEONATAL PULSE OXIMETRY

Pulse oximetry is a means of monitoring the saturation level of the **hemoglobin** in the blood. For example, a reading of 98% indicates that 98% of the hemoglobin available is bound to oxygen or saturated with oxygen. A machine uses infrared light to read the hemoglobin. Several things can affect the accuracy of this reading.

- The **perfusion status** of the neonate. If the infant is suffering from a condition that results in poor perfusion (hypovolemia, hypotension, etc.), the pulse oximetry reading will be inaccurate, as the machine will have difficulty reading the blood.
- **Phototherapy** used for jaundice will also cause inaccurate readings because, like the tool used in pulse oximetry, it is a light.
- Use of **dopamine**, a potent vasoconstricting drug, which causes problems reading the blood for oxygen levels if the veins are constricted, affecting blood flow.

Pulse oximetry is now a recommended screening tool for congenital heart defects. While not diagnostic, it provides information that can either rule out congenital heart defects or trigger further investigation.

NON-INVASIVE TRANSCUTANEOUS O_2/CO_2 MONITORING

Non-invasive transcutaneous O_2/CO_2 monitoring includes **skin oxygen tension ($TCPO_2$)** and **carbon dioxide tension ($TCPCO_2$)**. One or two leads are placed on the infant's skin over any part of the body that allows good contact. O_2 and CO_2 diffuse through the skin and monitors provide a digital display. If right-to-left shunting is suspected, then leads are usually placed on right shoulder and lower abdomen or leg (above and below the ductus arteriosus). The electrodes are calibrated (usually every 4 hours to ensure accuracy), and then heat (43-44 °C) the underlying skin, but they must be left in place for 15 minutes after calibration to ensure adequate heating of the skin. The electrodes can cause erythema (first-degree burns), so they should be repositioned every 2-4 hours. The electrodes should not be placed beneath the infant because the pressure against it can impede circulation.

CARDIOPULMONARY MONITORING

Cardiopulmonary monitoring includes **electrocardiogram (ECG)** and **respiratory sensors**. Usually, 3 chest ECG leads that record the electrical activity of the heart and sense respiratory movement are placed, and the patterns are recorded on a visual screen. Many computerized monitors have memory capability so that data can be analyzed out of real time. They can also be set to record certain events, such as periods of apnea. Alarm thresholds are set so that an alarm indicates dangerous changes. Apnea alarms should be both visual and auditory. False alarms may occur and should be thoroughly evaluated for a cause, such as loose leads or movement. Home monitors include records of compliance so that a review of data shows the time the monitor was actually in use. Home monitors are used for infants at risk for SIDS. Because of interference problems that might provide inaccurate readings, monitors should never be used as a sole evaluation of cardiopulmonary status. Observation and examination must be used to verify the infant's condition.

END-TIDAL CO_2 MONITORS

End-tidal CO_2 monitors are used to confirm correct placement of endotracheal tubes during intubation and to ensure adequate oxygenation. Both sidestream analysis with a double lumen endotracheal tube (ETT) and mainstream analysis within the ventilator circuit are used. Clinical assessment alone is not adequate.

Capnography is attached to the ETT and provides a waveform graph, showing the varying concentrations of CO_2 in real time throughout each ventilation (with increased CO_2 on expiration) and can indicate changes in respiratory status. A typical waveform rises with expiration (indicating CO_2 level), plateaus, and then falls with inspiration (and intake of oxygen). Changes in the height or shape of the waveform can indicate respiratory compromise. Pressure of end-tidal CO_2 ($PETCO_2$) is useful for neonates with normal lung function or in premature infants with mild-moderate lung disease, but results may be inaccurate if there is a large alveolar-arterial gradient.

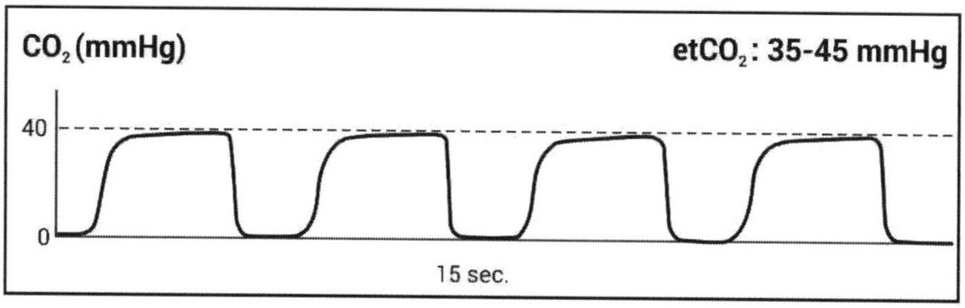

Neonatal Oxygen Administration

Principles of neonatal oxygen administration:

- Oxygen administration should be titrated to the need of the particular infant. The determining factor to titrate to should be PaO_2 levels as measured from arterial blood. Oxygen concentration should be titrated to keep the arterial PaO_2 level between 50 and 80 mmHg.
- Supplemental oxygen concentration should be initiated at 21% (30% in preterm infants) and then titrated up to prevent injuries from excessive oxygenation.
- Oxygen should never be given without some method of monitoring the level of oxygen in the infant's blood at all times, such as with pulse oximetry or arterial blood gas studies.
- Oxygen given to a neonate should always be humidified at 30-40%. Oxygen administered without humidification dries the nasal passages, increasing respiratory distress.
- Oxygen should also be warmed to 31-34 °C. Failing to warm the oxygen can cause cold stress for the infant.
- Any adjustments to the concentration of oxygen must be done slowly because an abrupt change can cause sudden vasoconstriction.

Oxygen Hood

Oxygen can be delivered through a clear **oxygen hood** (usually made of plastic) fitted over the infant's head. This type of delivery is appropriate for an infant who has a mild form of RDS and can maintain normal carbon dioxide levels in his blood, only needing supplemental oxygen. A blender that mixes the oxygen with water, thus humidifying it, is usually used with a hood. When the hood is being used for oxygen delivery, it is important that it fit the infant correctly. A hood too large will allow oxygen to escape and lower the concentration the infant is receiving, a hood too small will irritate the infant's skin at contact points. If the infant is to be held for feedings or otherwise removed from the hood, a secondary delivery tool should be available.

Nasal Cannula Delivery of Oxygen

A nasal cannula is used for the delivery of a neonate who has a long term need for oxygen and is starting to develop motor skills needing the mobility that a cannula allows. The cannula should be the correct size for the infant. The application of a cannula involves putting some kind of skin protection on the infant's cheeks, such as a piece of OpSite or some other kind of barrier. The tubing is then taped to this barrier to avoid skin irritation. The nares should be frequently assessed for patency. Infants are obligatory nose breathers (they must breathe through their nose) and if mucous or formula plugs the holes in the cannula, they will not be getting the concentration of oxygen they need. Suction the nares as often as needed to keep them clear.

Inhaled Nitric Oxide

Nitric oxide (NO) is an odorless, colorless gas that acts as a potent pulmonary vasodilator when it is inhaled and diffuses through the alveolar capillary membrane to the smooth muscle cells, reducing pulmonary vascular resistance, increasing blood flow through the lungs, and improving oxygenation. Because inhaled NO (iNO) works directly on the lungs, it reduces the risk of systemic hypotension. The only currently FDA-approved use for iNO is for the treatment of term or near-term neonates with acute hypoxic respiratory failure associated with persistent pulmonary hypertension. Although evidence does not support the use of iNO in neonates of less than 34 weeks' gestation, it is frequently used off-label for resuscitation of these preterm neonates. iNO is also sometimes used in perioperative treatment of neonates with pulmonary hypertension and hypoxia associated with congenital heart disease. Potential adverse effects includer methemoglobinemia, so neonates receiving iNO must be monitored carefully. iNO may be administered per conventional ventilator or high-frequency ventilator. If delivered by non-invasive ventilation, the dose received may be reduced by up to 50%. Weaning from iNO is necessary to prevent rebound pulmonary hypertension.

Non-Invasive Positive Pressure Ventilators

Nasal intermittent positive pressure ventilation (NIPPV) is a noninvasive method of respiratory support used in the treatment of respiratory distress syndrome for premature infants to avoid intubation and the risks of lung damage and bronchopulmonary dysplasia associated with mechanical ventilation. Other indications may include apnea of prematurity, bronchopulmonary dysplasia, and transient tachypnea of the newborn. NIPPV is used to augment CPAP and is delivered by nasal prongs or nasal mask. NIPPV delivers positive pressure to keep airways opens. Modes include CPAP, BiPAP, and NIPPV with synchronization. Monitoring includes vital signs, blood gases, and physical assessments. NIPPV may also be used as part of ventilator weaning following extubation to reduce the need for reintubation. Some studies have indicated that gaseous distention may occur if nasal prongs are incorrectly fitted to the neonate. Other complications include nasal injury and air leak syndromes. Weaning should be done slowly by reducing pressure levels and decreasing time spent on NIPPV.

Neurally-Adjusted Ventilatory Assist (NAVA)

Neurally-adjusted ventilatory assist (NAVA) is a spontaneous mode of ventilation that detects electrical activity from the phrenic nerve to the diaphragm (EAdi) through an orogastric catheter with sensors inserted into the esophagus. NAVA automatically synchronizes ventilatory assistance proportional to the neonate's breathing effort and ceases flow when the diaphragm relaxes. NAVA decreases the work of breathing, reduces the risk of ventilator-induced lung injury, improves synchronization, may reduce the need for sedation, and may be used invasively or noninvasively. Patient-specific parameters used to monitor and adjust ventilatory support include:

- **Edi peak**: maximum electrical activity of the diaphragm during inspiration
- **Edi min**: minimum electrical activity of the diaphragms at end of expiration
- **NAVA level**: overall level of inspiratory support provided
- **Trigger Edi**: threshold necessary to initiate a ventilatory support

Using the correct catheter size (based on length for infants 55 cm and over and length and weight for those under 55 cm) and insertion depth is essential. Indications for NAVA include respiratory distress syndrome, pulmonary hypertension, and central hypoventilation syndrome; however, it can be used in any condition that is treated with conventional ventilation.

MECHANICAL VENTILATION

ENDOTRACHEAL INTUBATION

The difficult airway of neonates makes choosing an age-appropriate **endotracheal tube** (ETT) very important. Generally, a 2.5 mm ETT is recommended for preterm neonates born at less than 28 weeks, a 3 mm ETT is recommended for neonates born between 28 and 24 weeks, a 3.5 mm ETT is recommended for neonates born between 34 and 38 weeks, and a 3.5 to 4 mm ETT is recommended for term neonates. Length-based tape (such as the Broselow Tape) can also be utilized for ETT size estimation in emergency situations. While uncuffed ETTs have been the traditional recommendation for newborns requiring intubation, cuffed ETTs that are low pressure and high volume have recently proven safe for neonates. Regardless, additional ETTs that are a size larger and a size smaller should be immediately available in the case of difficulty intubating.

An acceptable ETT leak is 15-20 cmH_2O pressure. The ETT may be inserted nasally or orally. Premedication (morphine or fentanyl and midazolam) is used to relieve stress on the neonate. Atropine may be given to block vagal response. ETT placement should immediately be verified by auscultation and radiograph, ultrasound, or disposable end-tidal carbon dioxide detectors. Esophageal intubation is indicated if no air exchange is detected bilaterally or if there is air sound over left upper abdomen. The tube may be too high if air sounds are diminished and too low if the right lung is better ventilated than the left.

POSITIVE PRESSURE VENTILATORS

Positive pressure ventilators assist respiration by applying pressure directly to the airway, inflating the lungs, forcing expansion of the alveoli, and facilitating gas exchange. Generally, endotracheal intubation or tracheostomy is necessary to maintain positive pressure ventilation. There are 3 basic kinds of positive pressure ventilators:

- **Pressure cycled**: This type of ventilation is usually used for short-term treatment in adolescents or adults. The IPPB machine is the most common type. This delivers a flow of air to a preset pressure and then cycles off. Airway resistance or changes in compliance can affect volume of air and may compromise ventilation.
- **Time cycled**: This type of ventilation regulates the volume of air the infant receives by controlling the length of inspiration and the flow rate. This type of ventilator is used almost exclusively for neonates and infants.
- **Volume cycled**: This type of ventilation provides a preset flow of pressurized air during inspiration and then cycles off and allows passive expiration, providing a fairly consistent volume of air.

HIGH FREQUENCY JET VENTILATION

High frequency jet ventilation (HFJV) (Life Pulse) directs a high velocity stream of air into the lungs in a long spiraling spike that forces carbon dioxide against the walls, penetrating dead space and providing gas exchange by using small tidal volumes of 1-3 mL/kg, much smaller than with conventional mechanical ventilation. Because the jet stream technology is effective for short distances, the valve and pressure transducer must be placed by the infant's head. Inhalation is controlled while expiration is passive, but the rate of respiration is up to 11 per second ("panting" respirations). HFJV may be used in conjunction with low-pressure conventional ventilation to increase flow to alveoli. HFJV reduces barotrauma because of the low tidal volume and low pressure. HFJV is used for numerous conditions, including evolving chronic lung disease, pulmonary interstitial emphysema, bronchopulmonary dysplasia, and hypoxemic respiratory failure. It reduces mean airway pressure (MAP) and the oxygenation index. Treatment with HFJV may reduce the need for ECMO.

High Frequency Oscillatory Ventilation

High frequency oscillatory ventilation provides pressurized ventilation with tidal volumes approximately equal to dead space at about 150 breaths per minute (bpm). Pressure is usually higher with HFOV than HFJV in order to maintain expansion of the alveoli and to keep the airway open during gas exchange. Oxygenation is regulated separately. HFOV has both an active inspiration and expiration, so the respiratory cycle is completely controlled. HFOV reduces pulmonary vascular resistance and improves ventilation-perfusion matching and oxygenation without injuring the lung, reducing the risk of barotrauma. HFOV is used for respiratory distress syndrome, persistent pulmonary hypertension of the newborn (PPHN) associated with meconium aspiration syndrome (MAS). Other indications are air leak syndromes, pulmonary interstitial emphysema, and congenital diaphragmatic hernia. Infants in respiratory distress may be placed on HFOV immediately after birth instead of on conventional ventilation to avoid pulmonary damage.

Review Video: Mechanical Ventilation
Visit mometrix.com/academy and enter code: 679637

Ventilator Management

There are many types of ventilators now in use, and the specific directions for use of each type must be followed carefully, but there are general principles that apply to all **ventilator management.** The following should be monitored:

- **Type of ventilation**: volume-cycled, pressure-cycled, negative-pressure, HFJV, HFOV, CPAP, Bi-PAP.
- **Control mode**: controlled ventilation, assisted ventilation, synchronized intermittent mandatory [allows spontaneous breaths between ventilator controlled inhalation/exhalation], positive-end expiratory pressure (PEEP) [positive pressure at end of expiration], CPAP, Bi-PAP.
- **Tidal volume** (T_v) range should be set in relation to respiratory rate.
- **Inspiratory-expiratory ratio** (I:E) usually ranges from 1:2 to 1:5, but may be outside of that range.
- **Respiratory rate** will depend upon T_v and $PaCO_2$ target.
- **Fraction of inspired oxygen** (FiO_2) [percentage of oxygen in the inspired air], usually ranging from 21-100%, usually maintained <40% to avoid toxicity.
- **Sensitivity** determines the effort needed to trigger inspiration.
- **Pressure** controls the pressure exerted in delivering T_v.
- **Rate of flow** controls the L/min speed of T_v.

VILI

Ventilation-induced lung injury (VILI) is damage caused by mechanical ventilation. It is common in acute distress syndrome (ARDS) but can affect any ventilation patient. VILI comprises 4 interrelated elements:

- **Barotrauma**: damage to the lung caused by excessive pressure
- **Volutrauma**: alveolar damage related to high tidal volume ventilation

- **Atelectotrauma**: injury caused by repetitive forced opening and closing of alveoli
- **Biotrauma**: inflammatory response

In VILI, essentially the increased pressure and tidal volume over-distends the alveoli, which rupture, and air moves into the interstitial tissue resulting in pulmonary interstitial emphysema. With continued ventilation, the air in the interstitium moves into the subcutaneous tissue and may result in pneumopericardium and pneumomediastinum, or rupture the pleural sac. This can cause tension pneumothorax and mediastinal shift, leading to respiratory failure and cardiac arrest. VILI has caused a change in ventilation procedures with lower tidal volumes and pressures used as well as newer forms of ventilation, HFJV and HFOV, preferred to mechanical ventilation for many patients.

Tracheostomy

A tracheostomy in the neonate is done in emergent situations, such as upper airway obstruction or abnormalities, and elective situations, such as for prolonged ventilation or subglottic stenosis related to endotracheal intubation. The tracheostomy tube should extend to 1 cm superior to the carina. Because of small size (2.5-3.0 cm inner diameter), neonatal tracheostomy tubes have no inner cannula and are usually not cuffed. Humidity must be provided by attaching the tracheostomy to a warmed humidified air source or use of heat-moisture exchangers. Suctioning to maintain patency is done every 4 hours with the suction catheter extending slightly below (3-5 mm) the tracheostomy tube, and the suctioning length should be prominently posted. There is no consensus on the use of saline instillation during suctioning. Tubes should be changed regularly, usually at least once weekly. Skin about the stoma should be inspected twice daily and drainage cleansed with saline or hydrogen peroxide/saline (if crusting). In some cases, a thin gauze or hydrocolloid dressing may be placed under the flanges.

Risk Factors with Administration of Oxygen/Ventilation

There are risk factors associated with administration of oxygen/ventilation:

- High oxygen concentration can result in **retinopathy of prematurity (ROP) and blindness**.
- The mechanical ventilation used to treat a neonate's respiratory disease exerts pressure on the vascular system feeding the lungs; this includes pressure on the pulmonary artery, which comes out of the heart. If this pressure on the pulmonary artery is great enough, **cardiac output can be lessened**. Lowering the positive pressure settings on the ventilator can alleviate some of this pressure, thus improving cardiac output. Cardiac output can also be supplemented by giving the infant an infusion of extra fluid. This helps to raise cardiac output by enough to compensate for the increased pressure from the ventilator pressures that the heart must overcome to keep the body well oxygenated.
- Oxygenation during resuscitation has been recommended to start at 21% (up to 30% in a preterm newborn) to prevent injuries that can occur from hyperoxygenation. During CPR, oxygen should be administered at 100%.

Chest Tube Insertion/Removal for Pneumothorax

Chest tubes are inserted in the neonate to treat pneumothorax causing cardiac or respiratory compromise or pleural effusion. **Transillumination** may be used to identify the area of pneumothorax but a **chest x-ray** is more accurate. An 8-12 Fr. chest tube is placed anteriorly for collections of air and posteriorly/laterally for fluid. The infant is supine with the arm at 90° on the insertion side. The insertion sites are

- **Anterior**: midclavicular line, second or third intercostal space
- **Posterior/lateral**: anterior axillary line, fourth, fifth, or sixth intercostal space

Lidocaine is instilled and an incision made over the rib below the target intercostal space. The tissue is spread and the pleura punctured above the rib with a hemostat, expelling air. The chest tube is inserted 2-3 cm for preterm infants and 3-4 cm for full-term infants. The purse-string suture is tightened and the chest tube attached to 2 or 3 bottles or a self-contained Pleur-evac underwater seal system. An x-ray is taken to confirm placement. The chest tube is removed quickly and pressure dressing applied if there is no bubbling for 24 hours and the radiograph is clear.

Pleur-Evac System

A chest tube is attached to a three-chamber system called a **Pleur-Evac.** As the name indicates, there are three separate chambers in this collection system:

- The first chamber is the **collection chamber**. This chamber is where the air and/or fluid that is being drained from the pleural space collects as a result of a pulmonary leak. Bubbling in this chamber is the result of air being pumped out of the pleural space and is expected.
- The second chamber is the **water seal chamber**; this chamber is where the water in an amount prescribed by the physician is placed to create the vacuum necessary to pull the fluid and/or air out of the pleural space. The amount of water placed in this chamber affects the amount of pressure and should be carefully monitored to make sure it remains at the ordered level. Bubbling in this chamber indicates a leak and must be investigated.
- The third chamber is the **suction chamber**, which is responsible for the suction that creates the pressure removing the air from the pleural space.

Needle Aspiration for Pneumothorax

Neonates receiving bag and mask ventilation or mechanical ventilation risk developing a **pneumothorax**. Signs of pneumothorax include rapid deterioration, poor oxygenation, tachypnea, increased work breathing, impaired circulation, unequal air entry into lungs, displaced apical heartbeat, and increased transillumination on the affected side. If the neonate's clinical status allows it, a chest x-ray will confirm the diagnosis. Air is removed by **needle aspiration.**

The **equipment** for needle aspiration:

- Oral sucrose
- 1% lidocaine
- Fentanyl
- 23- to 25-gauge scalp vein needle or 18- to 20-gauge angiocatheter
- 10 mL syringe
- 3-way stopcock attached to the syringe
- 70% isopropyl alcohol swab
- Sterile gloves

The **procedure** for needle aspiration is as follows:

1. Give oral sucrose.
2. Place infant in supine position.

3. Swab second and third intercostal spaces in midclavicular line with alcohol.
4. Infiltrate site with 1% lidocaine 0.5-1.0 mL.
5. Drape insertion site.
6. Give 250 mcg fentanyl over 2-3 minutes IV.
7. Insert needle directly into second or third intercostal space in mid-clavicular line until air is aspirated into the syringe.
8. Expel air through stopcock.

Chapter Quiz

Ready to see how well you retained what you just read? Scan the QR code to go directly to the chapter quiz interface for this study guide. If you're using a computer, simply visit the online resources page at **mometrix.com/resources719/ccrnneonatal** and click the Chapter Quizzes link.

Clinical Judgment: Endocrine and Hematology

Endocrine and Metabolic Complications

HYPOTHYROIDISM

Hypothyroidism is caused by a deficiency in production of the thyroid hormones (TH) T_4 and T_3. All newborns are screened for congenital hypothyroidism because of the severe consequences associated with lack of treatment and the ease of treatment with exogenous thyroid hormone. It may be congenital or acquired. **Congenital hypothyroidism** (formerly called cretinism) may manifest at birth or be delayed for years, but severe early onset can result in profound neurological deficit and intellectual disability if undiagnosed and treated:

- **Neonates***:* Widened posterior fontanel, hypothermia ≤95 °F, edema, respiratory distress, feeding difficulties, lethargy, delayed passage of meconium, prolonged physiologic jaundice, and vomiting
- **≤3 months of age**: Umbilical hernia, dry skin, constipation, enlarged tongue, lethargy, and minimal crying

Treatment includes oral TH replacement therapy. Prompt initiation of therapy is critical for congenital hypothyroidism in order to prevent developmental abnormalities. If symptoms of hypothyroidism are severe, therapy to reach appropriate levels of TH is initially given gradually over 3-4 weeks to avoid hyperthyroidism.

HYPERTHYROIDISM

Hyperthyroidism is caused by excess production of T3 and T4 thyroid hormones. Suppression of TSH may be present in neonates born to thyrotoxic mothers or those with genetic disorders, such as McCune-Albright syndrome. Hyperthyroidism may develop during the fetal stage, resulting in IUGR, fetal hydrops (non-immune), and fetal death. **Symptoms** of neonates include:

- Hyperkinesis
- Diarrhea
- Vomiting
- Failure to thrive or gain weight
- Tachycardia with increased pulse pressure
- Hypertension (systemic and pulmonary)
- Hepatosplenomegaly
- Thrombocytopenia
- Hyperviscosity syndrome
- Ophthalmic abnormalities
- Craniosynostosis

Treatment includes the use of antithyroid medications, such as propylthiouracil or methimazole, β-adrenergic blockers, and iodine. Digoxin may be necessary as well as glucocorticoids. Remission usually occurs in 20-48 weeks. In rare cases, thyroid ablation (thyroidectomy) may be necessary.

Inborn Errors of Metabolism

Inborn errors of metabolism comprise a wide range of genetic metabolic disorders, usually related to defects in gene coding for enzymes, resulting in toxic accumulations that interfere with metabolism. Disorders are classified according to the type of metabolic disorder and include:

- **Carbohydrates** (glycogen storage disease, fructose intolerance)
- **Proteins** (clotting defects, sickle cell, thalassemia, osteogenesis imperfecta, Marfan's)
- **Amino acids** (phenylketonuria, hyperammonemia)
- **Organic acid** (alcaptonuria)
- **Cholesterol/lipoprotein** (hyperlipoproteinemias, hypoproteinemias)
- **Mitochondrial** (Kearns-Sayre syndrome)
- **Porphyrin** (porphyria)
- **Defective DNA repair** (xeroderma pigmentosum)

Symptoms relate to the specific defect. Some symptoms are present in the neonate but others appear in childhood or adulthood, with some diseases life-threatening and others slowly progressive. Symptoms common to many disorders may include:

- Encephalopathy with poor feeding, lethargy, tachypnea
- Metabolic acidosis and/or hyperammonemia
- Hypoglycemia, hepatic dysfunctions with jaundice
- Dysmorphism (structural anomalies)
- Abnormal body odor or urine odor

Phenylketonuria

Phenylketonuria (PKU) is an inborn error of metabolism that results from a deficiency of the liver enzyme that changes phenylalanine to tyrosine (phenylalanine is a product that results when protein is digested). These infants are unable to digest protein. The symptoms of this disorder will show up sometime before 3 months if not caught in a screening. The first symptoms will be vomiting, poor feeding effort, and irritability. Later, if not treated, the infant will develop eczema and will have urine that smells musty. Once this condition is diagnosed, the infant must be put on a strict diet that restricts phenylalanine. Extensive family training must take place to educate the family about the diet. If the infant does not follow this diet restriction, intellectual disability will result. PKU screening within 7 days of birth is required in all 50 states.

Galactosemia

Galactosemia, an autosomal recessive disorder, is the most common inborn error of metabolism. In this disorder, the infant is lacking the enzyme that converts galactose to glucose. Because lactose is made up of galactose and glucose, the infant who cannot convert the galactose in lactose to glucose cannot tolerate lactose. Usually, the neonate is asymptomatic but develops symptoms rapidly. The clinical manifestations seen with galactosemia include jaundice, vomiting, diarrhea, inability to gain weight, and hypoglycemia. An infant with this condition that does not receive treatment can contract a serious gram-negative infection related to damage to the intestinal lining, and death may occur at 1-2 weeks. This condition must be treated by removing all lactose products and replacing the formula with soy or lactose-free formula. If left untreated, severe intellectual disability can result.

Adrenal Disorders of the Neonate

Congenital Adrenal Hyperplasia

Congenital adrenal hyperplasia (CAH) is an autosomal recessive defect that results in a cortisol deficiency, and is often accompanied by an aldosterone deficiency. 90 to 95% of CAH cases are due to a deficiency in 21-hydroxylase, the enzyme responsible for catalyzing two reactions in the adrenal glands:

- 17-Hydroxyprogestorne → 11-deoxycortisol → cortisol
- Progesterone → deoxycorticosterone → aldosterone

The cortisol deficiency results in shock, hypoglycemia, and circulatory collapse. The infant becomes dehydrated when CAH is accompanied by aldosterone deficiency (salt wasting), because of excessive loss of urinary sodium. Symptoms do not usually occur until the infant is 2 to 4 weeks old. Metabolic abnormalities of hyperkalemia, hyponatremia, hypoglycemia, and metabolic acidosis are present shortly after birth. Some infants have milder forms of CAH and are not diagnosed until later in life. Elevated levels of ACTH cause hypertrophy of the adrenal glands and increased production of androgens. Elevated androgens *in utero* virilize the female infant, so she has ovaries and uterus but external genitalia are often ambiguous.

Adrenal Insufficiency and Adrenal Hemorrhage

Adrenal disorders common to the neonate include the following:

- **Adrenal insufficiency** is the inadequate production of adrenal hormones (cortisol, aldosterone) because of adrenal or pituitary gland dysfunction. Clinical findings may be nonspecific but the condition is characterized by poor feeding, dehydration, hypoglycemia, hyponatremia, hyperkalemia, metabolic acidosis, hyperpigmentation, and hypotension. Treatment includes hormone replacement.
- **Adrenal hemorrhage** is associated with birth trauma, asphyxia, or sepsis. This may be asymptomatic or includes signs of adrenal insufficiency if 90% or more of the adrenal glands are destroyed, including electrolyte imbalances. Some neonates may present with anemia or late onset jaundice. An abdominal mass may be evident if bleeding is significant.

Ambiguous Genitalia

Ambiguous genitalia in the neonate can accompany the following conditions:

- **Congenital adrenal hyperplasia** (female): The adrenal glands are unable to produce glucocorticoids and mineralocorticoids (cortisol and aldosterone) but produce androgen, which is a male hormone. This results in virilization and an enlarged clitoris, which may resemble a small penis. The labia may be partially or completely fused, resembling a scrotum, and the vaginal orifice may be very small or obscured by the labia. Treatment with female hormones may aid in development of secondary sexual characteristics, but the brain was imprinted as male during development, typically leading to gender dysphoria.
- **5-alpha-reductase 2 deficiency:** This autosomal recessive disorder results in genetic males with the inability to convert testosterone to dihydrotestosterone (DHT), which is necessary for masculinization during fetal development, resulting in ambiguous or female-appearing external genitalia (micropenis, bifid scrotum, hypospadias), although internal reproductive organs are male.

- **Ovotestis** (formerly hermaphrodite): Both male and female reproductive organs are present in this condition, although there is considerable variation possible. A vagina may be present but is usually abnormal, penile length can vary but hypospadias is common, and the labia and scrotum vary widely. Most individuals with ovotestis will develop breasts at puberty.
- **Clitoromegaly** is a benign difference in the appearance of the clitoris, which is often enlarged and appearing to be a small penis. This may occur with neurofibromatosis, which should be ruled out.
- **Androgen insensitivity syndrome** is when genetically male neonates have a defect in androgen receptors that prevents response to testosterone and other androgens. External genitalia may appear as typical male or typical female, depending on the type:
    - Complete (CAIS): phenotype is female but no uterus or ovaries, vagina is short, testes are labial or inguinal.
    - Partial (PAIS-1): phenotype is primarily female with clitoromegaly, fused labia, urethra and vaginal openings or urogenital sinus
    - Partial (PAIS-2): phenotype is ambiguous with microphallus (<1 cm), bifid labia (appear scrotal), testes (descended or undescended), urogenital sinus or perineoscrotal hypospadias
    - Partial (PAIS-3: phenotype is primarily male with small or micropenis with perineal hypospadias, bifid scrotum, and testes (descended or undescended)
    - Minimal (MAIS): phenotype is male but undervirilized with normal appearing genitalia but impaired spermatogenesis and virilization at puberty

HYPOGLYCEMIA

Hypoglycemia is low blood sugar of 35 mg/dL or less during the first day after birth, or below 50 mg/dL thereafter. One neonate in every 25,000 experiences persistent **hypoglycemia**. Half of hypoglycemic neonates develop brain damage. The hypoglycemic patient may be asymptomatic or may have these symptoms: apnea, tachypnea, respiratory distress, vomiting, diminished oral intake, tachycardia, bradycardia, jitteriness, lethargy, brisk Moro reflex, seizures, coma, and temperature instability. Suspect hypoglycemia in these circumstances:

- Elevated insulin levels in the infant with a brittle diabetic mother
- Premature or SGA baby
- KATP-HI diffuse or focal disease, GDH-HI, or GK-HI genetic disorders
- Septic shock
- Hyperthyroidism
- Inadequate glucose stores in malnourished infants and poor feeders
- Hypoxemia or ischemia
- Ingestion of alcohol, beta blockers, or salicylates

Treatment initially involves a bolus of IV dextrose (0.2 g/kg over 5 to 10 minutes) with a continuous infusion to follow at 5 to 8 mg/kg per minute. If the hypoglycemia is secondary to hyperinsulinemic hypoglycemia, oral diazoxide is recommended at 5-20 mg/kg per day, 2-3 times a day. The doctor may also order hydrochlorothiazide, nifedipine, octreotide, and glucagon. Partial pancreatectomy is required if drugs are ineffective.

Causes and Risk Factors

Causes and risk factors for hypoglycemia include the following:

- **Decreased glucose availability**—Risk factors include preterm birth, glycogen storage diseases, intrauterine growth restriction, and prolonged fasting.
- **Increased glucose utilization**—Risk factors include cold stress and hypothermia, sepsis, labored breathing, perinatal asphyxia, Rh incompatibility, persistent neonatal hyperinsulinism, and maternal tocolytic drugs.
- **An umbilical artery catheter placed with the tip right above the pancreas**—delivers glucose directly to the pancreas and can stimulate too much insulin production.
- **Elevated insulin levels**—Risk factors include infant of diabetic mother (elevated glucose levels trigger increased insulin production), islet cell hyperplasia, abrupt cessation of IV glucose, exchange transfusion, and Beckwith-Wiedemann syndrome.

Acute Hypoglycemia/Hyperinsulinism

Acute hypoglycemia/hyperinsulinism can cause damage to the central nervous and cardiopulmonary systems, interfering with development of the brain and causing neurological impairment. **Causes** may include:

- Persistent hyperinsulinemic hypoglycemia of infancy (PHHI) in infants of diabetic mothers, usually apparent in the first 3 months
- Genetic defects in chromosome 11 (short arm)
- Severe infections, such as Gram-negative sepsis and endotoxic shock
- Maternal tocolytic administration

Symptoms in infants include:

- Blood glucose <40 mg/dL
- Central nervous system: seizures, altered consciousness, lethargy, and poor feeding with vomiting, myoclonus, respiratory distress, diaphoresis, hypothermia, and cyanosis

Treatment includes:

- Glucose/Glucagon administration to elevate blood glucose levels.
- Diazoxide inhibits release of insulin.
- Somatostatin to suppress insulin production.
- Nifedipine
- Careful monitoring. Surgical removal of 85-90% of pancreas may be needed for infants to reduce insulin but poses risk of diabetes.

Hypoglycemia Secondary to Glycogen Storage Disease

Glycogen storage diseases (GSD) are inherited enzyme deficiencies that prevent/inhibit glycogenolysis and release of glycogen. There are 10 different types, but I, III, and IV are most common. All are autosomal recessive defects. Glycogen is stored in the liver and muscles but cannot be accessed and builds up, eventually resulting in cirrhosis of muscles and organs (heart, liver, kidney). Infants present with hypoglycemia that does not respond to the administration of glucagon, enlarged liver, and failure to thrive. GSD infants require almost continuous enteral feeds to maintain their blood glucose levels. They are susceptible to episodes of damaging hypoglycemia that can cause seizures, apnea, hypothermia, hypotonia, and cyanosis. Some types can be treated with diet, monitoring of symptoms, and medications, but others have no effective treatment. Uric acid may accumulate, so medications to lower uric acid levels may be needed.

Hyperglycemia

Hyperglycemia is a value greater than 100 mg/dL glucose in the newborn and is often iatrogenic (caused by glucose infusion). Premature and very low birth rate infants receiving IV glucose are at greatest risk for developing **hyperglycemia** because these infants often have decreased insulin production or decreased insulin insensitivity. Congenital diabetes mellitus is rare and may either be transient or permanent in nature. One of the main dangers of hyperglycemia is dehydration from osmotic diuresis. The neonate's urine will contain glucose (glucosuria). Intracranial hemorrhage is associated with hyperglycemia. Decreasing the amount of IV glucose usually resolves hyperglycemia. Dehydration must be corrected with IV fluids, if necessary. Enteral feeds stimulate insulin production by the pancreas, so exogenous insulin is rarely required to control the infant's elevated blood sugar levels.

Excess IV Glucose

If excessive IV glucose is administered to a newborn, it will cause hyperglycemia to develop. Newborns utilize glucose at a rate of 4-8 mg/kg/min. Premature infants have a lower glucose tolerance, so start them at 4 mg/kg/min. Full term infants are started at 8 mg/kg/min. At levels greater than 150-180 mg/dL, osmotic diuresis occurs (glucose in the urine). The infant develops dehydration. Dextrose is the d isomer of glucose (d-glucose). In order to supply a 2-kg infant with 7 mg/kg/min of glucose using a solution of D10 (10% dextrose solution, 100 mg dextrose per mL) the following calculations are used:

$$\text{Required dextrose} = \left(7\frac{\text{mg}}{\text{kg}\cdot\text{min}}\right) \times (2\text{ kg}) = 14\frac{\text{mg}}{\text{min}}$$

$$14\frac{\text{mg}}{\text{min}} \times \frac{1\text{ mL}}{100\text{ mg}} = 0.14\frac{\text{mL}}{\text{min}}$$

$$0.14\frac{\text{mL}}{\text{min}} \times \frac{60\text{ min}}{1\text{ hr}} = 8.4\frac{\text{mL}}{\text{hr}}$$

IDM

Infants of diabetic mother (IDM) are exposed to elevated levels of glucose during their intrauterine development, as glucose freely crosses the placenta; the blood glucose level of the developing fetus mirrors that of the mother. The fetus increases production of insulin at around 20 weeks of gestation in response to the mother's elevated blood glucose. When the umbilical cord is cut, it abruptly disrupts the neonate's supply of glucose. The infant's greatest risk for hypoglycemia occurs 30-90 minutes after delivery. Because insulin levels are elevated in the fetus, the newborn may have an increased glucose need for several days to prevent hypoglycemia—as high as 10-15 mg/kg/min. Glucose is given as a continuous infusion to prevent the newborn from developing rebound hypoglycemia after a bolus of glucose. IDM infants show fewer symptoms of hypoglycemia when compared to other neonates and may also suffer from hypocalcemia, hypomagnesemia, and hyperbilirubinemia. Hypoglycemia is an easily treatable condition that, when left untreated, causes long-term neurological damage.

Infants of diabetic mother (IDM) often **present** with:

- Birth trauma secondary to cephalopelvic disproportion, including shoulder dislocation
- Hypoglycemia from sudden withdrawal of maternal glucose and elevated insulin in the infant
- Respiratory distress syndrome because elevated insulin inhibits surfactant production
- Polycythemia (excessive red blood cell production) and hyperviscosity because of elevated insulin and glucose increase the metabolic rate and oxygen consumption
- Iron deficiency because polycythemia leaches iron from the heart and brain
- Hyperbilirubinemia because of increased red blood cell destruction after birth
- Cardiovascular malformations, such as intraventricular hypertrophy with outflow tract obstruction, transposition of the great arteries, ventral septal defects, and coarctation of the aorta
- Congenital malformations, such as anencephaly, spina bifida, renal agenesis, and duodenal atresia
- Electrolyte abnormalities, including hypocalcemia and hypomagnesemia

Complications

There are several complications resulting from IDM, including:

- **Seizure activity** can occur in some of these infants due to the lack of sufficient fuel for the brain when the infant becomes hypoglycemic. Glucose is the fuel the brain needs to function properly, and when it is in short supply, the brain is essentially starved.
- **Shoulder dystocia** is a condition that is directly related to an infant that is large for gestational age (LGA) because of diabetes. Large babies will often experience shoulder dislocation at birth as they try to fit through the birth canal.
- **Thrombosis** sometimes forms in the kidneys (venous or arterial) as a result of a high hematocrit and increased viscosity of blood.
- **Increased diabetic risk**—2% of female and 6% of male IDMs will go on to develop juvenile type 1 diabetes.

Magnesium-Related Disorders of the Neonate

Hypomagnesemia in the neonate can result from prematurity, IUGR, and placental insufficiency as well as low maternal levels of magnesium. Hypomagnesemia may also result from increased magnesium loss associated with renal tubular acidosis, short bowel syndrome, and diarrhea, as well as insufficient magnesium in parenteral nutrition.

- Normal values: 1.6–2.6 mEq/L
- Hypomagnesemia: <1.6 mEq/L; critical value: <1.2 mg/dL

Signs and symptoms include irritability, tremors, hyperreflexia, seizure, cardiac arrhythmias, poor feeding, and apnea. Treatment is supportive and oral or IV magnesium according to severity.

Hypermagnesemia can result from maternal magnesium treatment, renal insufficiency, and excess magnesium intake (such as in parenteral nutrition).

- Hypermagnesemia: >2.6 mEq/L; critical value: >4.9 mg/dL

Signs and symptoms include respiration depression/apnea, bradycardia, hypotension, lethargy, poor sucking, flaccidity, hypotonia, decreased reflexes, GI hypomotility, and abdominal distention. Infants born to mothers receiving magnesium may require resuscitation at birth. Treatment includes adequate hydration, furosemide, and calcium gluconate to counteract effects and increased excretion.

Phosphorus-Related Disorders of the Neonate

Hypophosphatemia may occur in preterm and VLBW neonates because of inadequate storage, and this can result in metabolic bone disease with onset generally between 6 and 16 weeks because of bone demineralization. Other causes of hypophosphatemia include insufficient phosphorous in formula, maternal malnutrition, increased loss because of renal tubular disorders, refeeding syndrome, and some medications. Signs and symptoms include poor feeding, irritability, muscle weakness, and hypotonia. Treatment includes phosphate supplementation.

Hyperphosphatemia may result from renal insufficiency, over-supplementation, hypoparathyroidism (congenital or transient), and maternal hyperphosphatemia. Signs and symptoms include tetany (due to associated hypocalcemia), seizures, renal damage, calcium-phosphate precipitation in soft tissues, and oliguria. Treatment includes phosphate binders, limiting phosphate intake, hydration, diuretics, and calcium supplementation.

- Normal value: 0-5 days is 4.6–8.0 mg/dL
- Hypophosphatemia: <4.0–5.5 mg/dL
- Hyperphosphatemia: >6.5–8 mg/dL

Hematologic Complications

ABO Incompatibility

About 20–25% of pregnancies involve ABO incompatibility, usually with the mother type O and the fetus A or B. **Anti-A and anti-B antibodies** occur naturally when a woman is exposed to A and B antigens in foods or bacteria, so these antibodies can cross the placenta and result in **hemolysis of fetal RBC**; however, the antibodies are relatively large and do not enter the fetal circulation easily. If fetal blood leaks into maternal blood (a common occurrence), then smaller antibodies form and these can cross the placenta more easily. There is no difference in effect between the first pregnancy and subsequent pregnancies. There are rarely serious complications for the fetus, although the neonate may develop hyperbilirubinemia, so the infant should be observed carefully. Only in severe cases of hemolysis (rare), does the child require exchange transfusions. Anemia may develop in the weeks after delivery because of increased rate of RBC breakdown, so the neonate should be monitored with blood counts.

Maternal Rh Alloimmunization

Rh incompatibility occurs if the mother is Rh- and the father is Rh+, putting their infant at risk for hemolytic disease of the newborn (HDN) or Rh disease, (erythroblastosis fetalis). **Rh alloimmunization** (formation of antibodies against foreign antigens) can occur during abortion, abruptio placenta, amniocentesis, Cesarean section, chorionic villus sampling, cordocentesis, delivery, ectopic pregnancy, and toxemia. To prevent erythroblastosis fetalis, a woman who is Rh- with an Rh+ mate receives the serum anti-D immune globulin (**RhoGAM)**, containing anti Rh+ antibodies. The purpose of the antibodies is to agglutinate any fetal red blood cells that pass over into the mother's circulatory system and thus prevent the mother from forming antibodies against them that will attack the infant and sensitize her for future pregnancies. Testing and administration of RhoGAM is as follows:

- Order Rh(D) tests. If the mother is Rh- and the father is Rh+, then their infant is at risk for hemolytic disease of the newborn (HDN).
- Order an antibody screen of the mother's blood to find out if she acquired anti-D antibodies from a previous blood transfusion or pregnancy.
- The mother receives 300 mcg RhoGAM intramuscularly at 26–28 weeks of pregnancy and again within 72 hours after her delivery. Do not inject the infant or father. RhoGAM prevents Rh+ cells from the infant that have crossed over to the mother from causing her to create anti-D antibodies that will attack the infant and sensitize her for future pregnancies.
- Miscarriage, ectopic, abortion: At ≤12 weeks, the mother receives 50 mcg of MICRhoGAM. At ≥13 weeks, the mother receives RhoGAM as for pregnancy.

Blood-Loss Anemia

Blood loss is the most common cause of anemia in the neonate. Anemia is hematocrit or hemoglobin level >2 standard deviations below the mean for age. For a term infant, anemia is a hematocrit <45%. The loss of blood may be internal or external, and may occur in utero, during delivery, or post-delivery. **Treatment** may include packed red blood cell transfusions. Common **causes** of neonatal blood loss include:

Antenatal

- Abruptio placentae or placenta previa
- Fetomaternal transfusion (passage of fetal blood to the mother)
- Twin-to-twin transfusion, resulting in one twin with polycythemia and the donor twin with anemia

Perinatal

- Trauma to the placenta or umbilical cord
- Rupture of anomalous cord vessels
- Fetoplacental transfusion that occurs when the infant is positioned above the level of the placenta after delivery

Postnatal

- Internal hemorrhage, such as intracranial hemorrhage or cephalohematoma
- Damage to internal organs, such as the adrenal gland or liver
- Iatrogenic blood loss secondary to frequent laboratory sampling, a major cause of anemia in premature infants

Anemia of Prematurity

Anemia of prematurity (AOP) represents a pathologic exaggeration of the normal decrease in hematocrit that occurs in every newborn. AOP results from a combination of factors:

- **RBC production** decreases because the premature neonate's response to erythropoietin (EPO) has not matured. EPO is the main stimulus for RBC production. The normal progression of EPO production in the fetus is for the liver to initially be the primary site, with transfer to the kidney as the primary site of production in the full-term neonate. The liver is less responsive to hypoxia and allows for a lower threshold of anemia to progress until EPO production is increased. Lowest Hgb levels are usually at 2–3 months of age.
- **Premature RBCs have a shortened lifespan** when compared to the full-term neonate's because of decreased levels of intracellular ATP and enzyme activity.
- **Frequent blood draws** in premature neonates required for close monitoring deplete the blood supply.

Infants with signs of hypoxemia (poor feeling, tachypnea, tachycardia, pallor) may require transfusions.

Anemia of Red Blood Cell Destruction

Causes of anemia of red blood cell destruction are discussed below:

- **Intrinsic causes**—continued production of abnormal red blood cells that have a decreased survival time because of rare hereditary disorders:
  - **RBC enzyme defects**, such as G6PD deficiency, where hemolytic crisis occurs in response to drugs such as sulfonamide antibiotics, or infections
  - **RBC membrane defects**, such as hereditary spherocytosis, where abnormally-shaped red cells are prone to hemolysis
  - **Hemoglobinopathies**, such as thalassemia, which results in the reduced production of one of the protein chains that make up hemoglobin
- **Extrinsic causes**—temporary RBC destruction caused by some external stimulus:
  - **Immune hemolysis** from transfusion of an incompatible blood product (wrong Rh, ABO, or a minor blood group incompatibility)
  - **Acquired hemolysis** from infection, vitamin E deficiency, or poisoning

Polycythemia

Polycythemia is a hematocrit greater than 65%. An elevated hematocrit means that the blood has less plasma and more cellular elements, increasing the viscosity of the blood. Increased blood viscosity results in slowed blood flow and sludging of red blood cells. Small vessels become occluded with microthrombi, resulting in tissue or organ ischemia. **Clinical signs of polycythemia** include:

- **Dermatologic**: plethora and increased capillary refill time
- **CNS**: lethargy, irritability, abnormal cry, cerebrovascular hemorrhage, and seizures
- **Pulmonary**: respiratory distress, cyanosis, apnea, and the development of persistent pulmonary hypertension
- **Renal**: hematuria, oliguria, and renal vein thrombosis
- **Hematological**: thrombocytopenia secondary to the development of disseminated intravascular coagulation

- **Gastrointestinal**: abdominal distension, poor feeding, bloody stools, and necrotizing enterocolitis
- **Metabolic**: persistent hypoglycemia and hypocalcemia

Risk Factors

Polycythemia occurs in 4% of live-born infants. Its **etiologies** are divided into conditions that cause hypoxia and increased RBC production and those that cause abnormal transfer of RBCs to the neonate (hypertransfusion):

- **Hypoxia**
  - Disorders that disrupt normal placental function and decrease oxygen delivery to the fetus include preeclampsia, chronic placental abruption, maternal congenital heart disease, postdate pregnancy, and maternal smoking. Many of these are also associated with a growth-restricted neonate (IUGR).
  - Disorders that cause increased oxygen consumption by the fetus include infants of diabetic mothers and those with Beckwith-Wiedemann syndrome. Polycythemia occurs in 30–40% of neonates born to mothers with diabetes.
- **Hypertransfusion**
  - Delay in clamping the umbilical cord during delivery allows for increased blood volume to be transferred to the neonate.
  - Twin-twin transfusion creates one twin who is anemic and the second twin with an increased hematocrit in 10% of monozygotic twin pregnancies.

Exchange Transfusions

The infant with polycythemia requires a **partial exchange transfusion** with a plasma substitute in these situations:

- The hematocrit is greater than 65%, and the infant is symptomatic
- The hematocrit is greater than 70%, regardless of symptoms

Aliquots of the neonate's blood are replaced with isotonic saline to lower the hematocrit (Hct) to 50–55%. This formula calculates the volume of blood to be exchanged with an equal volume of saline:

$$\text{Exchange vol (mL)} = \frac{\text{initial Hct} - \text{desired Hct}}{\text{initial Hct}} \times \text{weight (kg)} \times 90\,\frac{\text{mL}}{\text{kg}}$$

The **procedure** is described below:

1. Withdraw no more than 5 mL of blood at a time from the umbilical artery or vein over 2–3 minutes.
2. Slowly infuse an equal amount of sterile normal saline.
3. Repeat the exchange until the desired volume of fluid is swapped.
4. Monitor the infant closely during the procedure.
5. Measure the hematocrit post procedure.

Thrombocytosis

Thrombocytosis is an increase in the platelet level >450,000/mcL; however, preterm infants often exhibit platelet levels of up to 600,000/mcL at 4–6 weeks. The normal reference range for platelets (thrombocytes) is 150,000–400,000/mcL. Thrombocytosis does not require specific treatment, but the underlying cause should be identified and treated. Neonates rarely have symptoms directly related to increased platelet count, but may experience cerebral ischemia with levels higher than 2,000,000/mcL. Treatment is aimed at the underlying cause. Almost all incidences of thrombocytosis in infants are secondary or reactive. **Common causes of thrombocytosis** in the neonate include:

- Infection
- Trisomy 21 (Down syndrome)
- Iron deficiency (often associated with chronic intrauterine blood loss from bleeding into a twin or GI bleeding)
- Congenital adrenal insufficiency
- Maternal abuse of narcotic drugs

Thrombocytopenia

Thrombocytopenia is a platelet count less than 150,000/mcL, caused either by decreased platelet production, increased platelet destruction, or a combination of both. Hematology labs use **mean platelet volume (MPV)**, a measure of the average platelet size, to differentiate the two. The MPV is normal if the cause is reduced production and elevated if the cause is accelerated destruction. Immature platelets are larger than normal and are released into circulating blood by the bone marrow when mature platelets are being destroyed. The lab may also differentiate the cause by a **retic count** (reticulated platelets are newly-produced platelets). If the retic count is elevated, then platelets are being destroyed, and if it is low, the production of platelets is suppressed. General guidelines for transfusing platelets depend on the clinical stability of the neonate. If the infant is stable, the attending physician considers a transfusion when the count is less than 25,000/mcL. If the infant is unstable, the attending physician considers a transfusion when the count is less than 50,000/mcL.

Fetal Onset, Early Onset, and Late Onset

Causes of **fetal onset** include:

- Alloimmune thrombocytopenia: The mother produces antibodies specific to antigens on the neonate's platelets, which cross the placenta, causing thrombocytopenia.
- Autoimmune thrombocytopenia: Mothers with idiopathic thrombocytopenia purpura or lupus produce antibodies against fetal platelets.
- Congenital infection—mediated: CMV, rubella, toxoplasmosis. Neonates with trisomy 18 or 21.

Causes of **early onset** (<72 hours) include:

- Placental insufficiency occurs in infants who are small for gestational age or with intrauterine growth restriction
- Perinatal asphyxia
- Disseminated intravascular coagulation (DIC)

Causes of **late onset** (>72 hours) include:

- Late onset sepsis
- Necrotizing enterocolitis

Hemophilia

Hemophilia is an inherited disorder in which the infant lacks adequate clotting factors. There are 3 **types**:

- Type A: Lack of clotting factor VII (90% of cases)
- Type B: Lack of clotting factor IX (about 5% of cases)
- Type C: Lack of clotting factor XI (affects both sexes, rarely occurs in the US)

Both Type A and B are usually X-linked disorders, affecting only males. The **severity** of the disease depends on the amount of clotting factor in the blood:

- Mild: >5% factor activity
- Moderate: 1–5% factor activity
- Severe: <1% factor activity

Severe neonatal hemophilia is often discovered when slow clotting is noted after circumcision or venipuncture. Approximately 1 to 2% of hemophiliacs have intracranial hemorrhage. Infants with severe hemophilia have a prolonged PTT, but normal PT values. Diagnosis is confirmed by Factor VIII and Factor IX tests.

Treatment includes:

- Desmopressin to stimulate production of clotting factor (if mild)
- Clotting factor or recombinant clotting factors (genetically-engineered)
- Plasma (Type C)

Neutropenia

Reduced neutrophils (neutropenia) indicate infection or bone marrow suppression. In neonates, the most common reasons for neutropenia are infection or stresses, such as respiratory distress syndrome, although it may be associated with congenital disorders, such as Shwachman-Diamond and Kostmann's syndrome. A segmented neutrophil nucleus (seg) is a mature cell. A banded nucleus (band) is immature. To calculate the absolute neutrophil count (ANC), the percentage of segs is added to the percentage of bands and multiplied by the total white blood cell count. A low ANC is more specific for identifying sepsis than an elevated ANC, but ANC by itself is a poor indicator of sepsis. **Normal neutrophil counts**:

- At birth the lower limit of normal is 1,750 cells/mm^3
- At 12 hours it rises to 7,200 cells/mm^3
- At 72 hours it falls to 1,720 cells/mm^3

The immature to total neutrophil ratio (I:T) is a better indicator of sepsis than ANC. An I:T ratio greater than 0.2 indicates sepsis. The formula for calculating the I:T ratio:

$$\text{I:T} = \frac{\text{immature neutrophils}}{\text{immature neutrophils} + \text{mature neutrophils}}$$

HYPERBILIRUBINEMIA

Hyperbilirubinemia, excess of bilirubin in the blood, is characterized by jaundice. Hyperbilirubinemia is evaluated according to the levels of direct (conjugated) bilirubin and/or indirect (unconjugated) bilirubin:

- **Direct/conjugated bilirubin** levels increase with blockage of bile ducts, hepatitis, or other liver damage, including drug reaction.
- **Indirect/unconjugated bilirubin** levels increase with anemias (such as hemolytic disorders) and transfusion reactions.

Four basic **types** of hyperbilirubinemia and jaundice:

- **Physiologic**: Common in newborns and usually benign, resulting from immature hepatic function and increased RBC hemolysis. Infants have larger red blood cells with a shorter life than adults, leading to more RBC destruction and resulting in an increased load of serum bilirubin, which the liver of the newborn cannot handle. Premature infants have an even greater physiologic jaundice as their RBCs live even shorter lives than the term infant's. Onset is usually within 24-48 hours, peaking in 72 hours for full-term or 5 days for preterm infants and declining within a week. Phototherapy is the indicated treatment.
- **Hemolytic**: Caused by blood/antigen (Rh) incompatibility with onset in first 24 hours. Preventive treatment is RhoGAM prenatally or post-natal exchange transfusion. This type of hyperbilirubinemia may also result from ABO incompatibility but rarely requires treatment other than phototherapy.
- **Breastfeeding associated**: Relates to inadequate calories during early breastfeeding with onset on 2-3 days. This slows the excretion of stool and allows bilirubin levels to rise. More frequent feeding with caloric supplements is usually sufficient, but phototherapy may be used for bilirubin 18-20 mg/dL.
- **Breast milk jaundice**: May result from human breast milk breaking down bilirubin and its being reabsorbed in the gut. Characterized by less frequent stools and onset in 4-5 days, jaundice peaks in 10-15 days but may persist for a number of weeks. Treatment involves discontinuing breastfeeding for 24 hours.

KERNICTERUS

Kernicterus (also called bilirubin encephalopathy) occurs when elevated serum bilirubin levels cause damage to the brain. The exact serum bilirubin level at which damage occurs is unknown. Premature infants are more susceptible to the development of kernicterus at lower serum bilirubin levels because of the immaturity of their blood-brain barrier, causing it to be more permeable to bilirubin than in full term infants. Disease processes, such as acidosis or meningitis, further lessen the competency of the blood-brain barrier. **Early signs of kernicterus** are divided into three phases:

- **Phase I:** Occurs during the first few days of life and is characterized by decreased alertness, hypotonia, and poor feeding.
- **Phase II:** The onset and duration of this phase is variable. Hypertonia of the extensor muscles develops. Infants may display opisthotonos (extreme hyperextension or arching of the back) and/or retrocollis (extreme arching of the neck).
- **Phase III:** This occurs generally after one week with the recurrence of hypotonia.

Review Video: Jaundice Icterus
Visit mometrix.com/academy and enter code: 339680

Phototherapy and Exchange Transfusion

Hyperbilirubinemia is often treated with **phototherapy** to prevent the need for exchange transfusion. For phototherapy, the infant is placed under lights to decrease bilirubin levels in the blood. The lights usually consist of a single tungsten halogen lamp or 4-8 white or blue fluorescent lights and a Plexiglas shield. The infant is placed under these lights with a protective mask covering the eyes to prevent retinal toxicity. The lights should be 15-20 cm above the infant. The lights convert bilirubin into a water-soluble compound that can be excreted by the liver into bile and eventually into the infant's stool. The success of phototherapy is directly related to the quantity of body surface area that is exposed to the lights, so the infant is clad only in a diaper to expose the most skin to the light as possible. Indications:

Weight	Serum Bilirubin Level
500-750 g	5-8 mg/dL
750-1000 g	6-10 mg/dL
1000-1250 g	8-10 mg/dL
1250-1500 g	10-12 mg/dL

Exchange transfusions may be used for hyperbilirubinemia. Blood <72 hours old is used to maintain potassium levels. Indications include:

Weight	Serum Bilirubin Level
500-750 g	12-15 mg/dL
750-1000 g	>15 mg/dL
1000-1250 g	15-18 mg/dL
1250-1500 g	17-20 mg/dL

There are many risks associated with exchange transfusions, including vascular complications, such as emboli or thrombosis, often related to umbilical catheters. Cardiac complications include dysrhythmias and overload, leading to arrest. Clotting disorders may result from over-heparinization (reversed with protamine sulfate). Electrolyte and glucose abnormalities as well as infection may occur.

Blood Component Therapy

Blood component therapy is described below:

- **Whole blood** has red blood cells (RBCs), white blood cells (WBCs), and platelets in their normal ratios. Whole blood is not a common neonatal blood transfusion product unless there is massive hemorrhage from trauma. Usually, its components are given individually to treat a specific condition.
- **Packed RBCs** are prepared by removing most of the plasma from blood, leaving a hematocrit of 70-90%. Use packed cells to treat anemia.
- **Leukocyte-poor RBCs** have more than 70% of WBCs removed by centrifuging, washing, or filtration. Much of the RBC mass is also lost. Leukocyte-poor blood products have less chance of passing on CMV infection or triggering a febrile reaction.
- **Washed RBCs** are cleaned with 0.9% sodium chloride to remove more than 95% of the nonviable RBCs and 80-90% of the WBCs. Washing is one method of producing leukocyte-poor RBCs.
- **Fresh frozen plasma** is comprised of 90-92% water, clotting factors, immunoglobulins, albumin, electrolytes, and enzymes and is used to add volume.

Blood Product Administration

In the NICU, **blood transfusions** are common, especially packed red blood cells. Blood should always be warmed to prevent hypothermia. Small volumes may be warmed passively by exposing to room temperature or heated isolette for 30 minutes prior to administration. Transfusions are given through peripheral IVs rather than umbilical lines except in extreme emergency. A filtered line should always be used for blood administration. During the transfusion, vital signs should be monitored and recorded every 15 minutes and the neonate carefully watched for any signs of a transfusion reaction. **Irradiated blood cells** are recommended for neonates <1200 mg and for those who are immunocompromised or receiving transfusions of granulocytes or exchange transfusions. Whole blood is not a common neonatal blood transfusion product unless there is massive hemorrhage from trauma. **Platelets** used for neonates to prevent cerebral hemorrhage with thrombocytopenia are collected from one donor instead of from pooled donations, suspended in plasma, and leukocyte depleted. Usual dose is 10-15 mL/kg given over 60-90 minutes.

Chapter Quiz

Ready to see how well you retained what you just read? Scan the QR code to go directly to the chapter quiz interface for this study guide. If you're using a computer, simply visit the online resources page at **mometrix.com/resources719/ccrnneonatal** and click the Chapter Quizzes link.

Clinical Judgment: Gastrointestinal, Renal, and Integumentary

Gastrointestinal Complications

Development of GI Tract

The **gastrointestinal (GI) tract** is anatomically complete by about 24 weeks gestation but functional development continues through 36-38 weeks:

- Fetal swallowing of amniotic fluid begins at about 11 weeks gestation.
- Peristalsis begins at 28-30 weeks. In the preterm infant, it is bidirectional, so milk is not propelled toward the stomach. With normal peristalsis, meconium should pass within 24 hours of birth, but this is delayed in preterm infants.
- The cardiac sphincter and neural control of the stomach are immature at birth, resulting in frequent regurgitation.
- Coordination of sucking and swallowing begins at 33-36 weeks.
- Enzymatic activity and ability to transport nutrients matures by 36-38 weeks.
- Salivary glands are inactive until 3 months.
- Lactase deficiency causes poor carbohydrate digestion, pancreatic lipase deficiency causes poor fat digestion (10-20% excreted), but protein digestion is good.
- Bowel sounds are evident 30-60 minutes after birth. Stomach capacity is 50-60 mL, and emptying time is 2-4 hours.

Short Bowel Syndrome

The neonate's small bowel is approximately 250 cm long. Most absorption of nutrients and vitamins takes place in the first 100-150 cm of the jejunum while the ileum absorbs vitamin B_{12} and bile acids. Infants with less than 100 cm of jejunum after surgical removal have significant malabsorption and require aggressive nutritional support. Infants with **short bowel syndrome** (SBS) have diarrhea, steatorrhea, bloating, anemia, electrolyte imbalances, malnutrition, and poor weight gain secondary to decreased absorption of nutrients and vitamins. The severity and exact nature of their symptoms depend on the amount and type of bowel that has been removed. Removal of significant portions of the ileum results in steatorrhea and poor absorption of fat-soluble vitamins (K, A, D, E) and vitamin B_{12}. Removal of significant portions of the jejunum results in poor absorption of calories, proteins, carbohydrates, and fats. Infants require careful monitoring of serum electrolytes, multivitamins, and a combination of parenteral and enteral nutrition. Over time, the small bowel adapts, increases its absorption, and grows in length.

Sucking and Swallowing Disorders

Sucking and swallowing disorders are very common in the preterm infant because of immaturity (coordination of sucking and swallowing occurs at 33-36 weeks) but may be caused in term infants by a number of conditions, including trisomy 21, FAS, cleft palate, central nervous system disorders (anoxia, hydrocephalus), congenital infection (rubella, cytomegalovirus), respiratory disorders (apnea, pneumonia, RDS), and cardiac or ENT anomalies. Typical characteristics of swallowing disorders include:

- Silent aspiration (not associated with cough or clearing airway)
- Laryngeal penetration (associated with lack of pharyngeal response)
- Nasopharyngeal reflux (especially common in preterm infants and may trigger apnea)

Pneumonia frequently develops in infants with sucking and swallowing disorders, so diagnosing the cause is critical. Observation is not sufficient because of the frequency of silent aspiration. Feeding infants in the upright position can reduce nasopharyngeal reflux. Tests include radiographic (videofluoroscopy) or fiberoptic evaluation of swallowing.

Hirschsprung's Disease

Hirschsprung's disease (congenital aganglionic megacolon) is failure of **ganglion nerve cells** to migrate to part of the bowel, usually the distal colon, so that part of the bowel lacks enervation and peristalsis, causing stool to accumulate, leading to **distention** and **megacolon**. There is a genetic predisposition to the disease that affects more males than females and is associated with trisomy 21 (Down syndrome).

Symptoms include:

- Failure to pass meconium in 24-48 hours
- Poor feeding
- Bilious vomitus
- Abdominal distension

Delayed diagnosis includes:

- Chronic constipation
- Failure to thrive
- Periods of diarrhea and vomiting
- With infection—severe prostration, watery diarrhea, fever, and hypotension

Treatment includes:

- Resection aganglionic section and perform colorectal anastomosis
- There are a number of procedures—Swenson, Duhamel, and Soave—but recently, minimally invasive laparoscopic or transanal approaches have proven successful

Gastroesophageal Reflux

Gastroesophageal reflux (GER) is involuntary regurgitation of stomach contents into the esophagus, usually caused by decreased tone in the lower esophageal sphincter in neonates, especially preterm.

Symptoms include:

- Frequent non-bilious regurgitation (especially after feeding, usually not associated with respiratory distress)
- Some neonates may have colicky symptoms, and some may cough, choke, wheeze or have periods of apnea

Treatment includes:

- **Regulating feeding**: Small, more frequent amounts, thickened with rice cereal. Continuous gavage rather than bolus may reduce reflux.
- **Positioning**: Prone positioning after feeding/eating reduces regurgitation (although some concern remains about SIDS with neonates). Placing the neonate in an upright position (avoiding slumping) after meals or carrying the neonate upright can help, but placing in infant seat position may increase intraabdominal pressure.
- **Medications:** Medications are only recommended in severe cases. Histamine-2 receptor blockers (famotidine) or proton pump inhibitors (omeprazole) may be used short term.
- **Surgery:** Considered for severe or life-threatening symptoms.

Malrotation/Volvulus

During weeks 4-8 of embryonic development, the GI tract is rapidly expanding and the abdominal cavity cannot accommodate it. Therefore, part of the intestinal loop buckles into the yolk stalk area, which will be the future umbilicus. As the intestinal loop buckles out of the abdomen, it begins a normal rotation of the bowel. As it continues to grow and returns to the abdomen during weeks 8-10, there is additional rotation occurring until it is situated into the anatomically correct position. Sometimes this rotation fails, and the result is a malrotation. **Malrotation** is a congenital defect in which the intestines are attached to the back of the abdominal wall by one single attachment, rather than a broad band of attachments across the abdomen, essentially suspending the bowels so they can easily twist, resulting in a **volvulus** (twisted bowel), cutting off blood supply. It may untwist but can lead to **bowel infarction.** Some children with malrotation have no symptoms, but most develop some of these **symptoms** by 1 year:

- Cycles of cramping pain about every 15-30 minutes
- Abdominal distension
- Diarrhea, bloody stools, or no stools
- Vomiting, occurring soon after crying begins, usually indicating small intestine obstruction; later vomiting usually indicative of large intestine blockage
- Tachycardia and tachypnea
- Decreased urinary output
- Fever

Treatment is by surgical repair.

Midgut Volvulus

A midgut volvulus is twisting of the bowel from the second portion of the duodenum to the mid-transverse colon around its mesenteric attachments. Signs depend on the extent of compromised blood flow to the bowel, blockage of lymphatic drainage, and obstruction of intestinal contents. **Signs** include bilious vomiting, gastric distension, rapid clinical deterioration, and shock. Midgut volvulus is usually secondary to congenital malrotation of the intestines. If this is the case, then it often presents during the first week of life, with complete obstruction and severe symptoms. Mortality rates range from 3-15%. The infant's prognosis depends on the amount of ischemic bowel and the length of time that elapsed before the volvulus was diagnosed and treated.

Imperforate Anus

Imperforate anus (anorectal malfunction) is a congenital abnormality in which the **rectum is absent, malformed, or displaced** from normal position. It may include disorders of the urinary tract. Imperforate anus occurs in 1 in 5000 births, more commonly in males than females.

Imperforate anus may include stenosis or atresia of the anus. There are 3 main **categories**, classified according to the relationship of the rectum to the puborectalis musculature:

- **Low anomalies:** no external opening, but rectum otherwise in normal position through the puborectalis muscle, with normal function and no connection to the genitourinary tract.
- **Intermediate anomalies:** rectum at or below the level of puborectalis muscle, anal dimple evident, and external sphincter in normal position.
- **High anomalies:** rectum ending above the puborectalis muscles, internal sphincter absent often with a rectourethral fistula in males or a rectovaginal fistula in females, and sometimes fistulas to the bladder or perineum.

Diagnosis, Symptoms, and Treatment

Imperforate anus is **diagnosed** by physical examination, digital or endoscopic examination, and contrast radiography with the infant inverted. An opaque marker at the anal dimple will outline the location of a pouch in relation to the normal position of the anus.

Symptoms include:

- Absence of anal opening, no meconium in 24-48 hours, Abdominal distension, and vomiting
- Rectovaginal fistula or rectourethral fistula (may not be evident at first because stool passes through fistula)
- Fistula between the rectum and the bladder with gas or fecal material possibly expelled through the urethra
- Displacement of the anus, with chronic constipation developing over time

Treatment includes:

Surgery performed in most cases, type depending upon extent of abnormality:

- With low anomalies, simple excision of anal opening
- Two- or three-step procedure for higher anomalies; colostomy first, with later reconstruction of the anus in the proper position, involving anoplasty and pull-through procedures
- Manual dilation to treat stenosis

Intestinal Atresia

When a portion of the bowel comes to a stop and then starts back up again forming a discontinuous or segmented bowel, this is called **intestinal atresia.** This condition usually relates to failures during the 5th to 10th week of fetal development, so it is often associated with other anomalies. The most common site for atresia to occur in the neonate is the duodenum. Atresia can also occur in the ileum, jejunum, colon, and even rarely the stomach. An atresia that occurs anywhere in the intestine except the duodenum is not associated with any other disorders. However, an atresia that occurs in the duodenum (the most common type) is usually (30% of the time) associated with other disorders such as trisomy 21, congenital heart disease, and VACTERL association. (VACTERL stands for **v**ertebral defects, **a**nal atresia, **c**ardiac defects, **t**rachea-**e**sophageal fistula, **r**enal anomalies, and **l**imb abnormalities.) The only treatment for intestinal atresia is surgical reconnection of the bowel.

Duodenal Atresia

Duodenal atresia occurs when the duodenum fails to correctly form in the fetus. Often, duodenal atresia is discovered prenatally via ultrasound examination. Neonates with **duodenal atresia** vomit within hours after birth. The vomitus may or may not be bilious, depending on the exact location of the defect. The infant may have a scaphoid abdomen and usually passes meconium. X-rays often show the "double-bubble" sign: The distended stomach is the first bubble and the distended duodenum proximal to the defect is the second bubble. One-third of all patients with duodenal atresia also have Down syndrome. An orogastric tube is immediately placed to relieve the Abdominal distension, and IV fluids and TPN nutrition are administered. When IV hydration is delayed, infants with duodenal atresia often develop hypokalemia, hypochloremia, and metabolic alkalosis. Definitive treatment is surgical repair.

Esophageal Atresia and Tracheoesophageal Fistula

Esophageal atresia often occurs with tracheoesophageal fistula (TEF). In esophageal atresia, the esophagus has a blind pouch and does not completely pass to the stomach. In TEF, an abnormal connection is present between the trachea and the esophagus. A congenital tracheoesophageal fistula (TEF) is present in 1 out of every 2,000-4,000 live births. There are 5 different **types of TEF**:

- **Esophageal atresia with distal TEF** (87%) is the most common type. The proximal esophagus ends in a blind pouch and the distal esophagus is connected to the trachea.
- **Isolated esophageal atresia without TEF** (8%), where the proximal esophagus ends in a pouch and there is no connection with the trachea.
- **Isolated TEF** (4%), where the esophagus is patent, traveling to the stomach with a fistula from the esophagus to the trachea. It is also called "H" type because of its resemblance to the letter H.
- **Esophageal atresia with proximal TEF** (1%), where the proximal esophagus connects with the trachea and there is no connection to the distal esophagus.
- **Esophageal atresia with proximal and distal TEF** (1%), where both the proximal and the distal esophagus connect with the trachea.

Infants born with tracheoesophageal fistula (TEF) are often diagnosed prenatally with ultrasound. TEF is often associated with polyhydramnios, as esophageal atresia prevents the fetus from swallowing amniotic fluid. Infants born with TEF have **symptoms** that include:

- Fine, white, frothy bubbles of mucous in the mouth and nose
- Copious secretions, despite suctioning
- Episodes of coughing, choking, and cyanosis that worsen with feeds
- Associated genetic anomalies, such as trisomy 13, 18, or 21
- Other digestive tract problems, heart problems, or kidney and urinary tract problems

Bowel Obstructions

Bowel obstruction occurs when there is a mechanical obstruction of the **passage of intestinal contents** because of constriction of the lumen, occlusion of the lumen, or lack of muscular contractions (paralytic ileus). Obstruction may be caused by congenital or acquired abnormalities/disorders:

Small Bowel Obstructions:

- Duodenal atresia
- Malrotation and volvulus
- Jejunoileal atresia
- Meconium ileus
- Meconium peritonitis

Large Bowel Obstructions:

- Hirschsprung disease
- Anorectal malformations
- Meconium plug syndrome

Symptoms include:

- Abdominal pain, distention, and rigidity
- Vomiting and dehydration
- Diminished or no bowel sounds
- Severe constipation (obstipation)
- Respiratory distress from diaphragm pushing against pleural cavity
- Shock, as plasma volume diminishes and electrolytes enter intestines from bloodstream
- Sepsis, as bacteria proliferate in the bowel and invade the bloodstream

Hypertrophic Pyloric Stenosis

Hypertrophic pyloric stenosis (PS) is obstruction of the pyloric sphincter between the gastric pylorus and small intestine, caused by hypertrophy and hyperplasia of the circular muscle of the pylorus so the enlarged tissue obstructs the sphincter. PS is more common in boys than girls and has a genetic predisposition. Onset of **symptoms** is usually >3weeks:

- Projectile vomiting (1-4 feet) usually shortly after eating but may be delayed for a few hours. Emesis may be blood-tinged but non-bilious
- Infant is hungry and eats readily, but shows weight loss and signs of dehydration
- Upper abdominal distension with palpable mass in epigastrium (to right of umbilicus)
- Visible left to right peristaltic waves

Diagnosis is based on ultrasound. Decreased sodium and potassium levels may not be evident with dehydration.

Treatment includes:

- Intravenous fluids to restore hydration and electrolyte balance
- Surgical pyloromyotomy: longitudinal incisions through the circular muscle fibers down to the submucosa to release the restriction and allow the muscle to expand

Meconium Plug Syndrome

Meconium plug syndrome (also called functional colonic obstruction) occurs when the first stool obstructs the intestinal tract and no other pathology is present. This will be evident in the first 24 to 48 hours of life, when the infant fails to pass the first meconium stool. Meconium plug syndrome usually occurs in full-term infants, infants of diabetic mothers, or infants with hypermagnesemia. The infant may have abdominal distension, poor feeding, and vomiting (often bilious in nature). An x-ray of the abdomen will show dilated loops of bowel. A contrast enema is diagnostic and helps differentiate from other causes of intestinal obstruction. It may also be therapeutic, causing the plug to pass. Infants usually do well after the plug has passed. A small percentage of infants initially identified as having meconium plug syndrome (5 to 10%) have Hirschsprung disease. The cause of meconium plug syndrome is thought to be immaturity of the ganglion cells of the colon.

Meconium Ileus Caused by Cystic Fibrosis

Cystic fibrosis is a congenital disease associated with the collection of thick mucus in the **lungs and intestines**. **Meconium ileus** is obstruction of the ileum with inspissated (thick) mucilaginous meconium that clings to the side of the narrowed lumen of the intestine and forms hard pellets (usually the first clinical sign of cystic fibrosis). The mucus interferes with the absorption of fat, protein, carbohydrates, and other nutrients, leading to malabsorption syndromes. **Diagnosis** is by abdominal x-rays to show air-to-fluid levels and contrast enemas to show obstruction.

Symptoms include:

- **Uncomplicated: abdominal distension, vomiting, no meconium in the first 24-48 hours**
- **Complicated** (may include volvulus, gangrene, perforations, or bowel atresia): pain, fever, erythema, and edema of abdominal wall consistent with peritonitis

Treatment includes:

- Contrast enema with water-soluble contrast (may relieve obstruction by emulsifying fecal material)
- 10-15 mL small volume enemas to flush stool, especially after contrast enema
- Enterotomy, with proximal instillation of wetting agent
- Resection of colon/fecal diversion for perforated or gangrenous bowel
- High protein diet with pancreatic enzyme supplementation

Necrotizing Enterocolitis

Necrotizing enterocolitis (NEC) is the most common gastrointestinal emergency in premature neonates. Seventy-five percent of neonates who develop NEC are less than 37 weeks gestation and weigh less than 2,000 grams. NEC is rare in healthy, full term infants. NEC is an acute necrosis (death of cells) in a bowel segment anywhere from the stomach to the rectum. Inflammation, bacterial invasion, and perforation often occur. NEC is fatal in up to 30% of cases. Risk factors other than prematurity and size should trigger careful observation. These risk factors include:

- **Prenatal**
  - Maternal age >35 years
  - Maternal cocaine use
  - Maternal infection requiring antibiotics
- **Perinatal**
  - Birth asphyxia
  - Respiratory distress syndrome
  - Systemic hypotension
  - Depressed 5-minute Apgar score
- **Postnatal**
  - Congestive heart failure
  - Use of hyperosmolar formula
  - Patent ductus arteriosus
  - Umbilical artery catheterization

The causes of necrotizing enterocolitis (NEC) are not completely understood, but it appears to be related to an ischemic episode, colonization by bacteria, and excess/rapid enteral feedings.

Symptoms include:

- Gastric retention, abdominal distension, and vomiting (bilious)
- Periods of apnea
- Occult or frank blood (25%) in stool
- Pneumatosis intestinalis (gas in intestinal wall) (75%)
- Portal venous gas (10-30%)
- Decrease in urinary output
- Jaundice
- Unstable temperature

Treatment includes:

- Cessation of oral feeding
- NG decompression
- Systemic antibiotics
- Correcting fluid and electrolyte imbalance
- Surgical repair with bowel resection may be necessary

Diastasis of Recti Muscles

Diastasis of the recti muscles is a postnatal maternal condition in which the abdominal muscles, specifically the rectus abdominis muscles (that have separated during pregnancy) remain separated. The pressure of the expanding fetus causes the connective tissue to stretch between the vertically running muscles and often after birth, the tissue slowly heals and the separation closes. When the connective tissue does not heal fully within 6 months, the gap can become permanent. This condition can lead to lower back pain, pain during intercourse, incontinence, or constipation in the mother. Diastasis of the recti muscles can be treated with specific physical therapy. Traditional abdominal crunches are avoided as a treatment because they may worsen the condition by making the muscles tighter in the separated position. Abdominal exercises during pregnancy are recommended as preventative measures. Surgical closure is a treatment option for extreme cases.

Neonatal Umbilical Hernia

Umbilical hernia is a skin-covered herniation of intestine and omentum through an abdominal wall defect near the umbilicus caused by an incomplete closure of the umbilical ring. The herniation may range from 1-5 cm in size and may be obvious on physical examination or felt on palpation. It may appear flat when the infant is supine but protrude when the infant is upright or crying. Approximately 1 in 6 infants are born with umbilical hernias. Symptoms are usually absent unless strangulation of the hernia occurs, and then the infant may cry with pain, feed poorly, vomit, and have an increase in temperature. The abdomen may become distended. In this case, emergency surgical repair must be done. Treatment usually involves just observing the hernia for complications as, in most cases, it will reduce on its own. If the hernia is still present at 3-4 years, a simple surgical repair of the hernia may be done.

Gastroschisis

Gastroschisis is extrusion of the non-rotated midgut through the abdominal wall to the right of umbilicus with no protective membrane covering matted, thickened loops of intestine. The abnormality is usually small, but the stomach and almost all of the small and large intestines can protrude. Because the intestines float without protection in amniotic fluid, there may be severe damage to the intestines with bowel atresia and ischemia. Gastroschisis is usually diagnosed with fetal ultrasound and is obvious at birth. These infants lose body temperature, fluids, and electrolytes and receive intravenous fluids. The exposed organs are covered with sterile plastic film for protection and to prevent fluid loss and a nasogastric feeding tube is inserted. Primary closure is done when the infant stabilizes for small abnormalities. Larger abnormalities may require stages with only part of organs returned to the cavity and the remaining covered with a Silastic pouch until the abdominal cavity grows and surgical repair can be completed.

Omphalocele

Omphalocele is a congenital herniation of intestines or other organs through the base of the umbilicus with a protecting amniotic membrane but no skin. The sac may contain only a loop or most of the bowel and the internal abdominal organs. This sac differentiates gastroschisis from omphalocele. Diagnosis is usually with fetal ultrasound.

Symptoms vary widely. Maintaining integrity of tissues by keeping exposed sac or viscera moist and providing intravenous fluids is important. Small omphaloceles are repaired immediately, but more extensive repair is usually delayed until the infant is stable if sac is intact. Silvadene cream toughens the sac, which is usually covered with a Silastic (plastic) pouch to protect the tissue. The abdomen may be unusually small, making correction difficult, so surgeons may wait 6-12 months while the abdominal cavity grows. Surgical repair may be done in stages over 8-10 days.

Lactation and Neonatal Nutrition

Digestion and Absorption

Digestion is the process by which food is converted into chemicals that are used by the body. These processes are immature at birth and most don't function until 3-6 months. Digestion begins in the mouth as milk is mixed with saliva, but salivary amylase, which begins the digestion of starch, has little effect on milk because milk passes into the esophagus and stomach quickly. Protein digestion begins in the stomach where hydrochloric acid acts on curds formed by the enzyme renin. The curds slow the progress of the milk to allow digestion. Pancreatic and liver enzymes further digest protein and fat in the small intestine. Infants cannot adequately absorb fat until 4-5 months or complex carbohydrates until 4-6 months. Simple carbohydrates break down into glucose and monosaccharides and fat into fatty acids and glycerol. Trypsin levels are sufficient to convert proteins into polypeptides and amino acids. **Absorption**, the transfer of digestive end products (electrolytes, vitamins, fluids, nutrients) into the circulation, takes place primarily in the small intestine and is facilitated by villi.

Nutritional Needs

Caloric Requirements of Neonates

The caloric needs of a neonate (pre-term or term) depend on postnatal age, activity, current weight, growth rate, thermal environment, and route of nutritional intake. Cold stress increases caloric requirements. Infants who receive parenteral nutrition need fewer calories, as they do not have any fecal loss, and the nutrients are not absorbed by the gastrointestinal tract. These are the general requirements for adequate growth:

- **Full-term infant**: 100-120 cal/kg/day
- **Premature infants**: 110-160 cal/kg/day
- Infants who are recovering from **surgery** or have a **chronic illness**, such as bronchopulmonary dysplasia (BPD): ≤180 cal/kg/day

Most human breast milk and unfortified formulas supply 20 calories per ounce. To ingest 120 cal/kg/day, an infant needs to ingest 6 ounces/kg/day of unfortified formula or human breast milk.

Special formulas designed for premature infants and fortifiers that can be added to human breast milk provide higher calorie contents per ounce (22-24 calories per ounce).

Protein Requirements

Neonates require adequate **protein** to sustain growth, with intake requirements depending on gestational age. A positive nitrogen balance exists when the intake of protein meets or exceeds the infant's requirements. A negative protein balance occurs when protein is provided in inadequate amounts, leading to catabolism (muscle breakdown). Generally, the USDA recommends newborns through 6 months of age receive 9.1 g/day of protein. Premature neonates have higher protein requirements relative to body weight than do full term infants:

- **Full term**: 2.0-2.5 g/kg/day
- **Preterm**: 3.5-4.0 g/kg/day

Preterm infants should be started on parenteral nutrition supplemented with protein as soon as possible to avoid negative protein balances. Special formulas designed for premature infants are available with elevated protein contents. Human breast milk fortifiers are also available to enhance the protein levels and caloric content of human breast milk for premature infants although the content of human breast milk adjusts automatically for the needs of preterm infants.

Carbohydrate and Fat Requirements

Nutritional requirements of carbohydrates and fats vary according to whether a neonate is full-term or preterm and the type of feeding (human breast milk, enteral, parenteral).

Lactose is the primary **carbohydrate** in human breast milk. A full-term neonate requires 60 g of carbohydrate daily for the first 6 months of life according to the USDA, and a preterm neonate requires 12-14 g/kg/day. Preterm infants may require supplemental glucose via infusion, starting at 6 mg/kg/min, and increased daily by 1 mg/kg/min, up to 12-13 mg/kg/min until blood glucose levels are stabilized and can be maintained by the neonate. Lactose is metabolized into galactose and glucose, the main energy source for the brain. Human breast milk is approximately 40% carbohydrates. Inadequate intake may result in hypoglycemia, while excess intake may result in weight gain and hyperglycemia.

Fats provide the primary energy source for neonates and should comprise at least 30% of calories but no more than 54%. Fat intake needs are 31 g/day for full-term neonates, according to the USDA, and 5-7 g/kg/day for preterm neonates. Because preterm neonates are more susceptible to essential fatty acid deficiency, they should be closely monitored, and administered IV 20% emulsion lipids (0.5-1.0 g/kg/day) if necessary, until stabilized. Fats provide energy for the body and contribute to the development of the CNS and tissue growth. Excess fat may contribute to weight gain, impaired cholesterol metabolism, and later cardiac morbidity. Deficiency may result in impaired development and dermatitis (from lack of adequate fatty acids).

VITAMINS

Nutritional requirements of vitamins are generally met with human breast milk or formula in the healthy neonate. Daily vitamin requirements vary according to the neonate's condition and whether preterm or term. **E**=Enteral, **P**=Parenteral.

Vitamin	Preterm/Term	Notes
A	**E**:700-1500/1250 IU **P**: 700-1500/2300 IU	**Deficiency**: Vision impairment/blindness, impaired growth, depressed immune system **Excess**: Poor feeding, weight loss, fever, diarrhea
C	**E**: 20-60/30-50 mg **P**: 35-50/80 mg	**Deficiency**: Impaired brain development, weakness, bleeding **Excess**: Diarrhea, skin irritation, GI upset
D	**E**: 400/300 IU **P**: 120-260/400 IU	**Deficiency**: Impaired skeletal growth, calcium malabsorption **Excess**: Hypercalcemia, dehydration, cardiac and renal impairment, bone loss, hearing impairment
E	**E**: 6-12/5-10 IU **P**: 2-4/7 IU	**Deficiency**: Peripheral neuropathy, retinopathy, IVH, spinocerebellar impairment, hemolytic anemia **Excess**: GI upset, bleeding
K	**E**: 0.05/0.2 mg **P**: 0.06-0.1/0.05 mg	**Deficiency**: Bleeding **Excess**: Hemolysis, hyperbilirubinemia
Vitamin B1 (Thiamine)	**E**: 0.2-0.7/0.3 mg **P**: 0.8-0.8/1.2 mg	**Deficiency**: Cardiovascular and neurological damage **Excess**: rash, tachycardia, irritability
Vitamin B2 (Riboflavin)	**E**: 0.3-0.8/0.4 mg **P**: 0.4-0.9/1.4 mg	**Deficiency**: Thyroid hormone insufficiency, stomatitis, hepatic and neurological impairment, anemia **Excess**: Vomiting, hypotension
Vitamin B3 (Niacin)	**E**: 5-12/5 mg **P**: 5-12/7 mg	**Deficiency**: GI upset, diarrhea, cognitive impairment **Excess**: Flushing, hives, hepatic impairment
Vitamin B6 (Pyridoxine)	**E**: 0.3-0.7/0.3 mg **P**: 0.3-0.7/1.0 mg	**Deficiency**: Impaired development of neurological system, seizures **Excess**: Peripheral nerve damage, respiratory distress, hypotonia, lethargy, GI upset
Vitamin B12 (Cobalamin)	**E**: 0.3-0.7/0.3 mg **P**:0.3-0.7/1.0 mg	**Deficiency**: Vomiting, diarrhea, hypotonia, lethargy, anemia, megaloblastic anemia **Excess**: Skin irritation, diarrhea, tachycardia, poor sleeping

MINERALS

Daily mineral requirements vary according to the neonate's condition and whether preterm or term. **E**=Enteral, **P**=Parenteral.

Minerals	Preterm/Term	Notes
Biotin	**E:** 6-20/10 mcg **P:** 6-13/20 mcg	Deficiency: Hypotonia, seizures, skin disorders, hearing loss, conjunctivitis, lethargy Excess: Hyperglycemia
Calcium	**E:** 210-250/130 mg/kg **P:**60-90/60-80 mg/kg	Deficiency: Jitteriness, irritability, stridor, tetany, high-pitched cry, seizures, and cardiac dysfunction Excess: Vomiting; constipation, hypertension, hypotonia, lethargy, seizures

Minerals	Preterm/Term	Notes
Chloride	**E:** 2-3/2-3 mEq/kg **P:**2-3/2-3 mEq/kg	Deficiency: Weakness, lethargy, irritability, impaired absorption of iron and vitamin B_{12} Excess: Metabolic acidosis
Chromium	**E:** 2-4/2 mcg/kg **P:** 0.2/0.2 mcg/kg	Deficiency: peripheral neuropathy, impaired glucose tolerance, muscle weakness, loss of weight Excess: Skin irritation
Copper	**E:** 100-150/75 mcg/kg **P:** 20/20 mcg/kg	Deficiency: Hypochromic anemia, bone demineralization, neutropenia Excess: Gastroenteritis, hepatic injury
Folate (Folic acid)	**E:** 50/25-50 mcg **P:** 40-90/140 mcg	Deficiency: Lethargy, pallor, tachycardia, low weight, general weakness Excess: GI upset, poor sleeping
Iodine	**E:** 4/7 mcg/kg **P:** 1.0/1.0 mcg/kg	Deficiency: Intellectual disabilities, hypothyroidism, thyroid enlargement Excess: Abdominal pain, fever, hypothyroidism, skin irritation
Iron	**E:** 1-2/1-2 mg/kg **P:** 0.09-0.2/0.1-0.2 mcg/kg	Deficiency: Anemia, lethargy, impaired development Excess: GI upset, tachycardia, hyperpnea, hypotension, seizures, coma, liver failure
Magnesium	**E:** 8-15/7 mg/kg **P:** 4-7/5-7 mg/kg	Deficiency: Tetany, seizure, coma, tachycardia, ventricular arrhythmias, respiratory depression Excess: Hypotonia, hyporeflexia, constipation, hypotension, apnea, vasodilatation/flushing
Manganese	**E:** 10-20/85 mcg/kg **P:** 1.0-1.0 mcg/kg	Deficiency: Weakness, hearing impairment Excess: Impaired iron absorption
Molybdenum	**E:** 2-3/2 mcg/kg **P:** 0.25/0.25 mcg/kg	Deficiency: Inability to metabolize sulfites, seizures Excess: growth restriction, diarrhea
Phosphorus	**E:** 112-125/45 mEq/kg **P:**40-70/40-45 mEq/kg	Deficiency: Impaired bone metabolism, muscle weakness, tremors, seizures, impaired immune response Excess: GI upset, tachycardia, hyperreflexia, tetany
Potassium	**E:** 2-3/2-3 mEq/kg **P:** 2-3/2-3 mEq/kg	Deficiency: Cardiac arrhythmias, ileus, and lethargy Excess: Cardiac arrhythmias (bradycardia, tachycardia, VF)
Selenium	**E:** 1.3-3/1.6 mcg/kg **P:** 1.5-2/2.0 mcg/kg	Deficiency: Impaired immune response Excess: Diarrhea, lethargy, respiratory depression
Sodium	**E:** 2-4/2-3 mEq/kg **P:** 2-3.5/2-3 mEq/kg	Deficiency: Apnea, irritability, twitching, weight gain, and seizures Excess: weight loss, irritability, lethargy, fever, seizures (late)
Zinc	**E:** 800-1000/830 mcg **P:** 400/250 mcg	Deficiency: Impaired growth, impaired immune response, dermatitis Excess: Vomiting and diarrhea, neurological damage

Human Breast Milk

Human breast milk is the food of choice for newborn infants. **Colostrum**, produced during the first few days after birth, is scant, thick, yellowish, and high in protein and antibody content. Colostrum stimulates the passage of meconium. **Transitional milk** (days 3-14) is thinner and white, with a composition closer to that of mature milk. By the second week, most mothers produce 23-27 ounces of bluish-white **mature human breast milk**. Most neonates nurse every 1-3 hours for 20-40 minutes. Benefits of human breast milk are as follows:

- Human breast milk provides appropriate amounts of carbohydrate, protein, fat, vitamins, minerals, enzymes, and trace elements.
- It contains maternal antibodies that help bolster the infant's immature immune system.
- Breastfed babies have reduced risks of eczema, asthma, obesity, and elevated cholesterol later in life.
- Breastfeeding enhances the bond between the mother and the infant by physical contact and promotes recognition of communication signals.
- The maternal cost is an extra 500 calories a day and extra water.
- It eliminates the possibility of kidney damage caused by incorrectly mixed formula.

Composition

Human breast milk has immunologic benefits that formulas lack, resulting in decreased morbidity in breastfed infants. Human breast milk contains these important substances:

- **Antibodies**: Secretory IgA to provide protection from respiratory, enteric, and viral pathogens
- **Primary nutrients:** Protein with whey-to-casein ratio of 60:40 (including IgM, IgG, lactoferrin, lysozyme, casein [40%], and fibronectin), carbohydrate (about 40% of total calories), and fat (free fatty acids)

The following are **secondary nutrients:**

- Nucleotides
- Vitamins A, C, D, E; vitamin D content ≤25 IU/L; supplement if ≤2 months of age
- Enzymes: anti-inflammatory and antibacterial properties, including lipase, which breaks down fat
- Growth factors
- Hormones: prolactin, cortisol, thyroxine, insulin, and erythropoietin
- Cells: beta-lymphocytes, macrophages (90%), neutrophil, T-lymphocytes, cytokines, interleukin 1b, 6, 8, 10, 12 (both inflammatory and anti-inflammatory properties)

Feeding

Feeding Cues

The infant gives a number of feeding cues to show hunger. Mothers should be taught to recognize these cues, as it's more difficult for a frantically hungry baby to latch on. These are some indications that the infant is hungry:

- Licking the lips
- Sucking motions of the mouth
- Rooting or bobbing of the head
- Keeping hands in fists
- Bringing hands near mouth or face
- Turning the head toward and trying to suck on a finger stroking the baby's cheek or lower lip
- Crying (usually the last indication)

Infants who are consistently not receiving adequate nutrition usually appear sleepy and listless. They often stop gaining weight or lose weight. Skin turgor may be poor. Urinary output and stools decrease. The infant may appear disinterested in nursing. On the other hand, an infant who is satisfied usually stops sucking and may turn the head away from the breast or resist nursing. The infant will appear relaxed and may doze. Some infants take short breaks while nursing and then resume.

Early Feeding Cues

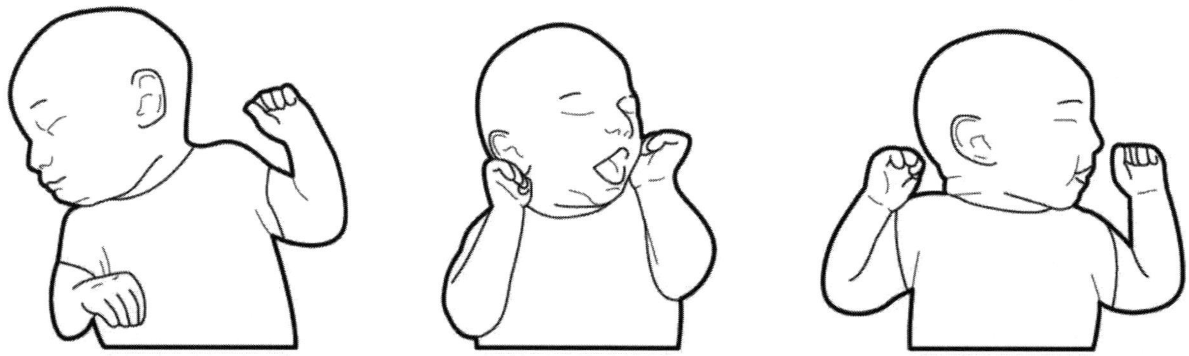

Mid-Active Feeding Cues

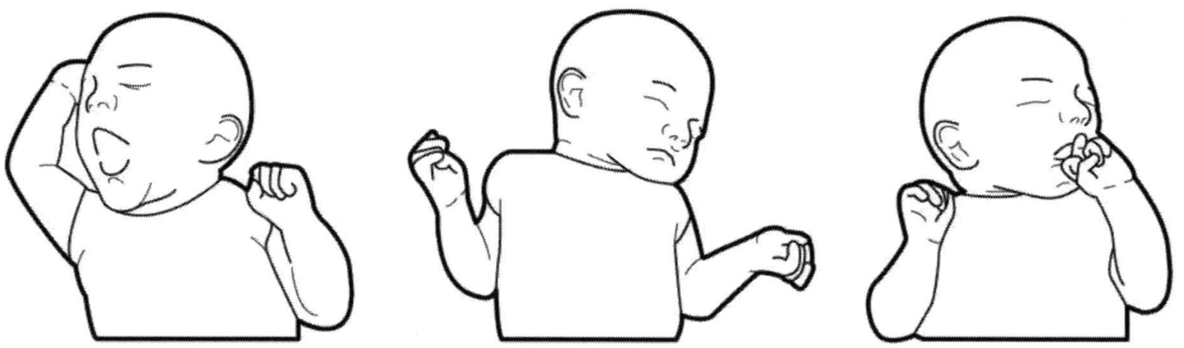

Late Feeding Cues

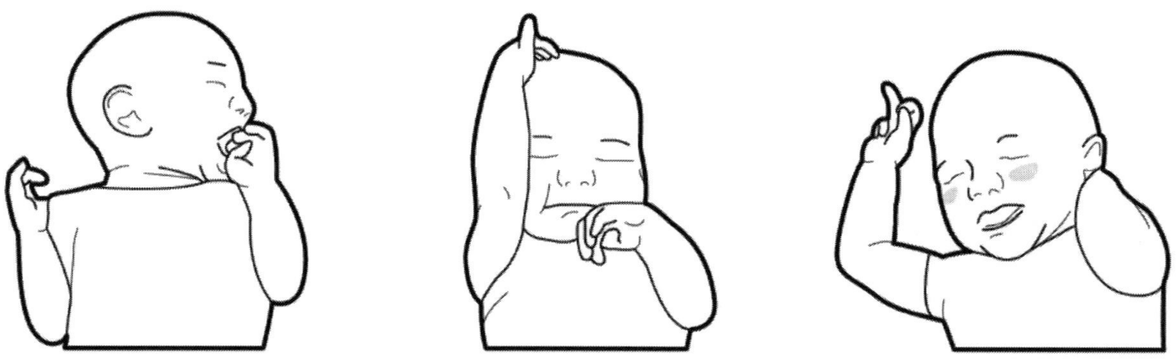

BREASTFEEDING FREQUENCY AND DURATION

Most infants initially nurse every 1-3 hours, but during **growth spurts** (2-3 weeks, 6 weeks, 3 months, and 6 months), the infant may nurse every half to one hour for 2-3 days, stimulating the breasts to increase production. Nursing usually takes 20-45 minutes, with 15-20 minutes on each side. Nursing should begin on the last breast used. Infants may nurse more frequently in the late afternoon and evening. Infants should be fed every 3 hours until they regain their birth weight, even if the infant must be awakened. Infants vary in **demand schedules**. Some eat 5-10 times over a 3-hour period and then sleep for about 4 hours. The schedule is less important than assuring that the child nurses **8-12 times** every 24 hours and appears satisfied. By 8-12 weeks, infants begin sleeping longer at night. Some may sleep through the night at 4 months, while others continue to nurse at night.

LATCHING ON AND LET-DOWN

Once the infant is in position, the mother should grasp the breast using a C-hold or U-hold (to make the breast firmer) and lean toward the baby, guiding the nipple toward the infant's mouth. Brushing the nipple against the infant's mouth usually causes the infant to open the mouth and lunge toward the breast. Then, the mother guides the nipple into the infant's mouth while pulling the infant toward the breast. The infant's lower lip should be low on the areola so the baby **latches** on to both the areola and the nipple.

Proper Latch

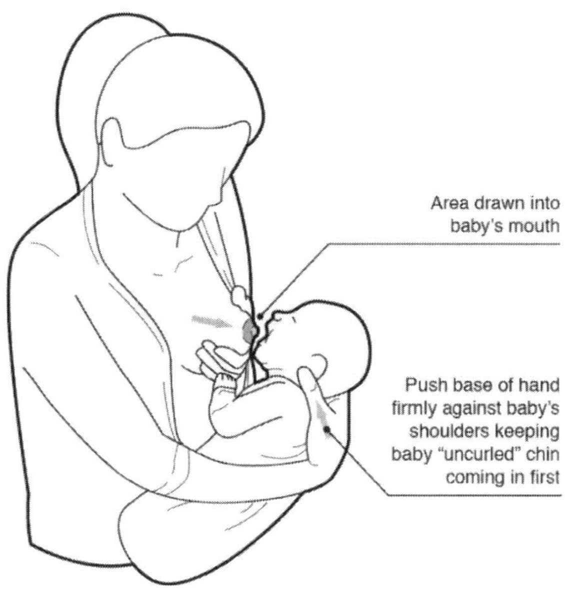

C-Hold

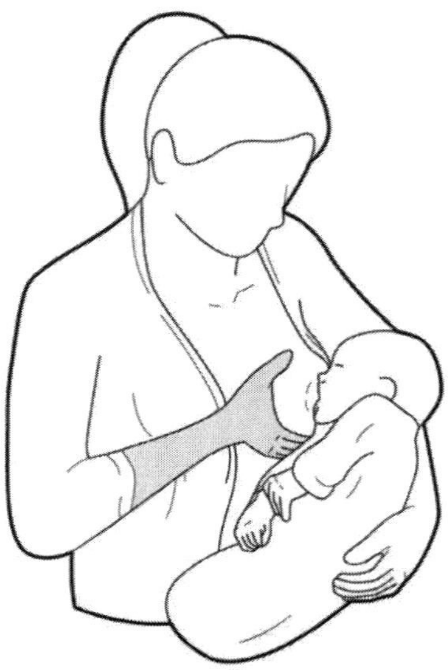

U-Hold

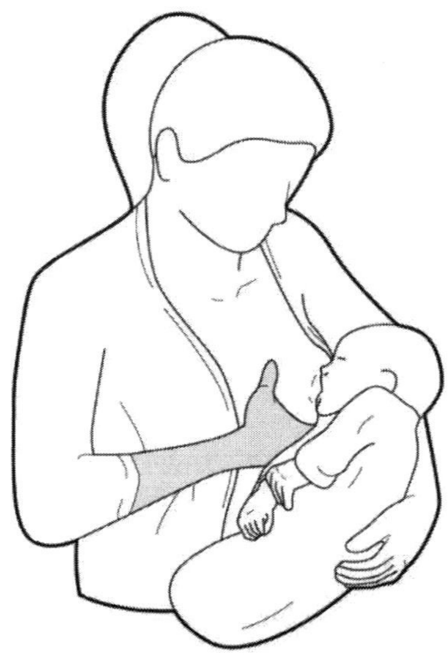

Suckling stimulates nerves in the areola and nipple, increasing production of prolactin and oxytocin, which in turn stimulate contraction of cells about the areola, causing milk to be ejected in a **"let-down"** (milk-ejection) reflex, which is sometimes associated with a tingling sensation, usually within a few minutes of nursing. It may take up to 2 weeks before letdown is efficient.

Problems Associated with Latch-On

Most problems associated with latch-on result from poor maternal technique and are easily resolved with demonstration and support:

- **Infant latches on to the end of the nipple,** resulting in pain and limited milk flow: The mother should learn to brush the nipple against the infant's lips until the baby opens the mouth completely before inserting the nipple.
- **Infant's mouth on just the nipple and not the areola**: The mother should use a C-hold or U-hold to guide the nipple into the infant's mouth, making sure that most of the areola (1.0-1.5 inches) is covered by the infant's mouth.
- **Inverted nipples**, making latching on difficult: If the nipple is so flat that the infant cannot easily latch on, using a silicone nipple shield for the first few minutes may help to elongate the nipple, at which point the shield should be removed because the shield doesn't allow adequate breast stimulation, and the infant must work harder to suckle.

Nipple Shields

Silicone nipple shields, which fit over the mother's nipple and areola, are sometimes used if a mother's nipples are inverted or flat, but they should not be used with cracked nipples if the mother can tolerate feeding. The breast does not receive adequate stimulation if the infant feeds with the shield in place, so milk production decreases and the baby may not be able to get adequate nutrition. Also, because the silicone nipple feels different from the breast, the infant may be reluctant to wean from the shield. If it is absolutely necessary to use a nipple shield for a flat or inverted nipple, it should be used only for the first few minutes, as even a flat nipple will usually elongate during that time. Then the rest of the feeding can be done without the shield.

Suck-Swallow Sequence

A neonate usually **sucks** and then **swallows** when the mouth becomes full. Each suck usually fills the mouth, a **suck to swallow ratio** of 1:1. Infants do not breathe while swallowing, so a 1:1 ratio means the child must breathe quickly, resulting in a rapid suck-hold breath and swallow-breathe sequence. During a swallow, the soft palate rises to block access to the nasal passages, the larynx rises, and the epiglottis covers the airway to prevent aspiration. If milk flow is inadequate, the child may need to suck twice for each swallow (2:1). If the flow is too fast, the child may need to swallow twice or more for each suck (1:2) and some milk may run down the pharynx and into the airway, resulting in aspiration. Or, the child may need to swallow so rapidly there is no time to breathe, and apnea may occur. A newborn usually sucks twice a second for about a minute and then about once per second as the milk flow increases.

Contraindications to Breastfeeding

Contraindications to breastfeeding include the following:

- **Infant with galactosemia**: The infant cannot properly metabolize the galactose in breast milk.
- **Maternal infections**: Active untreated HIV/AIDS, untreated tuberculosis, herpes simplex breast lesions, and untreated brucellosis may be transmitted to the neonate from the mother.
- **Maternal use of illicit substances**: Including cocaine, opioids, phencyclidine (PCP, aka angel dust), methamphetamines, and amphetamines. If their use is occasional, breastfeeding should be withheld for 24 hours after the most recent use. However, mothers on methadone, buprenorphine, and suboxone are usually encouraged to breastfeed.
- **Maternal use of alcohol**: Ideally, alcohol should be avoided because it is transmitted in the breast milk. If the mother limits her intake, alcohol should be avoided within 2 hours of breastfeeding.
- **Maternal medications**: Chemotherapeutic agents that affect DNA replication and cell division should be avoided. Avoid statins because they may interfere with the infant brain's needs for cholesterol to develop.
- **Maternal psychological factors**: If the mother suffers severe postpartum depression or postpartum psychosis, it may be safer for the neonate and the mother if the mother does not breastfeed.

Expressing and Storing Human Breast Milk

A mother can **express and store milk** for her infant if the infant is unable to nurse or if she must be separated from the infant. The most efficient method is to use a **bilateral electric breast pump**. The **pulsatile electric pump** provides adequate stimulation in the early postpartum period to establish and maintain the mother's milk supply, usually emptying the breasts within 15-20 minutes. If the child is not nursing, the pump should be used at least 8 times in each 24-hour period. Other methods of expressing milk include manual expression and use of a hand pump. Electric pumps usually have collection systems, so the milk flows into a bottle that can be used for feeding. Human breast milk can be stored for later use using the following guidelines:

- **Room temperature**: 4 hours
- **Refrigerated**: ≤4 days (best used within 48 hours)
- **Frozen**: 3-4 months in a separate-door freezer-refrigerator, and 6 months in a deep freezer at 0 °F

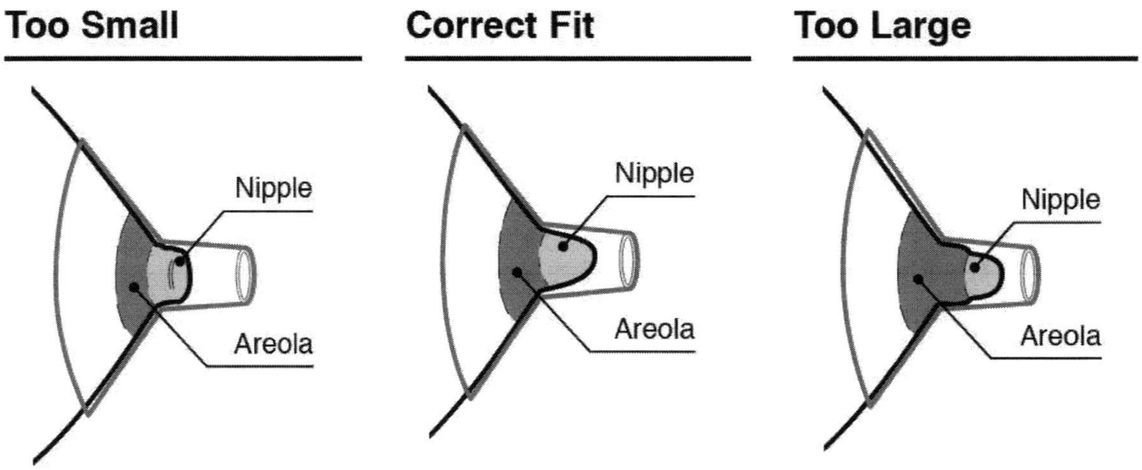

Supplemental Nursing System

Supplemental nursing systems allow the mother to provide supplemental nutrients or medication to the infant while breastfeeding. A typical system has a container for the liquid supplement and a tubing system with a tubing clamp to adjust flow. The tubing is taped to the breast and the end extends about 2-3 mm past the end of the nipple on the top, so the baby encloses both the nipple and the tubing in the mouth when nursing. The tubing should be under the baby's upper lip. Once the baby begins to nurse, the clamp is released so the supplement begins to flow. The bottom of the container is usually positioned level with the breast or slightly lower, so the child must suckle in order to gain the supplement. If the container is higher than the breast, the solution may flow too freely and may choke the child.

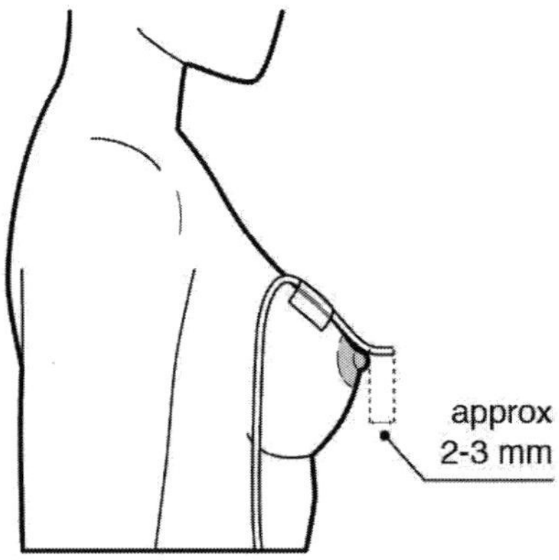

Donor Milk

While the mother's milk is most highly recommended for her newborn's nutrition, some mothers are not able to express sufficient milk for newborn growth and development. Low birth weight infants may also need more human breast milk than available. In these instances, the first recommendation for supplemental nutrition is donor milk, followed by formula. **Donor milk** has an association with lower rates of gut disorders (such as necrotizing enterocolitis) and other infections. Donor milk is generally collected by hospitals and nonprofit milk banks that receive human breast milk donations from mothers that overproduce milk. These mothers have been approved by their physician, by the infant's physician, and through a screening process to ensure the milk is safe to donate.

Infant Formulas

A wide variety of infant formulas are available, but there are 3 primary types:

- **Cow-milk-based formulas** (Enfamil, Similac, Good Start): These are appropriate for most infants. These are enriched with various components, including vitamins, minerals, iron, tyrosine, phenylalanine, and carnitine.
- **Soy-based formulas** (Isomil, ProSobee): These are appropriate for infants with primary lactose deficiency or galactosemia and those allergic to cow-milk-based formulas.
- **Therapeutic formulas** (Nutramigen, Pregestimil): Many preparations are available to meet special needs.

Formula may be purchased in ready-to-feed bottles or cans that require no preparation, liquid concentrate, or powder. Concentrate and powder require the addition of water, so a clean water supply and the ability to measure correctly are necessary to avoid inadequate or unsafe nutrition. Babies who are bottle-fed with formula usually feed less frequently than those who are breastfed. Neonates usually take 2-3 ounces of formula every 3-4 hours. Neonates require approximately 2.5 ounces of formula for each pound (0.5 kg) of weight within each 24-hour period.

Nutritional Value of Full Term Formula and Preterm Formulas

The nutritional value of full term formula and preterm formulas is discussed below:

- **Carbohydrates**: One gram of carbohydrates provides 3.4 calories. Carbohydrates provide approximately 1/3 of the caloric content in infant formulas. Lactose is the predominant carbohydrate. Premature infants may be deficient in the enzyme lactase (enzyme that breaks down lactose), so premature infant formulas utilize lesser amounts of lactose, combined with glucose polymers.
- **Lipids**: One gram of fat provides 9 calories. Lipids supply approximately 2/3 of the caloric content in infant formulas. Common sources of lipids include palm, soybean, coconut, and safflower oils. Premature infant formulas have a higher percentage of fat supplied as medium-chain triglycerides (MCT). MCTs can be absorbed without pancreatic lipase or bile salts that are deficient in premature infants.
- **Proteins**: One gram of protein provides 4 calories. Proteins provide less than 5% of the caloric content in infant formulas. Proteins provide amino acids that are used as building blocks for muscle and other tissues. Preterm formulas have higher protein content than term formula to help meet the increased growth requirements of preterm infants.

Special Preterm Formulas

Preterm formulas are designed with the special requirements of the premature infant in mind. These infants often have an increased caloric requirement to meet growth expectations. **Preterm formulas** differ from full-term formulas because they provide:

- 24 cal/oz as opposed to the 20 cal/oz found in human breast milk and in formulas for full-term infants.
- Increased levels of protein, vitamins, and minerals, particularly increased amounts of vitamin D, calcium, and phosphorus to prevent osteopenia of prematurity.
- Less lactose than term formulas, so they are less likely to cause diarrhea.

Human breast milk can be **fortified** with the addition of human breast milk fortifiers to achieve the same results. Infants are typically switched to a transitional or cow milk-based formula prior to discharge.

Fat-Soluble Vitamins in Formulas

Vitamins found in formulas are organic nutrients required in small amounts to maintain growth and normal metabolism. **Fat-soluble vitamins** include:

- **Vitamin A:** Important for growth and development of tissues as well as proper functioning of the immune system. Vitamin A supplementation in extremely low birth weight infants has been shown to reduce the incidence of bronchopulmonary dysplasia.
- **Vitamin D:** Required for adequate calcium and phosphorus absorption. Vitamin D deficiency leads to rickets (soft bones, bowed legs).
- **Vitamin E:** An antioxidant that is limited in preterm infants, making them susceptible to developing hemolytic anemia without proper supplementation.
- **Vitamin K:** Important in the clotting process. Infants receive an injection of Vitamin K shortly after birth to prevent hemorrhagic disease of the newborn.

Excessive fat-soluble vitamins A and D are toxic because they accumulate in adipose tissue and the liver. Water-soluble vitamins include thiamine (B_1), riboflavin (B_2), niacin (B_3), pantothenate (B_5), pyridoxine (B_6), cobalamin (B_{12}), C, biotin, and folic acid. Excessive water-soluble vitamins are excreted in the urine.

Enteral Feeding

Enteral (tube) feeding provides nutrition to infants with a functioning gastrointestinal tract but the inability to take an adequate amount of milk/formula orally. Ideally, human milk is provided for enteral feedings because it provides antimicrobial factors (IgA, leukocytes, complement, lactoferrin, lysozyme) lacking in formula. However, preterm infants don't grow at adequate rates on human milk alone, so human milk is usually supplemented with formula that contains additional carbohydrates, protein, fatty acids, vitamins, and minerals. Enteral feeding is indicated in infants requiring endotracheal intubation, or weak infants with an inability to suck, swallow, gag, or coordinate these activities (<34-36 weeks). Feedings may be continuous or intermittent (over 30 to 60 minutes). Feedings should be given slowly and tube position checked frequently to prevent aspiration. If feedings must be prolonged, oral aversion and gastroesophageal reflux may occur, so gastrostomy tube placement may be done. Oral feedings must be introduced slowly once per day, then once per 8 hours, every third feeding, every other feeding, and finally every meal.

Procedure

A feeding tube for enteral feeding should be measured (tip of ear to midpoint between xiphoid process and umbilicus) and marked before insertion. The infant should be swaddled and supine. Oral tubes are used for infants <1 kg and those with NCPAP, on a ventilator, or with a high need for oxygen. Nasal tubes are used for infants >1kg or those taking oral feedings or with a strong gag reflex. Short-term tubes (polyvinyl chloride) are changed every 24-72 hours and long-term tubes (polyurethane) every month. Prior to feeding, stomach contents are aspirated for assessment but then re-instilled to prevent electrolyte loss unless blood, bile, stool, or thick mucus is in aspirate. Feeding should be by gravity flow 5-8 inches above infant, usually over 30 minutes for intermittent feeding, and the tube should be cleared with 1-2 mL water at end. For continuous feeding, the placement of the tube and residual milk/formula should be checked every 2 hours. Usually, a 4-hour amount of milk/formula feeding is hung at one time.

Gavage Feeding

Gavage feeding per a nasogastric or orogastric tube is indicated for neonates who are preterm, critically ill, or unable to adequately swallow to obtain sufficient nutrition. Calories and nutrition provided are based on gestation, development, and laboratory findings (such as electrolytes). Typical caloric feedings:

- Preterm, 24-34 weeks: 15-20 g/kg/day.
- Preterm, 33-36 weeks: 14-15 g/kg/day.
- Full-term, 37-40 weeks: 7-9 g/kg/day.
- Full-term 0-3 months of age: 30 g/day.

Non-nutritive sucking should be provided during gavage feeding with the mother/caregiver holding the neonate with skin-to-skin (kangaroo care) contact during feeding if possible. The neonate has increased risk of gastroesophageal reflux if fed in the supine position, so prone or left lateral position with head elevated to 30 degrees during feeding is preferred. Additionally, one hour after feeding, position the neonate in the right lateral position for one hour followed by the left lateral position to facilitate gastric emptying.

Bolus vs. Continuous Feedings

Bolus gavage feedings are generally administered over a 15-30-minute period while continuous feedings are administered over a number of hours. There is not yet consensus as to which method is better and study results are often conflicting on the effects of each type, such as which method is most likely to increase apneic periods. Bolus feedings are generally more common but continuous feedings are becoming more popular and require less direct nursing time. Intermittent feedings are usually done with gravity flow and require constant attendance during feeding, but continuous feedings are usually provided with an automatic pump.

Bolus feedings:

- Simulates normal feeding patterns
- May cause metabolic instability
- Increases risk of gastroesophageal reflux
- May overwhelm immature GI system
- May improve splanchnic oxygenation

Continuous feedings:

- Improves feeding tolerance
- Promotes metabolic stability
- Decreases risk of gastroesophageal reflux
- May result in increased weight gain
- May increase risk of bacterial contamination
- May result in fat separation and decreased fat intake

Trophic Feedings

Trophic feedings (also called minimal enteric nutrition) are very small enteral feeds given soon after birth to extremely premature infants not expected to tolerate enteral feeds for several weeks. Studies have shown that trophic feeds prevent atrophy of the gut and enhance gastrointestinal maturation and small intestine motility. They may also protect the preterm infants from developing necrotizing enterocolitis (NEC). Trophic feeds can be started within 24-48 hours of birth in stable infants. The fluids of choice are colostrum, human milk, or preterm infant formula. Trophic feedings are non-nutritive (not designed to add significant calories or nutrition to the infant). Typical volumes are 1-2 mL/kg per feeding, with a total volume not to exceed 15 mL/kg/day.

Total Parenteral Nutrition

A preterm or compromised infant may not tolerate enteral feedings for several weeks, so the infant's nutritional needs are met with IV **total parenteral nutrition** (TPN). The goals of TPN are to:

- Provide normal metabolism
- Support growth without significant morbidity
- Prevent essential fatty acid deficiency
- Balance nitrogen
- Prevent muscle wasting (catabolism)

TPN is started after birth. Dextrose provides the majority of calories, but to avoid elevated blood glucose levels, dextrose is administered at 6mg/kg/min and increased to 10-12 mg/kg/min over several days. The infant's serum glucose is monitored regularly for hyperglycemia. Protein content is slowly increased over several days to 3-3.5 g/kg/day. Lipids, required for calories and the absorption of fat-soluble vitamins like A, D, and E, are started at 0.5 g/kg/day and increased to 3-3.5 g/kg/day. Other components of TPN include sodium, potassium, calcium, phosphorus, magnesium, trace elements, and vitamins. TPN may be administered through a peripheral IV line for <one week and a central line for longer periods.

Intravenous Lipids

Intravenous lipids are an important component of total parenteral nutrition (TPN) because they provide essential fatty acids, a concentrated calorie source (9 calories per gram of fat), and improve delivery of fat-soluble vitamins to infants who cannot tolerate enteral feeds. General guidelines for the administration of IV lipids are to start with 0.5/g/kg on the third day of life and advance slowly to a final administration rate of 3-3.5/g/kg/day by 7-10 days. Delivery of IV lipids should be continuous over 18-24 hours each day. Serum lipid levels should be monitored for hyperlipidemia. Potential **complications** include:

- Risk of kernicterus in infants with elevated unconjugated bilirubin (Free fatty acids displace bilirubin from albumin binding sites. Infusion of lipids should be at the lower level in infants with elevated unconjugated bilirubin.)
- Exacerbation of chronic lung disease
- Exacerbation of persistent pulmonary hypertension

TPN Complications

Complications of total parenteral nutrition (TPN) result from the presence of the intravenous access (usually a central line) and the development of cholestasis. Both of these events are more common in infants receiving TPN for longer than 2-3 weeks. The longer an infant receives TPN, the more likely complications will occur. Consequences of prolonged venous access include sepsis, thrombophlebitis, and extravasation of fluid into soft tissue with possible tissue necrosis. Premature infants have an immature hepatobiliary system. One hypothesis for the development of cholestasis is that a lack of fat in the duodenum leads to biliary stasis. Infants requiring TPN are often very ill, may have episodes of shock, or require surgical interventions, all of which contribute to the development of TPN-associated cholestasis. Jaundiced infants show an elevated direct bilirubin in blood serum. Treatment usually involves the discontinuation of TPN, along with the slow introduction of enteral feeds (if possible).

Supplementary or Complementary Feeding

Supplementary or complementary feeding with breastfed babies is usually discouraged because it may weaken the suckling reflex or cause the child to lose interest in breastfeeding, especially if a bottle is offered before breastfeeding is well established. To breastfeed, the child must latch on differently to the breast than to a bottle nipple, with the mouth opened more widely for the breast. Additionally, the tongue moves front to back when nursing (expressing milk) and up and down (squeezing the nipple) when feeding from a bottle. Changing from one to the other can be confusing for the infant, and some cannot adjust. Once the infant nurses well, usually after about 4 weeks, mothers who want to pump for supplementary feedings may try to slowly introduce the bottle. Neonates do not need water and should not be given juice or sugar water.

Dietary Supplements

Dietary supplements include:

- **Human milk fortifiers**: HMFs are added to human milk to improve nutritional values. Contains nutrients (protein, carbohydrates, fats), vitamins, and minerals. Some fortifiers are derived from cow's milk and others from human milk. Human milk fortifiers are generally used for preterm and VLBW (very low birth weight) neonates.
- **Glucose polymers**: Glucose polymers are derived from starches (such as rice and tapioca) and are alternatives to glucose used as nutritional supplements to increase carbohydrate intake. Glucose polymers and lactose are commonly found in formulas intended for preterm neonates.
- **Medium chain triglycerides**: This nutritional supplement is provided to preterm neonates in order to increase fat absorption to promote growth.
- **Probiotics**: Live bacteria and yeast supplements are added to feedings of preterm neonates to reduce the risk of necrotizing enterocolitis.

Iron Supplementation

The premature infant is especially susceptible to iron deficiency because of the lack of maternal iron transfer during the third trimester and the multiple blood samplings that occur with the extensive monitoring of the premature infant. To minimize the risk of iron deficiency anemia, premature infants fed human milk should be started on **iron supplementation** once they receive full enteral feeds. Studies have shown that premature infants fed a premature formula have better iron stores when that formula is supplemented with 15 mg/L of iron compared to those receiving formula with only 3 mg/L of iron. All formula-fed term infants should receive iron-fortified formulas. Breastfed term infants should be given iron supplementation when they are several months old.

Carnitine Supplementation for Premature Infants

Carnitine is a quaternary amino acid that is synthesized from methionine and lysine in the liver and kidney. Carnitine aids in the metabolism of long chain fatty acids by helping to transport them across the mitochondrial membrane. Carnitine is present in human milk and formulas in sufficient amounts. Infants who are born premature have low tissue stores of carnitine, as much of it is transferred to the fetus during the third trimester. Symptoms of carnitine deficiency include increased episodes of apnea, decreased muscle tone, and poor growth. Infants who are not being enterally fed and are receiving TPN may benefit from supplementation with carnitine because it makes them better able to metabolize fats.

Complications of Breastfeeding

Engorgement

Production of milk sometimes outstrips demand in the first 2-3 days as the mother is starting to nurse, and the breasts become **engorged** (enlarged, taut, and painful). The mother should be reassured that this is normal and can be relieved, as new mothers may feel they should stop nursing or be afraid they are doing something wrong. Nursing frequently (every 2-3 hours) and gently massaging the breast toward the nipple during nursing should reduce engorgement. If the areola is hard, some milk should be manually expressed to soften the areola before the infant latches on. Breast pumps and heat (except in a shower) may increase engorgement. Cold compresses, acetaminophen, or ibuprofen may provide relief. Engorgement usually recedes within 24-48 hours.

Insufficient Milk

Only about 1.5% of women are physiologically unable to produce **sufficient milk** for an infant. In almost all cases, the mother is simply not nursing correctly or frequently enough to stimulate milk production.

Blocked Milk Duct

A palpable, localized lump or an area of hard, swollen erythematous tissue usually indicates a **blocked duct**. Causes include nursing the baby in the same position or wearing a constricting or poorly-fitting bra. Painful, blocked ducts generally open within 24-48 hours, with symptoms receding, as opposed to mastitis which tends to worsen. Massaging the affected area while breastfeeding, manually expressing the breast during a warm shower, applying heat to the area, and using a breast pump to completely empty the breast after feeding may alleviate the blockage. Additionally, while breastfeeding on the affected side, the infant should be positioned so the chin points toward the blocked area, usually using the football position. If blockage is not alleviated, blocked milk ducts may progress to mastitis.

Mastitis

Indications that the breast has become infected (**mastitis**) with bacteria include induration, swelling, erythema, increasing fever, and acute pain. Without prompt treatment, painful abscesses may form. The infected area may be localized, sometimes appearing similar to blocked milk duct, or generalized, encompassing the whole breast. The mother may have chills and flu-like symptoms before obvious inflammation of the breast. Usually, the mother becomes infected from the infant, most commonly with *Staphylococcus aureus,* so breastfeeding does not endanger the neonate. Treatment includes antibiotics, usually penicillin G, dicloxacillin, or erythromycin, and nursing, pumping, or expressing on the affected side to prevent abscess formation. Applying heat or massaging the breasts in a warm shower may increase circulation. Pain relief includes alternating warm and cold compresses, and acetaminophen or ibuprofen.

Cracked Nipples

Nipples often become sore when the mother begins breastfeeding, but this typically lessens in a few days. However, **cracked nipples** may lead to infection. These are some of the causes:

- The baby latching on improperly to just the nipple and not the areola
- Use of drying lotions or soaps
- Use of a breast pump with too much suction
- Monilial infection from thrush in the baby's mouth

Sometimes changing the baby's **position** or rotating positions during nursing may reduce discomfort. Nursing should begin on the least sore nipple, as the infant nurses more strongly at first. The breasts should be cleansed only with water and a small amount of human milk applied to the nipple after nursing, unless the baby has thrush. One hundred percent USP modified **lanolin** (Lansinoh or PureLan) applied to the nipples may promote healing. It does not need to be removed for breastfeeding. Acetaminophen or ibuprofen may be taken 30 minutes before nursing. Nipple shields should be avoided if possible, as they interfere with latching on.

Renal and Genitourinary Complications

Renal Vein/Artery Thrombosis

A thrombosis that is not catheter-related, occurring predominantly in the neonatal period, is **renal vein thrombosis (RVT).** Upon diagnosis, the presence of a palpable abdominal mass, macroscopic hematuria, and thrombocytopenia are typically noted. Risk factors associated with RVT may include perinatal asphyxia, dehydration, maternal diabetes, as well as hereditary prothrombotic risk factors, though studies have shown the absence of the first three underlying factors in neonatal history. Therefore, it is considered good practice to screen children with thromboembolic diseases for prothrombotic risk factors. The diagnosis of RVT can also be confirmed with renal ultrasound, demonstrating enlarged and echogenic kidneys with loss or attenuation of corticomedullary differentiation, and the presence of calcification and thrombus outside of the kidneys, extending to the inferior vena cava. In addition, Doppler studies evaluate blood flow resistance, either venous or arterial, caused by intrarenal venous thrombosis. Finally, radionuclide scans can identify renal scarring and atrophy.

Treatment

Treatment of renal vein thrombosis (RVT) varies greatly among neonatal centers. Heparin therapy, with the use of low molecular weight heparin (LMWH), as opposed to unfractionated heparin, is likely to be initiated, often with the presence of inferior vena cava involvement and bilateral RVT. In contract, approximately 40 percent of neonates will be managed supportively without heparin therapy. Studies do not show a more favorable outcome in the prevention of renal atrophy or irreversible damage with or without heparin therapy. Supportive management in the acute phase of RVT by the multidisciplinary team of neonatologists, hematologists, nephrologists, and radiologists includes the maintenance of electrolyte and fluid balance, and renal replacement therapy, thereby treating acute renal failure (ARF). In addition, anticoagulant or fibrinolytic treatment may be initiated. On an ongoing basis, the need for monitoring of renal complications is imperative, to include hypertension, renal atrophy and functional loss, and chronic renal insufficiency.

Acute Renal Failure/Insufficiency in Neonates

Acute renal failure (ARF) or insufficiency is commonly found in the neonatal intensive care unit. Most neonates experience pre-renal failure due to underlying disease, recent heart surgery, or less commonly a congenital renal malformation. ARF is characterized by a sudden decrease in glomerular filtration rate (GFR), resulting in progressive retention of nitrogenous waste products and creatinine, and the loss of fluid and electrolyte homeostasis regulation. Early diagnosis of neonatal ARF is vital in order to preserve the neonate's renal function. At birth, a very low GFR is maintained in the kidney by the baby's own vasoconstrictor and vasodilator forces. This is normally sufficient for the newborn's growth and development of the kidney. However, the low GFR limits the newborn's ability to functionally adapt to endogenous and exogenous stresses, such as is seen with a low-birth-weight infant (less than 2.5 kg), predisposing the infant to ARF.

Treatment

Treatment of acute renal failure or insufficiency involves a conservative approach of adequate fluid and caloric intake in the neonatal intensive care unit, with ongoing daily monitoring and reevaluation of the fluid regimen, maintenance of acid-base balance and nutrition, and renal replacement therapy, if indicated. The latter is achieved by peritoneal dialysis, intermittent hemodialysis, or hemofiltration with or without a dialysis circuit. Although it is considered by some providers to be controversial, acute peritoneal dialysis (APD) may be initiated in the treatment of progressive renal failure, and is considered safe and effective by some recent studies. APD is reportedly successful in controlling hyperkalemia, fluid overload, and metabolic acidosis. Rapid exchanges during a short dwell time promoted maximum peritoneal permeability and transport. APD aids in managing the metabolic and hemodynamic imbalance present with ARF. Neonates can achieve a full recovery of renal function, but there may be complications such as peritonitis, leakage, hemoperitoneum, and hernia.

Polycystic Dysplastic Kidneys

Polycystic or multicystic dysplastic kidneys in the neonate refers to a condition in which the kidney has been replaced by multiple cysts due to abnormal fetal development, resulting in little to no normal kidney function. This condition can typically be detected via a prenatal ultrasound, and most likely occurs on the left side. Occasionally, this condition occurs bilaterally, which is grave as the kidney produces the amniotic fluid needed for developing the fetus' lungs in utero. The presence of one multicystic dysplastic kidney with a properly functioning other kidney will likely ensure that the required amount of amniotic fluid is maintained. However, there is approximately a 51 percent risk of an associated abnormality, such as vesicoureteral reflux, uretero-pelvic junction obstruction, or uretero-vesical junction obstruction, with the normal functioning kidney. Therefore, consultation with a pediatric urologist is necessary following birth to determine the treatment regimen.

Treatment Options for Complications

The three **complications** commonly found in the non-polycystic-dysplastic kidney (vesicoureteral reflux, uretero-pelvic junction obstruction, and uretero-vesical junction obstruction) are all surgically correctable via laparoscopic surgery, with a reduction in incision size and recovery time. Occasionally, these complications can have self-resolution. Prior to determining the proper treatment plan, radiological studies will be performed. These include a voiding cystourethrogram (VCUG), intravenous pyelogram (IVP), and a renal ultrasound (RUS). Currently, the majority of pediatric urologists recommend the monitoring of the kidney with serial RUS versus nephrectomy to remove the diseased kidney, as the diagnostic studies can help to pinpoint the exact diagnosis. Additionally, the risk of developing hypertension and malignancy is fairly low even if the kidney is not removed.

Urinary Outflow Tract Obstruction

In utero, the fetal urine forms the amniotic fluid, which is crucial for healthy lung development as it is swallowed by the fetus. If there is a blockage in the urinary system, a backup of urine results in dilation, which can be detected on the prenatal ultrasound. Various types of **blockage** preventing or slowing the urine from leaving the body include:

- Bladder outlet or urethral obstruction, most commonly due to an abnormal flap or tissue, or a posterior urethral valve.
- Bladder inlet or ureterovesical junction obstruction, or where the ureter connects the kidneys to the bladder.

- Kidney outlet or ureteropelvic junction obstruction, found between the kidney pelvis and the ureter, dilating the kidney's collection tubules.
- Ectopic ureter, an abnormal position of the ureter exiting the kidney or entering the bladder.
- Ureterocele, or a cyst that may cause obstruction at the end of the ureter.

Diagnostic Tests and Treatment

As **blockage of urine** can ultimately result in kidney damage, careful monitoring is prudent. Most often, one kidney is affected, leaving the undamaged kidney to function. Should both kidneys be affected, the decrease in urine production will likely result in decreased amniotic fluid and impaired lung development. Prenatal ultrasounds will monitor for amniotic fluid level changes, urinary system dilation, and any kidney changes. In addition, an amniocentesis with genetic counseling may be performed for mild hydronephrosis, which does not typically require surgery. Approximately half of babies with mild hydronephrosis will have resolution after birth. For severe and rare cases of urinary tract obstruction, such as the result of a posterior urethral valve, a catheter may be inserted into the fetal urinary system to aid in draining the urine into the amniotic sac. Early intentional delivery has not proven successful, but some neonates will undergo corrective surgery.

Hydronephrosis

Hydronephrosis is a dilated kidney that is swollen with urine. It most commonly results from a narrowed or blocked ureter, which under normal circumstances drains the urine into the bladder. This condition is more prevalent in male neonates than in females. **Prenatal hydronephrosis** is rarely diagnosed before it resolves by itself, or before the kidneys begin to compensate for the blockage. Prenatal ultrasounds can identify these cases that normally might not be detected until three or four years later when symptoms become obvious. Symptoms include nausea, vomiting, fever, swelling, and urinary difficulties. The presentation of symptoms depends on the severity of the case, as mild and occasionally moderate hydronephrosis may not present with symptoms at all. Severe hydronephrosis, if left untreated, is always accompanied by complications, such as kidney damage, infections, bleeding, and pain.

Treatment

The first action should be a prophylactic treatment to prevent a kidney infection that can result from the urine not adequately draining from the kidney. The preferred antibiotic selection is typically a low-dose with limited side effects. The pediatric urologist will determine the length of prophylactic treatment based on the results of diagnostic imaging studies, such as renal ultrasound. Surgical intervention is most likely considered for children with grade IV hydronephrosis. The overall goal of surgery is to relieve the uretero-pelvic junction (UPJ) obstruction. Pyeloplasty, or renal pelvic reconstruction\revision, is performed to decompress and drain the kidney to prevent recurrent infection and ultimately kidney damage. However, grades I, II, and III of hydronephrosis, as well as non-obstructive hydronephrosis, are not surgical candidates as these conditions will most likely resolve by themselves. The presentation of megaureters, or dilation due to ureterovesical junction abnormalities, typically does not require surgery either.

Hydrocele

A hydrocele is fluid in the scrotum or inguinal region. It co-occurs with an inguinal hernia in 10-20 infants per 1,000 live births. During fetal development, the testicles migrate from the abdominal cavity through the inguinal canal to the scrotum. A piece of peritoneum called the process vaginalis travels with the testicle into the scrotum. Normally, this extension of peritoneum closes and becomes a fibrous chord (tunica vaginalis), so there is no connection between the peritoneal cavity and the scrotum. If closure does not occur (patent process vaginalis), fluid accumulates in the scrotum. If the fluid collection comes and goes, then it is termed a communicating hydrocele. A non-communicating hydrocele is one where fluid is trapped in the scrotum after the process vaginalis closes. Physical examination reveals a bulge in the scrotum that may or may not be reducible. No bowel sounds should be audible with auscultation, which indicates a hernia. Transillumination of the scrotum reveals fluid retention.

Testicular Torsion

Two types of testicular torsion, or the twisting of the spermatic cord structures, are **extravaginal torsion**, which develops in the prenatal period and presents at birth, also associated with a high birth weight; and **intravaginal torsion**, which typically presents in older children, also referred to as a bell-clapper with its anomalous testicular suspension. Normally, the testes freely rotate within the scrotum via the tunica vaginalis. Extravaginal torsion occurs proximally to the tunica vaginalis, while intravaginal torsion occurs within the tunica vaginalis. Upon physical examination of the neonate, an affected testis will exhibit swelling, tenderness, and may appear to be high-riding. There may also be an absence of the cremasteric reflex. When torsion occurs, blood flow to the testis and epididymis may be interrupted. Salvage is more likely within 6-8 hours of noted torsion. However, testicular necrosis often develops when the torsion duration increases to 24 hours or longer.

Treatment

The management of **prenatal testicular torsion (PTT)** is controversial, with research lacking on the optimal approach and timing of intervention. For the neonate born with testicular torsion, surgical exploration with contralateral orchidopexy, or anchoring, is indicated following stabilization of the overall physiological status of the neonate, since imaging studies of neonatal bilateral torsion provide limited information. If the neonate born with a normal testis develops torsion, immediate exploration is warranted, with the preferred method being scrotal incision. Once the testis is examined for viability, any necrotic testis is removed, as the presence of necrotic tissue may trigger an autoimmune phenomenon and subsequent infertility. During surgery, any viable gonads are attached to the scrotal wall, to prevent recurrence of the torsion. Surgical exploration will also lend to ruling out additional possible diagnoses.

Undescended Testicles in Premature Infant

Cryptorchidism occurs when one or both of the testicles in the male infant fail to migrate from the abdominal cavity into the scrotum. Migration normally occurs sometime during 28-40 weeks gestation. Up to 30% of males born prematurely and 2-5% of those born full term, have an undescended testicle. When cryptorchidism is discovered on physical exam, it should be noted on the infant's chart. The parents should be reassured that it is not an immediate concern, as most testes will descend without therapy by 6 months of age. Those infants whose testes have not descended by 6 months of age may be treated medically with human chorionic gonadotropin or with surgery. A testicle that is allowed to remain in the abdominal cavity is at increased risk for malignancy, and adult men with undescended testicles have increased rates of infertility.

Hypospadias/Epispadias

The congenital defect with the urethral opening on the underside of the penis is **hypospadias**. The urethral opening typically presents near the tip of the penis; however, it may be located at the midshaft or base of the penis, or behind the scrotum. The penis is positioned in a downward curve, otherwise noted as ventral curvature or chordee. As a result, infants may commonly experience erections, as well as abnormal spraying of urine, the presence of malformed foreskin with the appearance of a "hooded" penis, and the necessity to sit down to urinate when older. Imaging studies may be indicated to rule out other associated congenital defects. In contrast, **epispadias** is much less common than hypospadias, with the urethral meatus dorsally displaced, and may be associated with exstrophy of the bladder in its severe form. Routine circumcision is contraindicated, as the penis appears splayed open lengthwise on the dorsal surface.

Treatment

In preparation for **surgical repair**, the foreskin should be preserved. Surgery is routinely performed prior to the beginning of elementary school, and can be performed as early as four months of age, typically at approximately eighteen months. Multiple surgeries may be required, with the straightening of the penis and the use of tissue grafts from the foreskin. Repeat or multiple surgeries may be indicated for correction of a returned abnormal curve of the penis, or to correct a fistula. If left untreated, urethral strictures and fistulas may form, and the growing boy will experience difficulty with toilet training and, in adulthood, difficulty with sexual intercourse. For the treatment of epispadias, surgical correction is also required. Parental education is imperative as parents must contact a pediatrician if they notice the presence of a curved penis with erection or an abnormal location of the urethral opening.

Vaginal Discharge

Neonatal vaginal discharge, or physiologic leukorrhea, is a normal occurrence in female newborns immediately after birth due to the drop in exposure to hormones that were present in the uterus. This discharge may be blood-tinged and should subside after a few months. The external genitalia (labia and surrounding area) can be cleaned with warm water (but without soap).

Vaginal discharge is concerning if it is accompanied by a foul odor or yellow/green coloration (which could indicate infection). Perfuse bleeding that continues after several months should also be investigated.

Integumentary Complications

Skin Development and Care

The **neonate's skin** comprises 4% of its body weight and is the largest organ, but it is still developing and doesn't reach maturity until adolescence or later:

- Neonatal skin is about 1 mm thick (2 mm at maturity) and has little subcutaneous fat, so thermoregulation is impaired, making the infant lose heat rapidly. The neonate's temperature must be maintained, but overheating must be avoided. The thinness of the skin increases chemical absorption, so care must be used when applying lotions, chemicals, or topical medications.
- The epidermis and dermis are loosely connected, increasing the danger of separation and blister formation with friction.
- Eccrine glands function and produce sweat but are immature and may not be adequate for temperature control, increasing the danger of overheating. Apocrine glands are small and nonfunctional.
- Melanin levels are low at birth, so skin is light-colored and more susceptible to damage from the sun. As such, infants must be shielded from direct sunlight.

Café Au Lait Spots

Café au lait spots (CAL) are flat skin lesions with increased melanin content and regular or irregular borders. If the CAL spots are faint, use a Wood lamp to make them easier to see. Fewer than 3 café au lait spots have no clinical significance. However, 6 or more café au lait spots with a diameter larger than 5 mm occur in 95% of patients with **neurofibromatosis type 1 (NF1)**, a disorder of chromosome 17. Lisch nodules on the irises and Crowe's sign (freckles on the axillae and inguinal area) corroborate the diagnosis of NF1. The pediatrician must be alerted that this child should receive future monitoring for the symptoms that occur with NF1, such as bowed legs, rib lesions, scoliosis, neurofibromas, glaucoma, and corneal opacification. Café au lait spots are also associated with tuberous sclerosis, McCune-Albright syndrome, ataxia-telangiectasia, Gaucher disease, basal cell nevus syndrome, and Fanconi anemia. CAL affects 18% of black infants, 3% of Hispanic infants, and 0.3% of white infants.

Hemangioma

Hemangioma is a bright red vascular tumor that occurs in 1-3% of neonates, especially in girls, preterm infants <1500 g, and those whose mothers had chorionic villus sampling. The head and neck are the most common sites. **Hemangiomas** may initially appear as a faint telangiectasia or red macule, but they proliferate rapidly during the first year, after which they go through a slow involution in which they decrease in size, usually complete in 95% by adolescence. Hemangiomas may be superficial, deep, or mixed and may involve skin as well as other organs. Complications, such as airway compromise, vision problem, ulceration, renal abnormalities, imperforate anus, and skeletal anomalies may occur as the hemangioma grows, depending upon adjacent structures. Imaging of hemangiomas is indicated only in infants that display evidence or possibility of underlying structural abnormalities. Treatment may include just monitoring or systemic or localized treatment with corticosteroids to slow proliferation. Oral propranolol is the first-line therapy for infantile hemangiomas in infants age 5 weeks to 5 months. Pulsed dye laser treatment is a common treatment to reduce proliferation.

Subcutaneous Fat Necrosis

Subcutaneous fat necrosis is a nodular skin lesion disorder that usually occurs ≤6 weeks of birth in full-term or post-term infants caused by necrosis of subcutaneous fatty tissue. Onset is usually between days 2-21. **Subcutaneous fat necrosis** is commonly associated with hypothermia, trauma to tissue from forceps, neonatal stress (various causes), and hypercalcemia. Single or multiple lesions may develop, ranging in size from about 1 cm in diameter to much larger, with erythema obvious over lesions. Lesions are usually rubbery and often distributed across the buttocks, upper legs, shoulders, upper back, upper extremities, and cheeks. In some cases, fluctuant lesions may open and drain or require aspiration. The lesions usually resolve over time with no treatment. Serum calcium should be monitored and hypercalcemia evaluated for cause and treated as necessary.

Ecchymosis, Petechiae, Hyperpigmentation, and Hypopigmentation

Ecchymosis (large blue-purple discolored bruising) and **petechiae** (pinpoint <1 mm hemorrhagic areas) may be the result of birth trauma, particularly difficult births, breech births, or forceps-assisted birth and is most noticeable on the presenting part. These types of bruising usually fade within 24-48 hours, but if they persist, they may indicate underlying pathology. **Ecchymosis** and petechiae can indicate clotting disorders and bleeding in the tissue, such as can occur with DIC. They may also be evidence of thrombocytopenia (especially diffuse petechiae) and vitamin K deficiency.

Hypopigmentation may be caused by a number of disorders, including PKU, Addison's disease, vitiligo, albinism, and herpes simplex virus. It may also result from post-inflammatory changes.

Hyperpigmentation, while rare in the newborn, can occur with severe toxoplasmosis infection, Addison's disease, liver disease, porphyria, pellagra, sprue, lentiginosis, and melanism. Untreated syphilitic lesions may cause hypo- or hyperpigmentation after regression.

Erythema Toxicum

Erythema toxicum is a skin eruption of erythematous papules, vesicles, and sometimes pustules that is essentially benign and occurs in ≥50% of newborns. It is a generalized rash that resembles that of herpes simplex, occurring on the face, limbs, and trunk (everywhere except the palms and soles of the feet). It usually occurs 2-3 days after birth. The lesions are surrounded by a mottled erythematous halo of about 0.5-1.5 cm. Individual lesions often appear and resolve within hours but new lesions occur. Lesions may be limited to a few on the face or may cover the body. Erythema toxicum is often associated with eosinophilia and occurs in the first few weeks of life before the immune system matures, so it is hypothesized that the rash may be an allergic response. The rash usually resolves in about 2 weeks without treatment.

Neonatal Pustular Melanosis

Neonatal pustular melanosis is a benign rash (vesicles and macules) that is present at birth in about 2.2% of white infants and 4.4% of black infants. Usually, in preterm infants, vesicles (2-4 mm) with milky fluid are present at birth and rupture, leaving a halo of white scaly tissue and a pigmented macule at the center. Erythema is not associated with this rash. Full-term infants may exhibit only the macular stage as the vesicles ruptured prior to birth. The pigmented discoloration fades with time but may persist for ≤3 months. The cause of neonatal pustular melanosis is not known. The rash may be localized and sparse or profuse (beneath chin, neck, upper chest, upper back, and buttocks). No treatment is indicated, and there appears to be no long-term sequelae, but the lesions must be differentiated from congenital herpes infection, especially if erythema is evident.

Preauricular Skin Tag

A preauricular skin tag is a small extension of skin located anterior to the ear. They may be single or multiple in number, and they may be pedunculated (attached by a narrow stalk) or sessile (flat). Occasionally, skin tags are associated with hearing loss and dysmorphic features in some congenital syndromes (e.g., cat eye syndrome). At one time, it was believed that a **preauricular skin tag** was an indication of renal anomalies, but this has not been supported by research. A skin tag with a narrow stalk may be simply ligated, but one with a thicker stalk should be removed by a surgeon, as the stalk may contain cartilage that extends into the subcutaneous tissue. Removal of a cartilaginous skin tag requires anesthesia.

Port-Wine Stain

A port-wine stain (capillary angioma) is a birthmark comprised of dilated capillaries below the epidermis. The lesion is usually on the face or neck and is light pink at birth but darkens with age. The lesion alone is benign, but it may be an indication of other disorders, such as Sturge-Weber syndrome (neurological disorder with seizures, paralysis, and glaucoma) or Klippel-Trenaunay-Weber syndrome (disorder with hypertrophy of bones and soft tissue as well as varicose veins and multiple port-wine stains), so the infant should be evaluated and have an eye examination, especially if the lesion is on the eyelids, as this is associated with glaucoma. Over time, the capillary angioma may thicken and form nodules, so early treatment is advisable. The most common treatment is laser therapy, which destroys the capillaries without damaging other tissue, usually done in infancy to prevent psychological trauma and to prevent changes in the skin, such as thickening.

Chapter Quiz

Ready to see how well you retained what you just read? Scan the QR code to go directly to the chapter quiz interface for this study guide. If you're using a computer, simply visit the online resources page at **mometrix.com/resources719/ccrnneonatal** and click the Chapter Quizzes link.

Clinical Judgment: Musculoskeletal, Neurological, and Psychosocial

Musculoskeletal Complications

Metatarsus Adductus

Metatarsus adductus ("toeing in") is the most common congenital disorder of the foot, occurring in about 1:1000 births. **Metatarsus adductus** is a convex curve turning the forefoot inward at the tarsometatarsal joint. Metatarsus adductus occurs equally in males and females and is common among siblings. It is believed the condition may be related to position in the uterus, and it is often associated with oligohydramnios. About 50% have bilateral metatarsus adductus, and 10-15% have hip dysplasia as well. In most cases, simple stretching exercises are the only needed therapy, and most cases resolve by 3 months. If the curvature is more than 15°, serial casting changed weekly may be necessary to maintain the foot in the correct position. Braces or special orthopedic shoes may be used after casting is completed.

Talipes Equinovarus

Talipes equinovarus (clubfoot) is a congenital abnormality of the foot that involves 3 types of **deformities**:

- Midfoot directed inferiorly (equinus)
- Hindfoot turns inward (varus)
- Forefoot adducts toward the heel and then turns superiorly in partial supination

Typically, the foot is small, the Achilles tendon shortened, and the lower leg muscles atrophied. The condition begins during the first trimester, so the foot position is very rigid at birth. Clubfoot occurs in about 1:1000 births with a male to female ratio of 2:1. About 50% of cases are bilateral. Cases vary in severity and some may be associated with other abnormalities, such as myelomeningocele. Diagnosis is often made on ultrasound (16-20 weeks) or at birth. The cause is unclear, but there appears to be a genetic component. Treatment is by long leg serial casting (changed every 1-2 weeks) begun shortly after birth. In some cases, surgery may be required (at 3-12 months) followed by casting and bracing.

Polydactyly and Syndactyly

Polydactyly is when the neonate has an extra digit on the hand or foot. This digit may be in the form of a small nub or may be a fully functional toe or finger. Usually, the digit attaches to the hand or foot with narrow tissue, though bone, nerves or muscles/tendons may be involved in the more complex cases. There are 3 types of polydactyly, based on the location: Preaxial (outside the thumb or big toe), postaxial (outside little finger or toe), and central (between other fingers or toes). Polydactyly is not generally associated with any other health problems but may occur with syndactyly. Treatment requires surgery to remove the digit.

Syndactyly is the fusing of two or more fingers or toes (fingernails may also be fused). Sometimes this fusion occurs at the bone, other times the skin, nerves, muscles or tendons are also fused. Syndactyly is often an inherited condition. Treatment is not always required, specifically in toes, if function is not limited. Often surgery is utilized to separate fingers unless nerves are shared, in which case separation may cause the fingers to lose function. In these cases, the fingers are left fused.

Achondroplasia

Achondroplasia is the most common cause of **dwarfism**, in which bone growth is inhibited as the result of an abnormal gene on **chromosome 4**. Achondroplasia can be inherited in an autosomal dominant fashion, but the majority of cases (75-80%) occur because of spontaneous mutations. Clinical features of achondroplasia apparent at birth include a long narrow torso with short arms and legs. The proximal segment of the limbs (upper arms and thighs) is disproportionately short. The head is large, with frontal bossing and midface hypoplasia. A small hump (gibbus) may be present in the mid-to-lower back. Mild, generalized hypotonia may be present. Monitor the infant's head size for the development of hydrocephalus. The pediatrician may order a skeletal survey to identify many of the skeletal features associated with achondroplasia and to help confirm the diagnosis.

Congenital Hip Dislocation

Congenital hip dislocation, also known as **developmental dysplasia of the hip or DDH**, is hip instability resulting from misalignment of the **femoral head** and **acetabulum**. Hip instability may present as dislocation, subluxation, or acetabular dysplasia (abnormal structural development of the joint). **Symptoms** may not be evident until after the neonatal period. The condition tends to worsen as the child grows. Involvement of the left hip is more common than the right. There appears to be a genetic tendency and an association with breech birth. **Signs at ≤3 months** include:

- Positive Barlow's test (Pressing on the knees to apply pressure to the head of the femur when hips are flexed causes posterior subluxation.)
- Positive Ortolani test (Hips rotated through range of motion cause a click at abduction as the femoral head slips.)

The AAFP recommends against using imaging for universal screening of DDH, but rather screening high-risk infants who are between 6 weeks and 6 months of age with a physical assessment that is otherwise normal. Radiography for the screening of DDH should be reserved only for children 4 months of age or older in this category.

Referral to an orthopedist is indicated for application of **Pavlik harness** for infants <3 months of age. Per AAFP guidelines, avoid tightly swaddling the legs and extending or adducting the hips.

Scoliosis

Scoliosis is a lateral (S-shaped) spinal curvature >10°. Curvature >30° produces marked deformity. The curvature of scoliosis may be structural or compensatory. Congenital scoliosis is increasing because of the survival of infants with preterm birth. About 10% of congenital scoliosis relates to abnormalities of the intervertebral/vertebral bodies, affecting the growth of the trunk, most commonly hemivertebra. The male to female ratio is 2.5:1, with about a third of the curvatures at the upper thoracic level with decreasing incidence down the spine (5% at lumbosacral area). Thoracolumbar curvatures carry the worst prognosis. About 20-50% of cases have other spinal cord abnormalities, and 30-60% of these have other anomalies, such as VACTERL association (a condition assigned when a child is diagnosed with birth defects in three or more body parts).

Impairment of pulmonary function is a major complication. Bracing is a successful treatment for <10% of cases, but it may be used early to prevent further curvature in preparation for later surgery.

Apert Syndrome

Apert syndrome is an autosomal dominant (or new mutation) disorder that results in craniosynostosis (early fusion of some bones of the skull). Apert syndrome is characterized by:

- **Craniosynostosis**: abnormal shape of head and facial features, midface hypoplasia (which may result in breathing disorders) such as prominent forehead, wide-set or bulging eyes, flattened nasal bridge, beak nose, sunken facial appearance; the neonate may have a narrow palate, with or without a cleft
- **Syndactyly**: webbing of fingers and toes, short radially-deviated thumbs, hands are described in terms of appearance: spade, mitten, or rosebud
- Intellectual impairment/developmental delays
- **Various anomalies**: hearing loss, dentition problems, vision impairment, cervical spine abnormalities

Apert syndrome occurs equally in male and female neonates, and incidence correlates with advanced paternal age. Complications include increased intracranial pressure, corneal scarring, respiratory distress, aspiration pneumonia, and neurological deficits. Treatment is multidisciplinary and includes surgical interventions (often done in stages), ongoing monitoring, and supportive therapies as the child ages, including speech therapy, educational support, and occupational therapy.

Crouzon Syndrome

Crouzon syndrome is an autosomal dominant syndrome (mutations in FGFR2 gene or a new mutation) that results in craniosynostosis (early fusion of some bones of the skull) and other abnormalities. Crouzon syndrome is characterized by the following:

- Craniosynostosis: results in characteristic facial appearance
- Midface hypoplasia: concave appearance, underdeveloped upper jaw
- Shallow eye sockets with bulging eyes (proptosis)
- Hypertelorism: widely-spaced eyes
- Prominent nasal bridge: beaked nose
- Dental anomalies: teeth misaligned and other abnormalities
- Malformations of middle ear: hearing problems
- Cleft lip or palate may occur

Complications include increased intracranial pressure, intellectual impairment, vision impairment, corneal scarring, aspiration pneumonia and other respiratory problems resulting from airway changes. Treatment includes surgical interventions and supportive therapies. If abnormalities in the cranial vault are corrected surgically, relieving pressure on the brain and other structures, the neonate may develop normal intellect, hearing, and vision. Life span is typically near normal with early intervention and support.

Neurological Complications

Neonatal Neurosensory Capabilities

A neonate is born with the following neurosensory capabilities:

- **Hearing**: The neonate's crying after birth clears middle ear mucus and the eustachian tubes, and hearing becomes acute with hearing thresholds similar to adults and children. Because hearing deficit is one of the most common congenital abnormalities, all infants should be assessed for hearing.
- **Vision**: The neonate's vision is about 10-30 times less acute than that of an adult, but the infant has peripheral vision, can fixate at 8-14 inches, and can accommodate to large objects. The neonate is able to perceive shapes, colors, and faces.
- **Tactile sense**: The neonate has a good sense of touch and reacts emotionally to tactile stimulation.
- **Smell**: The neonate has a strong sense of smell after nasal passages clear and will react to the smell of milk or turn away from strong smells.
- **Pain**: Neonates experience pain, and pain prevention/management should be part of neonatal care.

Perinatal Asphyxia

Perinatal asphyxia is the cause of many problems after birth. Perinatal asphyxia is defined as an event that alters the exchange of gas (oxygen and carbon dioxide) during labor or delivery. This interference with gas exchange leads to a decrease in the amount of oxygen delivered to the fetus along with an increase in the level of carbon dioxide the fetus is exposed to. This gas imbalance causes the fetus to switch from normal aerobic metabolism to anaerobic metabolism. Fetal distress results, which then leads to increased fetal heart rate, release of meconium into the amniotic fluid, and lowered pH. Infants experiencing birth asphyxia will often present at birth with APGAR scores that are less than 5. Symptoms of birth asphyxia include:

- **Mild**
  - Overly alert for the first 45 minutes to one hour following birth (infants are normally sleepy after about 15 minutes following birth)
  - Pupils dilated
  - Respiratory rate and heart rate both slightly increased
  - Newborn reflexes and muscle tone normal
  - Oxygen may be administered
- **Moderate**
  - Hypothermia as evidenced by low body temperature
  - Hypoglycemia as glucose stores are used up trying to supply organs needed energy
  - Pupils are constricted
  - Signs of respiratory distress evident
  - May experience seizure activity at 12-24 hours of age
  - Lethargy (floppy infant)
  - Bradycardia
- **Severe** (Requires close monitoring in a NICU)
  - Pale color related to the inability of the heart to perfuse the body
  - Cerebral edema related to apnea episodes and/or intracranial hemorrhage

Resuscitation will vary according to the infant's condition, but warming the infant, stabilizing the glucose level, and providing oxygen or EMCO (in severe cases) may be indicated.

HIE

Hypoxic-ischemic encephalopathy (HIE) results when oxygen supply to the brain is impaired. A common cause of HIE is perinatal asphyxia. The degree of insult to the neonate depends on the severity of the ischemic event. HIE is typically divided into three categories based on the Sarnat Scoring System:

- **Mild HIE**: Characterized by increased muscle tone with brisk deep tendon reflexes and mild distal flexion. The infant may also exhibit poor feeding, irritability, and excessive sleepiness. These abnormalities generally resolve after 3-4 days.
- **Moderate HIE**: Characterized by significant hypotonia and lethargy with diminished deep tendon reflexes and distal flexion. Moro and grasp reflexes may be absent. Seizures may occur. Full recovery may still occur after 1-2 weeks.
- **Severe HIE**: Generalized hypotonia/flaccidity with depressed deep tendon reflexes, decerebrate posturing, and coma. The infant may not respond to physical stimulus. Breathing may be irregular and the infant requires ventilatory support. Basic neonatal reflexes may be absent. Pupils may be dilated and fixed. Generalized seizure activity is present and may be difficult to treat.

Risk Factors and Treatment Options

Neonatal **risk factors** for hypoxic-ischemic encephalopathy include:

- Cardiac arrhythmias
- pH <7.10 (umbilical artery), indicating acidosis during delivery
- Meconium-stained amniotic fluid
- Apgar <7 at 5 minutes after birth or <4 for more than 5 minutes
- Seizures during the first 24 hours
- Neurological dysfunction as demonstrated by coma, lethargy, irritability, hypotonia, and/or altered reflexes
- Symptoms of multiple organ damage: Cardiac damage, indicated by reduced contractility with hypotension; renal damage, indicated by oliguria; and damage to the intestinal tract, indicated by poor peristalsis, delayed gastric emptying, and the development of necrotizing enterocolitis

Identifying infants at risk and instituting treatment may decrease neurological impairment. **Treatment** is focused on supportive care and may include:

- Phenobarbital given in high doses after birth decreases seizures and improves long-term outcome.
- Calcium channel blockers may improve cerebral blood flow during ischemia.
- Mild to moderate hypothermia for 5-72 hours may decrease damage; studies are in progress.
- Intubation and mechanical ventilation for neonates with severe HIE.

Subdural and Subarachnoid Cranial Hemorrhages

Subdural hemorrhage between the dura and the cerebrum, usually from tears in the cortical veins of the subdural space, tends to develop more slowly and can result in a subdural hematoma. If the bleeding is acute and develops within minutes or hours of injury, the prognosis is poor. Subacute hematomas that develop more slowly cause varying degrees of injury. Subdural hemorrhage is a common injury related to birth trauma and child abuse, although it can result from coagulopathies or aneurysms. Symptoms of acute injury may occur within 24-48 hours, but subacute bleeding may not be evident for up to 2 weeks after injury. Symptoms may include bradycardia, tachycardia, hypertension, and alterations in consciousness. Subdural taps may suffice for infants, but some infants will require surgical evacuation of the hematoma.

Subarachnoid hemorrhage may result from childbirth (one of the most common causes) or from shaken impact syndrome. The presenting symptom may be seizures, and other symptoms are similar to those of subdural hematoma. Symptoms worsen as ICP rises.

Subgaleal Hemorrhage

Subgaleal hemorrhage occurs when the emissary veins that connect the scalp veins to the dural sinuses rupture, allowing blood to accumulate between the scalp and the periosteum. Most subgaleal hemorrhages are associated with trauma caused by vacuum or forceps-assisted delivery. Additional risk factors include large neonates, cephalopelvic disproportion, coagulopathy (vitamin K, factor VII, or factor IX deficiencies), and prolonged labor (especially the second stage). Because the bleeding is usually slow, symptoms may not occur until 8 to 10 hours after birth, although they may occur abruptly with severe bleeding. Indications may include increased head circumference, ecchymosis, hyperbilirubinemia, falling hematocrit, and neurological compromise, including seizures, pallor, loss of tone, and increased cardiac and respiratory rates. As the bleeding increases, a palpable mass that crosses suture lines becomes evident, and the neonate may exhibit signs of shock related to hypovolemia. Some will develop DIC. Those at risk must be monitored carefully, the head circumference should be measured frequently, and the physician should be notified immediately of any abnormal findings.

Intraventricular Hemorrhage

Intraventricular hemorrhages (IVH) are common in premature neonates less than 32 weeks estimated gestational age. IVH presents within the first 72 hours of life in 90% of affected neonates, and within the first 24 hours in 50% of cases. Depending on the amount and location of bleeding seen on cranial ultrasound, IVH is **graded** as follows:

	Anatomy	Severity
Grade I	The hemorrhage is limited to the germinal matrix (subependymal region).	Mild (5% death rate; 5% motor or cognitive impairment)
Grade II	The hemorrhage extends 10-40% into the lateral ventricles on sagittal view, but has not dilated them significantly.	Moderate (10% death rate; 30-40% motor or cognitive impairment)
Grade III	The hemorrhage extends 50% or more into the lateral ventricles with significant ventricular dilation.	Severe (27-50% death rate; 35% motor or cognitive impairment)
Grade IV	The hemorrhage extends into brain tissue.	Periventricular hemorrhagic infarction (80% death rate; 90% motor or cognitive impairment)

SYMPTOMS AND TREATMENT

IVH is also categorized based on **symptoms**:

- **Asymptomatic**: 25-50% of IVH infants are asymptomatic or have only a fall in hematocrit and anemia, but ultrasound shows an IVH.
- **Saltatory**: Infants are pale or ashen and have gradual neurological deterioration (attention, movements, level of consciousness, eye movements).
- **Catastrophic**: Acute onset of decreased level of consciousness, bulging fontanel, cranial nerve abnormalities, decerebrate posturing, and hypotension with drop in hematocrit.

IVH **treatment** must be approached with extreme caution. Infants should be closely monitored, with serial cranial ultrasounds recommended twice a week. If ventricular dilatation continues, then CSF drainage is required using serial lumbar punctures or a temporary ventricular drain. A more permanent shunt may be required for persistent cases.

CRANIOSYNOSTOSIS

Types of craniosynostosis (early fusing of the skull) include the following:

- **Sagittal craniosynostosis** (scaphocephaly) is the fusion of the sagittal suture at the top of the skull, front to back, resulting in a long narrow skull. This typically has little impact on development of the brain but may result in increased intracranial pressure (ICP). This is the most common form. Of craniosynostosis.
- **Coronal craniosynostosis** is the fusion of one or both sutures that extend from each ear to the top of the skull, resulting in a wide, short skull. If both sides fuse (brachycephaly), the forehead may bulge forward. If one size fuses (plagiocephaly), the nose and eye socket on the affected size are affected. May result in vision impairment and increased ICP.
- **Metopic craniosynostosis** (trigonocephaly) is the fusion of the suture from top of nose to anterior fontanel and sagittal suture, causing a triangular forehead and associated with developmental delays and cognitive impairment
- **Lambdoid craniosynostosis** (posterior plagiocephaly) is the fusion of the suture along the back of the head. One side of head may be flat, ears at different levels, and head tilted laterally. This does not typically affect brain development but can cause vision impairment.

Complex craniosynostosis affects multiple sutures and is often part of genetic syndromes, such as Crouzon and Apert. It is associated with increased ICP, cognitive impairment, developmental delays, and other

PERIVENTRICULAR LEUKOMALACIA

Periventricular leukomalacia is necrosis of the brain's white matter (described as "white spots") in the area surrounding the ventricles of the brain, likely due to inadequate oxygenation or blood flow to the area. It occurs most often in preterm infants born before 32 weeks of gestation or in very low birth weight (VLBW) infants. The necrosis can be identified on ultrasound and is associated with poor outcomes. If bilateral occipital cysts are present, this is a reliable predictive factor for cerebral palsy. With VLBW infants, a more diffuse pattern of white spots can be seen on magnetic resonance imaging scans. Additional risk factors include twin-twin transfusion syndrome, hypocarbia, infections (e.g., antenatal and postnatal), intraventricular hemorrhage, and necrotizing enterocolitis. Signs and symptoms vary depending on the severity of the injury but can include motor impairments, developmental delays, visual impairment, cognitive impairment, seizures, and cerebral palsy (typically spastic diplegia). Periventricular hemorrhage is a frequent complication. There is no treatment other than supportive care.

Hydrocephalus

Hydrocephalus occurs when there is an imbalance between production and absorption of cerebrospinal fluid in the ventricles, resulting from impaired absorption or obstruction, which may be congenital or acquired. There are **primarily 2 types** of hydrocephalus that affect infants:

- **Communicating**: CSF flows (communicates) between the ventricles but is not absorbed in the subarachnoid space (arachnoid villi).
- **Noncommunicating**: CSF is obstructed (non-communicating) between the ventricles with obstruction, often stenosis of the aqueduct of Sylvius but it can occur anywhere in the system.

In early infancy, before closure of cranial sutures, head enlargement is the most common presentation while brain damage occurs later as pressure causes damage to the central nervous system. **Early infancy symptoms** include bulging, non-pulsating fontanels (usually anterior) with increasing head circumference, dilated scalp veins, separating sutures, and positive Macewen sign (resonance on tapping near the frontal-temporal-parietal juncture), irritability, seizures, vomiting, and setting-sun sign (the upper eyelids retract and the eyes turn downwards due to pressure on the mesencephalic tegmentum and paralysis of upward gaze).

Causes

Hydrocephalus can be acquired or congenital. Approximately 75% of neonates with intraventricular hemorrhage (IVH) develop hydrocephalus. **Congenital hydrocephalus** is present at birth and can occur due to:

- **Aqueductal stenosis**, the most common cause, when the cerebral aqueduct connecting the third and fourth ventricles is blocked by an infection (toxoplasmosis, mumps, syphilis, or cytomegalovirus), tumor, hemorrhage, or developmental narrowing, and fluid accumulates in the third ventricle
- **Spina bifida**, where 80-90% of infants born with meningocele or myelomeningocele also have hydrocephalus.
- **Arnold-Chiari malformations** in the base of the brain where the spinal column joins the skull, characterized by parts of the cerebellum protruding through the foramen magnum into the spinal canal, which interferes with the normal flow of CSF.

Treatment

Hydrocephalus is diagnosed through CT and MRI, which help to determine the cause. Treatment may vary somewhat depending upon the underlying disorder, which may also require treatment. For example, if obstruction is caused by a tumor, surgical excision to directly remove the obstruction is required. Generally, however, most hydrocephalus is treated with **shunts**:

- **Ventricular-peritoneal shunt**: This procedure is the most common and consists of placement of a ventricular catheter directly into the ventricles (usually lateral) at one end with the other end in the peritoneal area to drain away excess CSF. There is a one-way valve near the proximal end that prevents backflow but opens when pressure rises to drain fluid. In some cases, the distal end drains into the right atrium.
- **Third ventriculostomy**: A small opening is made in the base of the third ventricle so CSF can bypass an obstruction. This procedure is not common and is done with a small endoscope.

NEURAL TUBE DEFECTS

The neural tube is the embryonic structure that eventually forms the brain and spinal cord. **Neural tube defects** (NTD) are a spectrum of congenital disorders involving the meninges covering the spinal cord. Mild forms are asymptomatic. Severe cases are incompatible with life. Diagnosis is often made in pregnancy by ultrasound or by an elevated level of alpha-fetoprotein in the amniotic fluid or in the mother's serum. Causes are multifactorial, with both genetic and environmental components. **Risk factors** for NTD include:

- Poor diet lacking in folic acid
- Family history of a NTD in a parent or sibling
- Maternal obesity with poorly controlled diabetes
- Maternal use of valproic acid or carbamazepine during pregnancy
- Increasing core temperature 3-4 °F (2 °C) through saunas, hot tubs, or fever

Studies have shown that if the mother ingests 400 micrograms of folic acid daily before and during pregnancy, it protects the fetus from developing an NTD.

TYPES

The neural tube defects, spina bifida and myelomeningocele, are often used interchangeably, but there is a distinction. Spina bifida is a neural tube defect with an incomplete spinal cord and often missing vertebrae that allow the meninges and spinal cord to protrude through the opening. There are **5 basic types**:

- **Spina bifida**: Defect in which the vertebral column is not closed with varying degrees of herniation through the opening.
- **Spina bifida occulta**: Failure of the vertebral column to close but no herniation through the opening, so the defect may not be obvious.
- **Spina bifida cystica**: Defect in closure with external sac-like protrusion with varying degrees of nerve involvement.
- **Meningocele**: Spina bifida cystica with meningeal sac filled with spinal fluid.
- **Myelomeningocele**: Spina bifida cystica with meningeal sac containing spinal fluid and part of the spinal cord and nerves.

PHYSICAL ASSESSMENT OF NEONATES WITH NEURAL TUBE DEFECTS

Neural tube defects (i.e., congenital malformations of the nervous system with incomplete closure of the neural tube during embryonic development) result in anomalies of the brain, spine, and/or spinal cord. Physical assessment includes:

- General: Measure vital signs and observe for signs of lethargy, irritability, or distress.
- Neural tube defect: Note the site and dimensions of defect and the type of lesions:
  - Anencephaly: The skull may be partially or completely absent, the brain may be exposed, and the face is usually intact.
  - Spina bifida occulta: Subtle external signs over the spine (e.g., birthmark, indentation, hair tuft, nevi, lipoma).
  - Meningocele: A fluid-filled sac containing meninges protrudes through the spinal defect.
  - Myelomeningocele: The same as meningocele, but the sac contains meninges and neural tissue.

- Cranial: Head circumference, palpate fontanels for bulging, and look for splayed sutures (indicate increased intracranial pressure). Assess the cranial nerves by observing facial and eye movements and the sucking reflex.
- Neurological function: Check motor movement and muscle tone, note paresis or paralysis, response to tactile stimuli, check deep-tendon reflexes and primitive reflexes.
- Musculoskeletal: Assess spinal alignment, limb deformities (clubfoot, hip dislocation), range of motion.
- Urogenital: Assess anal wink and the bulbocavernosus reflex—signs of urinary retention.

MYELOMENINGOCELE

Myelomeningocele, which involves spina bifida cystica with a meningeal sac containing spinal fluid and part of the spinal cord and nerves, comprises about 75% of the total cases of spina bifida. There are numerous **physical manifestations**:

- **Exposed sac** poses the danger of infection and cerebrospinal fluid leakage; so surgical repair is usually done within the first 48 hours although it may be delayed for a few days, especially if the sac is intact.
- **Chiari type II malformation** comprises hypoplasia of the cerebellum and displacement of the lower brainstem into the upper cervical area, which impairs the circulation of spinal fluid. It may result in symptoms of cranial nerve dysfunction (dysphonia, dysphagia) and weakness and lack of coordination of upper extremities.
- **Neurogenic bladder** is common and may require the Credé maneuver for infants and later intermittent clean catheterization.
- **Fecal incontinence** is common and is controlled with diet and bowel training as the child gets older.
- **Musculoskeletal abnormalities** depend upon the level of the myelomeningocele and the degree of impairment but often involve the muscle and joints of the lower extremities and sometimes the upper. Dysfunction often increases with the number of shunts. Scoliosis and lumbar lordosis are common. Hip contractures may cause dislocations.
- **Paralysis/paresis** may vary considerably and be spastic or flaccid. Many children require wheelchairs for mobility although some are fitted with braces for assisted ambulation.
- **Seizures** occur in about a quarter of those affected, sometimes related to shunt malfunction.
- **Hydrocephalus** is present in about 25-35% of infants at birth and 60-70% after surgical repair with ventriculoperitoneal shunt. Untreated, the ventricles will dilate and brain damage can occur.
- **Tethered spinal cord** occurs when the distal end of the spinal cord becomes attached to the bone or site of surgical repair and does not move superiorly with growth, causing increased pain, spasticity, and disability and requiring surgical repair.

ANENCEPHALY

Anencephaly is a neural tube defect in which the **embryological neural tube**, which forms the brain and spinal cord, fails to close at the **cephalic (head) end**, resulting in an infant without most of the brain, skull, or scalp, so that the top of the head is open. The eyes bulge forward. Because the forebrain is missing, the child has no cognitive ability or sensation of pain. A rudimentary brain stem may be present, supporting reflexive breathing and cardiac function, but the child's condition is not compatible with life. Most are stillborn, and others live a few hours or days. There is no treatment possible other than supportive care until death. The condition is often diagnosed with ultrasound. An ethical dilemma exists about the use of these infants' organs for donation, with some authorities believing that viable organs should be harvested before brain death.

Encephalocele

Encephalocele is a neural defect that involves a bony defect and herniation of the brain and/or cerebrospinal fluid through part of the skull in a skin-covered sac. In the United States, most commonly the mass is midline in the occipital and occasionally the frontal area. The **encephalocele** may be as large as the skull or may look like a small nasal polyp. In many cases, other abnormalities may exist, so thorough examination, including angiography and MRI, are usually required. Often, the part of the brain that herniates is disorganized, so the condition may be associated with cognitive impairment, although in mild cases the child has normal mentation. Surgical repair to place the herniated mass inside the skull and to repair the bony defect is the standard treatment. If the sac is left in place, the skin can erode, resulting in meningitis.

Neonatal Seizures

Causes

Causes of neonatal seizures are listed below, roughly in order of frequency:

- **Hypoxic-ischemic encephalopathy** after a difficult or traumatic delivery
- **Metabolic abnormality**:
  - Low levels of glucose, calcium, or magnesium
  - Elevated or low levels of sodium
- **Infections**:
  - Bacterial meningitis caused by Group B strep, *E. coli, S. pneumoniae*, or Listeria
  - Viral encephalitis caused by herpes simplex, cytomegalovirus, or enterovirus
- **Cerebrovascular accidents**:
  - Intraventricular hemorrhage
  - Subarachnoid hemorrhage
  - Subdural hematoma
  - Sinus thrombosis
- **Seizure syndromes**:
  - Epileptic encephalopathies (early myoclonic or early infantile)
  - Benign neonatal seizure syndromes, such as benign familial neonatal convulsions, benign idiopathic neonatal seizures, or benign sleep myoclonus

Types

Seizures indicate an abnormality of the central nervous system and are differentiated by their associated abnormal movements:

- **Subtle seizures** are more common in full-term infants, who present with feet pedaling, chewing, apnea, eye movements, or a blank stare.
- **Tonic seizures** are more common in preterm infants, who present with tonic flexion or extension of the limbs, which may be focal (one limb) or generalized.
- **Clonic seizures** occur primarily in full-term infants, indicate a focal cerebral injury, and involve slow, clonic movements (1-3 movements per second), often in one extremity or on one side of the body.
- **Myoclonic seizures** are rare in neonates and may be focal, multi-focal, or generalized, with rapid jerking movements of the extremities.

Treatment depends upon identifying underlying cause but may include glucose (if related to hypoglycemia), phenobarbital (drug of choice), fosphenytoin, and phenytoin.

Review Video: Seizures
Visit mometrix.com/academy and enter code: 977061

Initial Management

Seizures in the neonate require immediate treatment to avoid brain injury from hypoxia and hypoglycemia:

- Glucose (10% solution) if indicated for hypoglycemia with bolus 2 mL/kg and maintenance ≤8 mL/kg.
- Provide supplemental oxygen and ventilation.
- Give a loading dose of phenobarbital (20 mg/kg IV); if the initial loading dose is ineffective, give an additional 10-20 mg/kg IV.
- Draw STAT blood glucose and electrolyte levels.
- Correct electrolyte abnormalities such as low calcium, magnesium, and sodium.
- Give a maintenance dose of 4-6 mg/kg of phenobarbital IV every 12-24 hours.
- Monitor blood pressure and respiratory status frequently, because large doses of phenobarbital cause respiratory and cardiac depression.
- Give fosphenytoin, phenytoin, and lorazepam per order if seizures are uncontrolled.

Jitteriness

Jitteriness (tremor of chin and extremities) occurs in about half of neonates within the first few days of life and may persist intermittently when the child is excited or crying for ≤2 months. Jitteriness may also be present with drug withdrawal, hypoglycemia, hypocalcemia, and encephalopathy. Jitteriness must be differentiated from seizures, which may have a similar appearance. **Characteristics of jitteriness** include:

- There is a lack of ocular deviation or other abnormalities.
- Gentle restraint halts jitteriness.
- Stimulation elicits jitteriness.
- Clonic jerking has both fast and slow elements.
- Autonomic changes involving the heart rate, respirations, and blood pressure are not present.
- EEG is normal.

Jitteriness is distinct from shuddering, a 10-15 second period of fast tremors that may recur ≤100 times daily. Both jitteriness and shuddering are benign conditions that require no treatment.

Monitoring Neonatal Brain Activity Using aEEG

Amplitude-integrated electroencephalography (aEEG) is a continuous method of monitoring brain function and seizure activity in critically ill or preterm neonates, especially those with suspected hypoxic-ischemic encephalopathy. For the aEEG, usually 2–4 electrodes are placed on the scalp to record brain waves. The signals are processed and compressed to emphasize the brain wave amplitude over time. The tracing on the screen is time-compressed so that several hours of brain activity are displayed on a single screen. Abnormal aEEG patterns include:

- Burst suppression: low activity (suppression) with bursts of high activity, representing severe brain injury.
- Continuous low voltage: low amplitude, representing significant brain dysfunction
- Isoelectric: flat tracing, no detectable brain activity
- Repetitive spikes/sharp waves: seizure activity

If an abnormal aEEG pattern develops, then a cEEG (continuous electroencephalography) is often done because it provides more comprehensive information about brain activity. The cEEG is usually done for 24 hours or longer with 19–21 scalp electrodes applied.

Near-Infrared Spectroscopy (NIRS) Monitoring

Near-infrared spectroscopy (NIRS) is a noninvasive device to measure tissue oxygenation and hemodynamics, primarily cerebral, renal, and intestinal oxygenation in neonates. The NIRS device emits near-infrared light that passes through the tissue and is absorbed by different tissues at different wavelengths. Sensors detect the amount of light absorbed and calculate concentrations of oxyhemoglobin and deoxyhemoglobin. NIRS measures oxygen saturation at 2–3 cm below the sensors, so deeper tissues may not be assessed accurately. NIRS is used most commonly to assess cerebral oxygenation but is also used to detect hypoxia and to assess perfusion, such as during cardiac surgery. NIRS can be used to guide interventions for neonates with hypoxic-ischemic encephalopathy. Normal regional oxygen saturation (rSO_2) in cerebral tissue is 55–85%. Lower than normal rSO_2 is associated with hypoxia while higher than normal rSO_2 indicates hyperoxia and risk for retinopathy of prematurity.

Therapeutic Hypothermia

Therapeutic hypothermia for the neonate is used for neuroprotection to prevent neonatal asphyxia leading to severe hypoxic-ischemic encephalopathy. The temperature of deep brain structures is lowered to 33-34 °C through the whole body, hypothermia or head cooling only (CoolCap). **Therapeutic hypothermia** should be initiated within 6 hours after resuscitation for neonates ≥35 weeks with moderate to severe HIE. Other indications include fetal heart disorders, fetal anemia, meconium in amniotic fluid, SGA, LGA, and maternal prenatal hypoxemia. Criteria includes asphyxia as evidenced by Apgar ≤5 after 10 minutes. The goal of hypothermia is to reach the target temperature within 60 minutes. Cooling is typically carried out for about 72 hours followed by 12 hours of rewarming. The neonate must receive sedation and ventilatory support to ensure oxygen levels and ventilation are adequate. The neonate must be monitored carefully (ECG, BP, oxygen saturation, $ETCO_2$). The heart rate normally decreases about 15 bpm per 1 °C decrease, so bradycardia may occur. Temperature must be constantly monitored and temperature alarms set. EEG and neurological monitoring may be necessary because almost half of infants with HIE have seizures during cooling, especially during the first 48 hours. Fluids are limited to 40-60 mL/kg/day.

Psychosocial Complications

Family Types

Some of the different types of families are described below:

- **Nuclear**: This **husband-wife-children** model was once the most common family type but is no longer the norm. In this model, the husband is the provider, and the mother stays home to care for the children. This makes up only about **7%** of current American families.
- **Dual career/dual earner**: This model, where **both parents work**, is the most common in American society, including about **66%** of two-parent families. One parent may work more than another, or both may work fulltime. Income disparities may affect family dynamics.
- **Childless**: **10-15%** of families have no children because of **infertility** or **choice**.
- **Extended**: These may include **multigenerational families** or **shared households** with friends, parents, or other relatives. Childcare responsibilities may be shared or primarily assumed by an extended family member, such as a grandparent.
- **Extended kin network**: Two or more nuclear families live close together, share goods and services, and support each other, including sharing childcare. This model is common in the Hispanic community.
- **Single-parent**: This is one of the fastest-growing family models. Typically, the mother is the single parent, but in some cases, it is the father. The single parent may be widowed, divorced, or separated, but more commonly, has never married. In cases of divorce or abandonment, the child may have minimal or no contact with one parent, often the father. Single parents often face difficulties in trying to **support and care for a child** and may suffer **economic hardship.**
- **Stepparent**: Because of the high rate of divorce, stepparent families are common. This can result in **stress** and **conflict** when a new child enters the picture. There may be jealousy and resentment on the part of siblings and estranged family members. In some cases, families work together to achieve harmony and provide added support to children.
- **Binuclear/co-parenting**: In this model, children share time between two primarily nuclear families because of **joint custody agreements**. While this may at times result in conflict, the child benefits from having a continued relationship with both parents.
- **Cohabiting**: **Unmarried heterosexual couples** live together. The relationships within this model may vary, with some similar to the nuclear family. In some cases, people are in committed relationships and may avoid marriage because of economic or personal reasons. A planned child may strengthen the relationship, but an unplanned child may cause conflict.
- **Gay/lesbian**: Whether gay and lesbian couples marry or cohabit, they create families in non-traditional ways. For example, lesbian couples may use sperm donors. Gay couples often adopt. Children in these families may face social pressures because of their parents' lifestyles.

Surrogacy and Gestational Carriers

With traditional surrogacy, the surrogate is the biological mother, who donates her egg to the intended parents. The egg is fertilized, usually through intrauterine insemination, with the intended father's or donated sperm. With gestational surrogacy, the surrogate has no genetic ties to the fetus and is referred to as a gestational carrier. Gestational surrogacy is most common in the United States and is less legally complex. The embryo may be created through in vitro fertilization using donated eggs and sperm or with the eggs and/or sperm of the intended parents. States have differing laws regarding surrogacy. Some states allow the surrogate to receive financial compensation, whereas others prohibit compensation and may criminalize such arrangements.

Prospective parents can find their own surrogates, but many others use agencies that specialize in surrogacy contracts and match surrogates to intended parents. Surrogacy is very costly, typically ranging from $90,000 to $150,000, but it can be even higher. The issue of parentage also varies by state. In some states, the intended parents are listed as the legal parents on the birth certificate, while other states require postbirth adoption of the infant by the intended parents. Some states also require at least one parent to be genetically linked to the child.

Foster Parents

In some cases, a newborn is released to foster parents rather than to the birth parents if the birth parents are unable or are not allowed to care for the infant. For example, if a mother is incarcerated or actively using drugs, child protective services workers may remove the infant from the parents' custody. Foster parents are trained and licensed by the states to provide temporary care of an infant until the infant can be reunified with the birth family or another permanent placement, such as adoption, is made. Foster parents are compensated by the states, which also provide health insurance, usually Medicaid. Foster parents receive a monthly stipend; a clothing allowance; and support services, such as case management. If foster care is provided by relatives of the infant, such as the grandparents, this is referred to as kinship care. Foster parents are responsible for providing clothing, shelter, and emotional support and keeping medical appointments, attending court hearings, and facilitating visitations with the birth parents. If the infant cannot be reunified with the birth parents, the foster parents often can adopt the child.

Maternal Attachment Process

By the time of birth, most mothers have developed an emotional connection with their infants and demonstrate a number of typical steps in the **maternal attachment process**.

- **Touching**: The mother usually begins by lightly touching the infant's extremities with her fingertips and running her palm over the baby's trunk. This exploration of the infant can proceed very quickly in minutes, or be more tentative and take days. Early skin-to-skin contact with the infant tends to accelerate this process.
- **En face positioning**: The mother increases the amount of face-to-face eye contact with the infant, typically holding the infant close to her face and responding to eye contact by speaking in a sing-song, high-pitched tone (baby talk).
- **Responding**: The mother tends to respond verbally to sounds the infant makes.

Initially, the mother may feel separate and distant from the child, especially if she doesn't feel an immediate bond, and she should be reassured that these feelings are normal.

Acquaintance

During the acquaintance period, the first few days, responding helps the mother to recognize **clues** the child is giving about needs, such as hunger. The mother's ability to respond to those needs strengthens the bond and helps her gain confidence in her parenting ability. During this time, the infant is also learning to recognize **routines**, such as nursing when held toward the breast.

Mutual Regulation

During this phase, which may vary in duration, the mother is learning to **balance** the needs of the infant against her own needs, and she may have some negative feelings, such as resenting her lack of sleep or feeling frustrated by the infant's crying. The mother may be afraid to express any negative feelings, fearful that people will think she is a "bad" mother, but these feelings are normal and are likely to continue until the mother and infant reach a mutual balance. The ability of the mother and infant to recognize each other's cues and respond to them is termed **reciprocity**.

MATERNAL ATTACHMENT/BONDING ASSESSMENT

Assessment of maternal attachment/bonding should be done prior to discharge so that any issues and needed interventions can be discussed. In doing the assessment, the nurse evaluates the mother's:

- Progression in touching and face-to-face eye contact with extended times and indications of attraction, such as verbally responding to the infant and cuddling the infant. If there has been no progression, the nurse should assess contributing environmental, cultural, and social factors that may be interfering.
- Consistency in caring for the infant and seeking knowledge about and validation of her infant care; adjusting care to the needs of the infant. Sensitivity to infant's needs, such as recognizing discomfort or hunger quickly and exhibiting pleasure at infant's response to her efforts.
- Pleasure in the infant, expressed by calling the infant by name, noting family traits/characteristics, showing overt happiness. If the mother shows displeasure or apathy, this may indicate poor attachment, but might also indicate that the mother is experiencing pain or weakness.

PATERNAL ATTACHMENT

Paternal attachment, referred to as engrossment, occurs in many ways similar to maternal attachment. The father may feel pride and wonderment at the child and develop a strong sense of nurturing. Early and frequent contact with the infant promotes engrossment, so the nurse should ensure that the father is not overlooked after delivery but is able to hold, touch, and respond to the child as soon as possible.

SIBLING AND FAMILY ATTACHMENT

Siblings should be allowed to visit the mother and infant as early as possible and be encouraged to hold or care for the infant as appropriate for their ages. Siblings sometimes feel left out or overshadowed by the new infant, so it's important that the parents take time to talk to the siblings and give them attention as well. Grandparents and other family members also form attachments to the infant and should be included.

SIBLING RESPONSES/INTERVENTIONS

If there are abnormalities or complications with the neonate, this may cause stress to the **siblings**. Younger children may be hostile and older children ashamed. They may feel guilty about their responses, and they may feel neglected as parents go through the stages of grief and are unable to provide the support that the siblings need. In some cases, parents may express their concern by focusing their anxiety on one of the siblings, becoming hypercritical. In these cases, staff may need to intervene by discussing observations with the parents and encouraging other family members to provide support to the siblings. Parents' groups that involve the entire family can be very helpful. Whenever possible, children should be included in education and demonstrations and encouraged to ask questions. Age-appropriate books and other materials that explain medical conditions and treatments should be available for siblings.

PREPARATION OF SIBLINGS FOR BIRTH OF INFANT

Preparation of siblings prior to the birth of an infant can decrease anxiety and sibling rivalry by helping the children feel that they are participants in the process and are valued. Children should be prepared for physical changes in the mother, changing family dynamics, and infant care. Formal classes may be available for children ages 3-12 to help them identify and express their concerns, and to teach them about pregnancy and childcare. Booklets, books, and videos are also available.

The parent or teacher may use dolls to demonstrate childcare and allow the children to practice holding and caring for the baby. When possible, children should have contact with an infant, such as that of a friend or family member. Children may help to decorate the infant's room or prepare a welcome gift, such as a drawing or toy. Children should be told who will care for them during labor and delivery and should visit the mother and infant as soon after delivery as possible.

Barriers to Parent-Infant Interaction

There are many **barriers to parent-infant interaction**, especially with preterm infants or those with genetic disabilities or birth defects that require prolonged hospitalization or treatment. Barriers include:

- **Physical separation**: When the infant cannot be held or fed, when the child is transported to a different facility outside of the area, or when the mother is discharged and the infant remains hospitalized, attachment can be difficult to form.
- **Lack of clear understanding of handicaps or developmental problems**: Lack of infant response is sometimes interpreted as rejection, and parents may be frightened by abnormalities.
- **Attitude of medical staff**: Negative attitudes may cause the parent to grieve rather than attach to the child. Staff members need to encourage the parents to become involved in the child's care and to provide stimulation. Staff often needs to demonstrate care to parents, who may be intimidated by the infant's condition and medical needs.
- **Environmental overload**: The equipment (alarms, ventilators, monitors) and environmental constraints (no chairs) may overwhelm parents.

Cultural/Lifestyle Factors Affecting Family Integration

Values

Values based on attitudes, ideas, and beliefs often connect family members to common **goals**. However, these values may be influenced by many **external factors**, such as education, social norms, and attitudes of peers, other family, and coworkers, so values may change and impact family integration.

Roles

In some families, roles are clearly defined by **gender** and **task** (homemaker and breadwinner), but the roles blur or are **shared** in many families, and in some cases, the father becomes the primary caregiver while the mother works. Other common roles include peacemaker, nurturer, and social planner. How these roles are perceived and actualized affects the manner in which a child is integrated into the family.

Decision-Making

Family power structures vary widely, but in many families, **power** rests with one person who makes ultimate decisions and whose opinions affect other family members. In cultures with a strong emphasis on tradition, power often lies with the father, a grandparent, or another family member. However, it should not be assumed that the families of a given cultural background will always have the same power structure. Instead, power may be **shared** or it may rest with either the mother or the father.

Socioeconomic

Employment trends, marriage rates, and economic trends all affect **family integration**. Many people have become unemployed and are unable to support their families, resulting in severe **stress**, which may be exacerbated by the arrival of a new child. The divorce rate is high, leaving many parents with inadequate funds to support a child. Even if both parents are employed, the cost of living continues to escalate, including the cost of caring for a child.

MOTHER RELINQUISHING CHILD FOR ADOPTION

A mother relinquishing her child for **adoption** may have feelings of ambivalence and sadness. Many who relinquish their infants for adoption are young and unmarried. Adoptions may be closed or open, so procedures will vary. In some open adoptions, the adoptive parent(s) may accompany the mother and participate in the birth, with the birth mother relinquishing the child immediately after birth. In this case, the adoptive parents should be treated as the actual parents of the child, while staff should recognize the needs of the birth mother and provide for her emotional and physical support. In other cases, the child is first relinquished to an agency, such as Social Services, which then places the child. If possible, prior to the birth, the birth mother should indicate how she wants to handle the birth. Some want to hold and spend time with the child; others do not. The birth mother should be in a single room, rather than with other mothers, to protect her privacy.

Abuse and Neglect

Indicators of Abuse That May Be Identified in the Patient History

The healthcare provider should always be aware of the presence of any **indicators** that may present a potential for or an actual situation that involves **abuse**. These indicators may present in the **patient's history**. Some examples of indicators concerning their primary complaint may include the following: vague description about the cause of the problem, inconsistencies between physical findings and explanations, minimizing injuries, long period of time between injury and treatment, and over-reactions or under-reactions of family members to injuries. Other important information may be revealed in the family genome, such as family history of violence, time spent in jail or prison, and family history of violent deaths or substance abuse. The patient's health history may include previous injuries, spontaneous abortions, or history of pervious inpatient psychiatric treatment or substance abuse.

During the collection of the patient history, the financial history, the patient's family values, and the patient's relationships with family members can also reveal actual or potential **abuse indicators**.

- The **financial history** may indicate that the patient has little or no money or that they are not given access to money by a controlling family member. They may also be unemployed or utilizing an elderly family member's income for their own personal expenses.
- **Family values** may indicate strong beliefs in physical punishment, dictatorship within the home, inability to allow different opinions within the home, or lack of trust for anyone outside the family.
- **Relationships** within the family may be dysfunctional. Problems such as lack of affection between family members, co-dependency, frequent arguments, extramarital affairs, or extremely rigid beliefs about roles within the family may be present.

During the collection of the patient history, the sexual, social, and psychological history of the patient should be evaluated for any signs of actual or potential abuse.

- The **sexual history** may reveal problems such as previous sexual abuse, forced sexual acts, sexually transmitted infections (STIs), sexual knowledge beyond normal age-appropriate knowledge, or promiscuity.
- The **social history** may reveal unplanned pregnancies, social isolation as evidenced by lack of friends available to help the patient, unreasonable jealousy of significant other, verbal aggression, belief in physical punishment, or problems in school.
- During the **psychological assessment** the patient may express feelings of helplessness and being trapped. The patient may be unable to describe their future, become tearful, perform self-mutilation, have low self-esteem, and have had previous suicide attempts.

Observations That May Indicate Abuse

During the initial assessment, observations may also be made by the provider that can provide vital information about actual or potential abuse. **General observations** may include finding that the patient history is far different from what is objectively viewed by the provider or that there is a lack of proper clothing or lack of physical care provided. The home environment may include lack of heat, water, or food. It may also reveal inappropriate sleeping arrangements or lack of an environmentally safe housing situation. Observations concerning **family communications** may reveal that the abuser answers all the questions for the whole family or that others look to the controlling member for approval or seem fearful of others. Family members may frequently argue, interrupt each other, or act out negative nonverbal behaviors while others are speaking. They may avoid talking about certain subjects that they feel are secretive.

Indicators of Abuse That May Be Evident During the Physical Assessment

During the **physical assessment** the provider should always be aware of any **indicators of abuse**. These indicators may include increased anxiety about being examined or in the presence of the abuser; poor hygiene; looks to abuser to answer questions for them; flinching; over or underweight; presence of bruises, welts, scars or cigarette burns; bald patches on scalp for pulling out of hair; intracranial bleeding; subconjunctival hemorrhages; black eye(s); hearing loss from untreated infection or injury; poor dental hygiene; abdominal injuries; fractures; developmental delays; hyperactive reflexes; genital lacerations or ecchymosis; and presence of STIs, rectal bruising, bleeding, edema, or poor sphincter tone.

Domestic Violence

Men, women, elderly, children, and the disabled may all be victims of **domestic violence**. The violent person harms physically or sexually and uses threats and fear to maintain control of the victim. The violence does not improve unless the abuser gets intensive counseling. The abuser may promise not to do it again, but the violence usually gets more frequent and worsens over time. The provider should ask all patients in private about abuse, neglect, and fear of a caretaker. If abuse is suspected or there are signs present, the state may require **reporting**:

- Give victims information about community hotlines, shelters, and resources.
- Urge them to set up a plan for escape for themselves and any children, complete with supplies in a location away from the home.
- Assure victims that they are not at fault and do not deserve the abuse.
- Try to empower them by helping them to realize that they do not have to take abuse and can find support to change the situation.

Review Video: Domestic Violence
Visit mometrix.com/academy and enter code: 530581

Assessment of Domestic Violence

According to the guidelines of the Family Violence Prevention Fund, **assessment** for domestic violence should be done for all adolescent and adult patients, regardless of background or signs of abuse. While females are the most common victims, there are increasing reports of male victims of domestic violence, both in heterosexual and homosexual relationships. The person doing the assessment should be informed about domestic violence and be aware of risk factors and danger signs. The interview should be conducted in private (special accommodations may need to be made for children <3 years old). The manager's office, bathrooms, and examining rooms should have information about domestic violence posted prominently. Brochures and information should be available to give to patients. Patients may present with a variety of physical complaints, such as headache, pain, palpitations, numbness, or pelvic pain. They are often depressed and may appear suicidal and may be isolated from friends and family. Victims of domestic violence often exhibit fear of spouse/partner, and may report injury inconsistent with symptoms.

Steps to Identifying Victims of Domestic Violence

Identifying and assisting victims of domestic violence involves the following steps:

1. **Inquiry**: Non-judgmental questioning should begin with asking if the person has ever been abused—physically, sexually, or psychologically.
2. **Interview**: The person may exhibit signs of anxiety or fear and may blame himself or report that others believe he is abused. The person should be questioned if she is afraid for her life or for her children.
3. **Question**: If the person reports abuse, it's critical to ask if the person is in immediate danger or if the abuser is on the premises. The interviewer should ask if the person has been threatened. The history and pattern of abuse should be questioned, and if children are involved, whether the children are abused. Note: State laws vary, and in some states, it is mandatory to report if a child was present during an act of domestic violence as this is considered child abuse. The provider must be aware of state laws regarding domestic and child abuse, and all healthcare providers are mandatory reporters.
4. **Validate**: The interviewer should offer support and reassurance in a non-judgmental manner, telling the patient the abuse is not his or her fault.
5. **Give information**: While discussing facts about domestic violence and the tendency to escalate, the interviewer should provide brochures and information about safety planning. If the patient wants to file a complaint with the police, the interviewer should assist the person to place the call.
6. **Make referrals**: Information about state, local, and national organizations should be provided along with telephone numbers and contact numbers for domestic violence shelters.
7. **Document**: Record keeping should be legal, legible, and lengthy with a complete report and description of any traumatic injuries resulting from domestic violence. A body map may be used to indicate sites of injury, especially if there are multiple bruises or injuries.

Injuries Consistent with Domestic Violence

There are a number of characteristic **injuries** that may indicate domestic violence, including ruptured eardrum; rectal/genital injury (burns, bites, or trauma); scrapes and bruises about the neck, face, head, trunk, arms; and cuts, bruises, and fractures of the face. The pattern of injuries associated with domestic violence is also often distinctive. The bathing-suit pattern involves injuries on parts of body that are usually covered with clothing as the perpetrator inflicts damage but hides evidence of abuse. Head and neck injuries (50%) are also common. Abusive injuries (rarely attributable to accidents) are common and include bites, bruises, rope and cigarette burns, and welts in the outline of weapons (belt marks). Bilateral injuries of arms/legs are often seen with domestic abuse. Defensive injuries are indicative of abuse.

Defensive injuries to the back of the body are often incurred as the victim crouches on the floor face down while being attacked. The soles of the feet may be injured from kicking at perpetrator. The ulnar aspect of hand or palm may be injured from blocking blows.

Maternal and Family Grief

Types of Grief

Anticipatory grief occurs when a child is diagnosed with a terminal illness. The parent begins to mourn over the loss of the child before he or she expires.

Delayed grief occurs when the grieving process is postponed months to years after the loss of a child. Initially, the parent may not be able to grieve appropriately because of an inability to cope, or the pressing need to care for other family members.

Incongruent grief occurs when the mother and the father are out of sync in their grieving process, creating a source of stress and conflict in the marriage. It may be due to the differences in how men and women grieve:

- Some parents are more expressive about their loss and more emotional. These individuals are more likely to look for support from others.
- Other individuals grieve in a more solitary and cognitive manner. These individuals are generally more oriented to fact-gathering or problem-solving.

Incongruent grief may also exist because the **bond** that develops between a pregnant woman and the developing fetus is unique and generally very intense. The mother's bond begins before the birth of the child, while the father often forms a strong bond after the birth of the child.

Factors That Influence Grieving Families

The emotions that individuals and families experience with the loss or severe illness/disability of an infant are varied and dependent on many **factors that influence grief**:

- **Cultural influences**: Different cultures have their own practices and beliefs concerning sickness, death, and dying, and varying rituals and ceremonies for processing loss.
- **Family system**: The family's composition, the roles of its various members, and its economic circumstances affect its expression of grief. A large family with extended community support processes grief differently from a single mother living far from home.
- **Siblings**: The impact on other children in the family must be considered, in addition to the impact on the parents.
- **History of loss**: Many diseases have a genetic component, and this may not be the first child to be affected.

Minimizing Dilemmas Surrounding Severe Illness of an Infant

Dealing with neonates who are severely ill and not likely to survive is distressing to the staff responsible for their care. Caregivers can have dilemmas concerning adequate pain control, do not resuscitate (DNR) status, the family's cultural norms and religious beliefs that differ from their own, or grieving parents. Studies have shown that formal palliative care teams can help with issues that families face and with staff concerns. Specific procedures that may help staff deal with dying neonates include:

- Formal training in palliative care
- Assigning nurses who are comfortable with administering palliative care to dying neonates whenever possible
- Debriefing meetings shortly after a traumatic death or event to allow staff concerns to be discussed
- Consistent procedures established concerning organ donation

Interventions for Specific Circumstances

Parents may need extra support in circumstances that lead to grief:

- **Chronic sorrow**: If grief is prolonged and the individual does not seem to be able to move forward, the individual should be encouraged to talk about feelings and express grief openly and to seek outside support, such as a therapist or support group.
- **Death of a twin or other multiple**: The parents should be allowed to hold the child if possible and encouraged to name the child, talk about the child, and express feelings of loss. Some parents may want to keep a tangible memory, such as a clipping of hair or a handprint or footprint of the child. Some may benefit from a support group.
- **Repeated obstetric loss** (recurrent abortion, still birth, preterm delivery): The losses should be acknowledged by those caring for the parents ("I'm so sorry...") and the parents encouraged to express feelings about their loss.

Helping Families Deal with Their Dying Infant

The loss of an infant is an incredibly difficult time for families. In order to provide **compassionate care for the grieving family**, follow these steps:

- Recognize and acknowledge their emotions.
- Provide a private area for family members to gather.
- Allow the family members to take pictures or gather other mementos of the infant (identification bracelets, etc.).
- Discuss possible end-of-life care.
- Acknowledge that the grieving process can be a lifelong process and that each individual experiences grief in a different manner.
- Ensure the family is aware of counseling services provided by the hospital.
- Give the family contact information for local grief support groups.

Review Video: The Five Stages of Grief
Visit mometrix.com/academy and enter code: 648794

Pathologic/Complicated Grief Responses

Pathologic/Complicated grief occurs when the grieving process does not become resolved over time. The person continues to have intrusive thoughts and severe emotions for a period of greater than 6 to 12 months and typically has sleep disturbances, shows lack of interest in activities, withdraws from others, and feels severely lonely. With complicated grief, the person is at risk of comorbidities, such as depression and PTSD. **Types of complicated grief** includes:

- **Absent**: The person shows little emotion or response to grief but may experience a delayed grief reaction months or years later.
- **Chronic**: Prolonged grief that persists for years with little resolution, often associated with a codependent relationship.
- **Conflicted**: The person has ambivalent feelings about the deceased and may have little emotion initially but may feel delayed and increased grief associated with feelings of guilt.
- **Traumatic**: Associated with traumatic loss that did not allow any time to prepare. Some may react with anger or guilt.

Palliative Care for Children

Palliative care is providing pain relief and comfort to the neonate who is not responding to current methods of treatment and has a poor prognosis. The goal of palliative care is to achieve the best possible quality of life for the patient and his or her family. Consider the cultural and spiritual beliefs of the family during this difficult time. In its *Policy Statement of Palliative Care for Children,* the American Academy of Pediatrics recommends the following guidelines:

- Respect for the dignity of patients and family
- Access to compassionate and competent care
- Support for the caregivers
- Improved professional and social support
- Continuing improvement through research and education
- The availability of an interdisciplinary pediatric palliative care team 24 hours a day

Chapter Quiz

Ready to see how well you retained what you just read? Scan the QR code to go directly to the chapter quiz interface for this study guide. If you're using a computer, simply visit the online resources page at **mometrix.com/resources719/ccrnneonatal** and click the Chapter Quizzes link.